Industrial and Applied Mathematics

The *Industrial and Applied Mathematics* series publishes high-quality research-level monographs, lecture notes and contributed volumes focusing on areas where mathematics is used in a fundamental way, such as industrial mathematics, bio-mathematics, financial mathematics, applied statistics, operations research and computer science.

More information about this series at http://www.springer.com/series/13577

David D. Hanagal

Modeling Survival Data Using Frailty Models

Second Edition

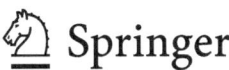 Springer

David D. Hanagal
Symbiosis Statistical Institute
Symbiosis International University
Pune, Maharashtra, India

ISSN 2364-6837   ISSN 2364-6845 (electronic)
Industrial and Applied Mathematics
ISBN 978-981-15-1180-6   ISBN 978-981-15-1181-3 (eBook)
https://doi.org/10.1007/978-981-15-1181-3

Mathematics Subject Classification (2010): 62F15, 62N01, 62N86, 65C60, 62H86, 62G05, 62F03, 37M05

This Springer imprint is published by the registered company Springer Nature Singapore Pte Ltd.
The registered company address is: 152 Beach Road, #21-01/04 Gateway East, Singapore 189721, Singapore

Dedicated to the Memory of My Loving Father

Preface

This book discusses the concepts of frailty models for survival analysis, including their recent methodology and applications. There are several books on survival data, that is, data concerning the time to some event. In the standard case, the event is death, but the topic is much broader. This book, however, covers frailty models for survival data. It also features eight datasets whose analysis is carried out using the R statistical package which has free open access for everyone. Covering fundamental concepts to advanced applications, this book is of value to scientists, research students, and teachers.

Survival data measures time to a certain event. This event is a transition from one state to another. In survival analysis, the event may be death, occurrence of disease (or a complication), time to an epileptic seizure, time it takes for a patient to respond to a therapy, or time from response until disease relapses. The problem of analyzing time to event data arises in a number of applied fields, such as medicine, biology, public health, epidemiology, engineering, economics, and demography. Although the statistical tools presented are applicable to all these disciplines, this book focuses on applying the statistical tools to biology and medicine.

The first three chapters are devoted to the basic concepts of survival analysis. Chapters 4–10 are based on shared frailty models, and Chaps. 11–14 are based on bivariate and correlated frailty models. Chapter 1 presents nine datasets on survival times with covariates and an introduction to survival analysis. Chapter 2 presents some important parametric distributions and their corresponding regression models with examples by using R. Chapter 3 discusses nonparametric Kaplan–Meier estimation and Cox's proportional hazard model, graphical plotting with examples by using R. Chapter 4 gives the concept of frailty, and Chap. 5 presents important frailty models. Chapter 6 presents different estimation procedures such as EM and modified EM algorithms. Chapter 7 gives data analysis of six datasets discussed in Chap. 1 by using R. Chapter 8 presents logrank tests and CUSUM of chi-square tests for testing frailty. Chapter 9 gives shared gamma frailty models with generalized Weibull, generalized log-logistic, generalized Rayleigh, weighted exponential, and extended Weibull as the baseline distributions. This chapter also presents the Bayesian estimation procedure and analyzes kidney infection data. Chapter 10 presents gamma frailty models based on reversed hazard with generalized log-logistic type I and type II, modified inverse Weibull, exponentiated Gumbel, modified inverse Weibull, and generalized inverse Rayleigh as the baseline distributions. This chapter also presents the Bayesian estimation procedure and analyzes Australian twin data. Chapter 11 presents different estimation procedures in bivariate frailty models, and Chap. 12 gives several kinds of correlated frailty models and their estimation procedures. Chapter 13 presents correlated gamma frailty and correlated inverse Gaussian frailty models with different baseline distributions and analyzes kidney infection data. Chapter 14 gives correlated gamma frailty models based on reversed hazard and analyzes Austrian twin data.

I thank the reviewers for their valuable suggestions and comments. I would also like to thank my wife, Anjali, for her support while writing this book. Finally, I am fully responsible for any errors remaining in this book. The views expressed are those of the authors noted in the bibliography. Readers are encouraged to give suggestions and comments for further improvisation. They can write to me at david.hanagal@gmail.com or david_hanagal@yahoo.co.in.

Pune, India   David D. Hanagal

Contents

About the Author

David D. Hanagal is Honorary Professor at the Symbiosis Statistical Institute, Symbiosis International University, Pune, India. He was previously a professor at the Department of Statistics, Savitribai Phule Pune University, India. An elected fellow of the Royal Statistical Society, UK, he is an editor and on the editorial board of several respected international journals. He has authored two books and published over 125 research publications in leading journals. With 30 years of research experience, he is an expert on writing programs using SAS, R, MATLAB, MINITAB, SPSS, and SPLUS. He also has worked as a visiting professor at several universities in the USA, Germany, and Mexico, and delivered a number of talks at conferences around the globe. His research interests include statistical inference, selection problems, reliability, survival analysis, frailty models, Bayesian inference, stress–strength models, Monte Carlo methods, MCMC algorithms, bootstrapping, censoring schemes, distribution theory, multivariate models, characterizations, repair and replacement models, software reliability, quality loss index, and nonparametric inference.

List of Figures

List of Tables

Part I
Basic Concepts in Survival Analysis

Chapter 1
Introduction to Survival Analysis

1.1 Introduction

Survival data is a term used for describing data that measure the time to a certain event. In survival analysis, the event may be death, occurrence of disease (or complication), time to an epileptic seizure, time it takes for a patient to respond to a therapy, or time from response until disease relapse (i.e., disease returns). In demography, the event can be entering marriage. The event is a transition from one state to another. Death is a transition from state alive to the state dead. Occurrence of disease is a transition from the state of being healthy to a state of presence of disease. Marriage is the transition of being unmarried to being married. For an epileptic seizure, an event is a transition from the seizure-free state to the state of active seizure.

Time to an event is a positive real-valued variable having continuous distribution. It is necessary to define the starting time point, say 0, from which times are measured. When we measure age, the starting time point maybe the date of birth. For studying the occurrence of disease, the time scale is the known duration of the disease. Here the known duration is the time since diagnosis of the disease. For the drug trial, the starting time is the time of the start of treatment.

The problem of analyzing time to event data arises in a number of applied fields, such as medicine, biology, public health, epidemiology, engineering, economics, and demography. Although the statistical tools we present are applicable to all these disciplines, our focus is on applying the statistical tools to biology and medicine. In this chapter, we present some examples drawn from these fields that are used throughout the text to illustrate the statistical techniques.

In biomedical applications, the data are collected over a finite period of time and consequently the "time to event" may not be observed for all the individuals in our study population (sample). This results in what is called "**censored**" data. That is, the "time to event" for those individuals who have not experienced the event under study is **censored** (by the end of study). It is also common that the amount of follow-up for the individuals in a sample varies from subject to subject. The combination of

© Springer Nature Singapore Pte Ltd. 2019

D. D. Hanagal, *Modeling Survival Data Using Frailty Models*,
Industrial and Applied Mathematics, https://doi.org/10.1007/978-981-15-1181-3_1

censoring and differential follow-up creates some unusual difficulties in the analysis of such data that cannot be handled properly by the standard statistical methods. Because of this, a research area in statistics has emerged which is called "**Survival Analysis**".

A common feature of these data sets is that they contain either censored or truncated observations. Censored data arises when an individual's life length is known to occur only in a certain period of time. Well-known censoring schemes are *right censoring*, where it is known that the individual is still alive at a given time; *left censoring*, where it is known that the individual has experienced the event of interest prior to the start of the study; or *interval censoring*, where the only information is that the event occurs within some interval. Truncation schemes are *left truncation*, where only individuals who survive a sufficient time are included in the sample and *right truncation*, where only individuals who have experienced the event by a specified time is included in the sample.

1.2 Bone Marrow Transplantation (BMT) for Leukemia

Data set on bone marrow transplantation for Leukemia of 137 patients at the Ohio State University Bone Marrow Transplantation Unit was studied by Avalos et al. (1993). The data set is also available in Klein and Moeschberger (2003). Bone marrow transplant treatment is a standard method for acute Leukemia. Patients with three disease types are acute myelocytic leukemia (AML) with low and high-risks and acute lymphoblastic leukemia (ALL). The prognosis for recovery may depend on risk factors known at the time of transplantation, such as the patient's age and sex (1-Male, 0-Female). Patients may develop acute or chronic diseases. The patient's age, sex, and disease group (1-ALL, 2-AML low risk, 3-AML high-risk) were considered as covariates. The following is the description of Table 1.1 with only six patients.

```
g--Disease Group
     1-ALL
     2-AML Low Risk
     3-AML High-Risk
T1 -- Time to Death or on Study Time
T2 --Disease Free Survival Time (Time to Relapse, Death or End of Study)
I1 -- Death Indicator
     1-Dead 0-Alive
I2 -- Relapse Indicator
     1-Relapsed, 0-Disease Free
I3--Disease Free Survival Indicator
     (1-Dead or Relapsed, 0-Alive Disease Free)
TA--Time to Acute Graft-Versus-Host Disease
IA--Acute GVHD Indicator
     (1-Developed Acute GVHD 0-Never Developed Acute GVHD)
TC--Time to Chronic Graft-Versus-Host Disease
IC--Chronic GVHD Indicator
```

```
      1-Developed Chronic GVHD 0-Never Developed Chronic GVHD
TP--Time to Return of Platelets to Normal Levels
IP--Platelet Recovery Indicator
      1-Platelets Returned to Normal, 0-Platelets Never Returned to Normal
Z1--Patient Age in Years
Z2--Donor Age in Years
Z3--Patient Sex
      1-Male, 0-Female
Z4--Donor Sex
      1-Male, 0-Female
Z5--Patient CMV Status
      1-CMV Positive, 0-CMV Negative
Z6--Donor CMV Status
      1-CMV Positive, 0-CMV Negative
Z7--Waiting Time to Transplant in Days
Z8--FAB
      1-FAB Grade 4 or 5 and AML, 0-Otherwise
Z9--Hospital
      1-The Ohio State University, 2-Alferd, 3-St. Vincent, 4-Hahnemann
Z10--MTX Used as a Graft-Versus-Host- Prophylactic 1-Yes 0-No
```

1.3   Remission Duration from a Clinical Trial for Acute Leukemia

Freireich et al. (1963) report the results of a clinical trial of a drug 6-mercaptopurine (6-MP) versus a placebo in 21 children with acute leukemia. The trial was conducted at 11 American hospitals. The random variable of interest consists of remission times (in weeks) of the patients assigned to treatment with 6-MP drug or a placebo during remission maintenance therapy. After having been judged to be in a state of partial or complete remission for the primary treatment with prednisone, a patient was paired with a second patient in the same state. One randomly chosen patient in each pair received the maintenance treatment 6-MP and the other a placebo. It was assumed that deaths at a given time always preceded censoring at the same time, and other

Table 1.1 Bone marrow transplantation data

g	T1	T2	I1	I2	I3	TA	IA	TC	IC	TP	IP	Z1	Z2	Z3	Z4	Z5	Z6	Z7	Z8	Z9	Z10
1	2081	2081	0	0	0	67	1	121	1	13	1	26	33	1	0	1	1	98	0	1	0
1	1602	1602	0	0	0	1602	0	139	1	18	1	21	37	1	1	0	0	1720	0	1	0
1	1496	1496	0	0	0	1496	0	307	1	12	1	26	35	1	1	1	0	127	0	1	0
1	1462	1462	0	0	0	70	1	95	1	13	1	17	21	0	1	0	0	168	0	1	0
1	1433	1433	0	0	0	1433	0	236	1	12	1	32	36	1	1	1	1	93	0	1	0
1	1377	1377	0	0	0	1377	0	123	1	12	1	22	31	1	1	1	1	2187	0	1	0

Table 1.2 Remission duration from a clinical trial for acute leukemia

Pair	Status	Time (TP)	Time (T6)	Replace indicator
1	1	1	10	1
2	2	22	7	1
3	2	3	32	0
4	2	12	23	1
5	2	8	22	1
6	1	17	6	1

ties were broken by randomization. Success (failure) was defined to occur in the ith pair if the time from remission to relapse or censoring for the patient on 6-MP (placebo) exceeded the time to relapse for the patient on placebo (6-MP). The trial was stopped once the number of successes or failures had reached significance. Out of 21 patients in the treatment group, 9 failed during the study period and 12 were censored. In contrast, none of the data are censored in the placebo group; that is, all 21 patients in the placebo group went out of remission during the study period. The data set contains a single covariate x with value 0 or 1 indicating remission status (0 = partial, 1 = complete). The description of the data is reported in Table 1.2 with six patients only. One can get the entire Table from Freireich et al. (1963).
col 1: Pair
col 2: Remission status at randomization (S) (1 = partial, 2 = complete)
col 3: Time to relapse for placebo patients, weeks (TP)
col 4: Time to relapse for 6-MP patients, weeks (T6)
col 5: Relapse indicator (RI) (0 = censored, 1 = relapse) for 6-MP patients
Note: All placebo patients relapsed.

1.4 Times of Infection of Kidney Dialysis Patients

Nahman et al. (1992) reported the data on time to first exit-site infection (in months) in patients with renal insufficiency, 43 patients utilized a surgically placed catheter (Group 1), and 76 patients utilized a percutaneous placement of their catheter (Group 2). The description of the data is reported in Table 1.3 with six patients. One can get the entire Table from Nahman et al. (1992).

col 1: Time (in months) to Infection (T)
col 2: Infection Indicator (I) (0-No, 1-Yes)
col 3: Catheter Placement (P) (1-Surgically, 2-Percutaneously)

Table 1.3 Times to infection of kidney dialysis patients

Time	Indicator	Catheter placement
1.5	1	1
3.5	1	1
4.5	1	1
4.5	1	1
5.5	1	1
8.5	1	1

1.5 Kidney Infection Data

The following data set is presented in McGilchrist and Aisbett (1991). The kidney infection data set consists of times to the first and second recurrences of infection at the point of insertion of the catheter in 38 kidney patients using a portable dialysis machine. For each patient, first and second recurrence times (in days) of infection from the time of insertion of the catheter until it has to be removed owing to infection is recorded. Infections can occur at the location of the insertion of the catheter. The catheter is later removed if infection occurs and can be removed for other reasons, which we regard as censoring. So, survival times for patients given maybe first or second infection time or censoring time.

After the occurrence or censoring of the first infection sufficient (ten weeks interval) time was allowed for the infection to be cured before the second time the catheter was inserted. So, the first and second recurrence times are taken to be independent apart from there common frailty component. The survival times from the same patient are likely to be related because of frailty describing the patient's effect.

The data set consists of three risk variables age, sex ($0 =$ male and $1 =$ female), and disease type GN, AN, and PKD where GN, AN, and PKD are short forms of Glomerulo Neptiritis, Acute Neptiritis, and Polycystic Kidney Disease. The infection times from each patient share the same value of the covariates. Table 1.4 shows the first and second recurrence times with recurrence indicator variable (0-censored,

Table 1.4 Kidney infection data

Pat	Time1	Ind1	Time2	Ind2	Age	Sex	GN	AN	PKD
1	8	1	16	1	28	0	0	0	0
2	23	1	13	0	48	1	1	0	0
3	22	1	28	1	32	0	0	0	0
4	447	1	318	1	31.5	1	0	0	0
5	30	1	12	1	10	0	0	0	0
6	24	1	245	1	16.5	1	0	0	0

Table 1.5 Litters of rats data

Litter number	Indicator	Time	Status
1	1	101	0
1	0	49	1
1	0	104	0
2	1	104	0
2	0	102	0
2	0	104	0

1-recurrence) and covariates age, sex (0-male, 1-female), and three indicator variables GN, AN, and PKD for six patients only. One can get the entire Table from McGilchrist and Aisbett (1991).

1.6   Litters of Rats Data

Mantel et al. (1979) reported the data on litters of rats. The experiment involved 50 male and 50 female litters, consist of three rats within each litter. One rat in each litter was treated with putative carcinogen and the other two served as control animals. The data recorded are the time to tumor appearance. Censoring was induced by death from other causes, as well as by the end of the study after 104 weeks. The sample of male rats was heavily censored because there were only two male rats that developed tumors. Table 1.5 contains four columns, the first column is the litter number (even litter numbers are male rats, odd litter numbers are female), the second column is treatment indicator, the third column is follow-up time, and the last column is status (1-tumor, 0-censored due to animal death). Table 1.5 gives the description of the data for the first two litters only. One can get the entire Table from Mantel et al. (1979).

1.7   Kidney Dialysis (HLA) Patients Data

Batchelor and Hackett (1970) reported 16 cases of badly burned patients. Because different patients had varying number of grafts in the study, it will be referred to as the "unbalanced data set". Each patient was given a number of skin grafts from a variety of donors and the time to graft rejection was recorded. The covariate was the quality of kidney dialysis (HAL) matching, indicated by 1 for the good and 0 for the poor. The censoring indicator is 1 for censored and 0 when the graft was rejected. Table 1.6 shows the description of the data with three patients only. The entire Table can be obtained from Batchelor and Hackett (1970).

Table 1.6 Kidney dialysis patients data

Patient	Time	Censor Ind	HAL
1	37	1	1
1	29	1	0
2	19	1	1
2	13	1	0
3	57	0	1
3	57	0	1

1.8 Diabetic Retinopathy Data

Here, we consider the data set obtained from the Diabetic Retinopathy Study reported by Huster et al. (1989). Patients with diabetic retinopathy in both eyes and visual acuity of 20/100 or better in both eyes were eligible for the study. The 197 patients in this data set represented a 50% simple random sample of the patients with "high-risk" diabetic retinopathy.

One eye of each patient was randomly selected for laser treatment and the other eye was observed without treatment. For each eye, the event of interest was time to onset of blindness from the initiation of treatment recorded in months. Survival times in this data set are the actual time to blindness in months, minus the minimum possible time to the event (6.5 months). Therefore, for getting actual data we have added 6.5 months to each available survival time. The first component of the bivariate survival times is the time to blindness (measured from a suitable experimental starting time point) in the untreated eye and the second component is the time to blindness in the treated eye.

The status is an indicator (0-censored, 1-failed). We have considered two covariates in the analysis, one is laser type (0-xenon, 1-argon) and the second is the type of diabetes (0-juvenile, 1-adult) denoted by X_1 and X_2, respectively. Therneau and Grambsch (2000) analyzed this data using gamma and Gaussian frailty models.

Out of the 197 patients, 159 patients experienced some form of censoring. Survival times of both eyes were censored for 80 patients. Both eyes of these patients were censored at the same time but the censoring times varied across patients. The treated eyes alone were censored for 63 patients and the censoring times were greater than or equal to the failure times of the untreated eyes. The reverse happened for only 16 patients. The remaining 38 patients experienced failures in both eyes, of which simultaneous failures were observed in 6 patients. The partial data is given in Table 1.7 with six patients.

Table 1.7 Diabetic retinopathy data

SI	LT	TE	Age	TD	OT	ST	TT	OU	SU	TU
5	2	2	28	2	9	0	46.23	9	0	46.23
14	2	1	12	1	8	0	42.5	6	1	31.3
16	1	1	9	1	11	0	42.27	11	0	42.27
25	2	2	9	1	11	0	20.6	11	0	20.6
29	1	2	13	1	9	0	38.77	10	1	0.3
46	1	1	12	1	9	0	65.23	9	1	54.27

```
1: Subject id(SI)
2: laser type(LT): 1 = xenon, 2 = argon
3: treated eye(TE): 1 = right 2 = left
4: age at diagnosis of diabetes(Age):
5: type of diabetes(TD): 1 =  juvenile (age at dx < 20), 2 = adult
6: Outcome for the treated eye(OT): risk group: 6-12
7: status(ST): 0 = censored, 1 = blindness
8: follow-up time for treated eye(TT):
9: Outcome for the untreated eye(OU): risk group: 6-12
10: status(SU): 0 = censored, 1 = blindness
11: follow-up time for untreated eye(TU):
The risk group variable was used to define the 'high-risk' samples.
```

1.9 Myeloma Data

Krall et al. (1975) analyzed data from a study on multiple myeloma in which re-searchers treated 65 patients with alkylating agents. Of those patients, 48 died during the study and 17 survived. In the data set Myeloma, the variable Time represents the survival time in months from diagnosis. The variable status consists of two values, 0 and 1, indicating whether the patient was alive or dead, respectively, at the end of the study. If the value of status is 0, the corresponding value of Time is censored. The variables thought to be related to survival are levels of LogBUN (log(Blood Urea Nitrogen) at diagnosis), HGB (hemoglobin at diagnosis), Platelet (platelets at diagnosis: 0 = abnormal, 1 = normal), Age (age at diagnosis in years), Log-WBC (log(WBC) at diagnosis), Frac (fractures at diagnosis: 0 = none, 1 = present), LogPBM (log percentage of plasma cells in bone marrow), Protein (proteinuria at diagnosis), and SCalc (serum calcium at diagnosis). The interest lies in identifying important prognostic factors from these nine explanatory variables. The partial data is presented in Table 1.8 with six patients.

Table 1.8 Myeloma data

T	S	LBUN	HGB	P	Age	LW	F	LPBM	Pr	SC
1.25	1	2.2175	9.4	1	67	3.6628	1	1.9542	12	10
1.25	1	1.9395	12.0	1	38	3.9868	1	1.9542	20	18
2.00	1	1.5185	9.8	1	81	3.8751	1	2.0000	2	15
2.00	1	1.7482	11.3	0	75	3.8062	1	1.2553	0	12
2.00	1	1.3010	5.1	0	57	3.7243	1	2.0000	3	9
3.00	1	1.5441	6.7	1	46	4.4757	0	1.9345	12	10

```
Time(T)
Status(S)
LogBUN(LBUN)
HGB
Platelet(P)
Age
LogWBC(LW)
Frac(F)
LogPBM(LPBM)
Protein(Pr)
SCalc(SC)
```

1.10 Australian Twin Data

Duffy et al. (1990) presented Australian twin data. The data consists of six zygote categories. We consider the subset of the data with zygote category 4. The data consists of males gender only and consist if 350 pair of twins with 9 and 11 censored in twin 1 and twin 2, respectively. An individual having age at onset less than 11 is considered as left censored observations. The data has information on the age at appendectomy of twins. The genetic factor or environmental factor involved in the risk of appendectomy is the frailty variable. Here there is a common covariate age for both T_1 and T_2 and one covariate each for T_1, T_2, i.e., the code for presence or absence of appendectomy as 1 and 0. The partial data is presented in Table 1.9 with six families.

Table 1.9 Australian Twin Data

Id	Twin age	Age-onset (T1)	Age-onset (T2)	Append-1	Append-2
134	53	8	9	1	1
152	22	22	22	0	0
176	26	26	26	0	0
178	46	46	46	0	0
198	22	11	22	1	0
206	27	18	25	1	1

```
Family Id
Age of Twin
Age at onset(T1)
Age at Onset(T2)
Appendectomy-1
Appendectomy-2
```

1.11 Definitions and Notations

1.11.1 Survival Function

The basic quantity employed to describe time-to-event phenomenon is the **Survival Function** $S(t)$, and it is defined as:

$$S(t) = P[T > t] = \text{ the probability an individual survives beyond time } t.$$

Since a unit either fails, or survives, and one of these two mutually exclusive alternatives must occur, we have

$$S(t) = 1 - F(t), \quad F(t) = 1 - S(t),$$

where $F(t)$ is the cumulative distribution function (CDF). If T is a continuous random variable, then $S(t)$ is a continuous, strictly decreasing function. The survival function is the integral of the probability density function (pdf), $f(t)$, that is

$$S(t) = \int_t^{\infty} f(x)dx$$

Thus,

$$f(t) = -\frac{dS(t)}{dt}.$$

1.11.2 Failure (or Hazard) Rate

The failure rate is defined as the instantaneous rate of failure (experiencing the event) for the survivors to time t during the next instant of time. It is a rate per individual of time. The next instant the failure rate may change and the individuals that have already failed will play no further role since only the survivors count.

The failure rate (or hazard rate) is denoted by $h(t)$ and is defined by the following equation

$$h(t) = lim_{h \to 0} \frac{P[t \leq T \leq t + h | T \geq t]}{h}$$

$$= \frac{f(t)}{S(t)} = \text{the instantaneous (conditional) failure rate.}$$

The failure rate is sometimes called a "conditional failure rate" since the denominator $S(t)$ (i.e., the population survivors) converts the expression into a conditional rate, given survival past time t.

Since $h(t)$ is also equal to the negative of the derivative of $ln\{S(t)\}$, we have the useful identity:

$$S(t) = \exp\left\{-\int_0^t h(t)dt\right\}.$$

If we let

$$H(t) = \int_0^t h(t)dt$$

be the **Cumulative Hazard Function**, we then have $S(t) = e^{-H(t)}$. Two other useful identities that follow from these formulas are:

$$h(t) = -\frac{d\ ln\ S(t)}{dt}$$
$$H(t) = -\ ln\ S(t)).$$

Bathtub curve:

People have calculated empirical population failure rates as units age over time and repeatedly obtained a graph such as shown in Fig. 1.1. Because of the shape of this failure rate curve, it has become widely known as the "Bathtub" curve.

The initial region that begins at time zero when a baby is born, the mortality rate is high and gradually decreases after one year. This region is known as the **Early Failure Period** (also referred to as **Infant Mortality Period**, from the actuarial origins of the first bathtub curve plots).

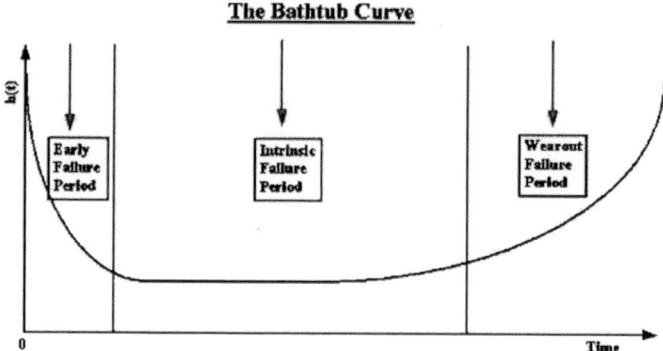

Fig. 1.1   Bathtub failure rate curve

Next, the failure rate levels off and remains roughly constant for (hopefully) the majority of the useful life of an individual. This long period of a level failure rate is known as the **Intrinsic Failure Period** (also called the **Stable Failure Period**) and the constant failure rate level is called the **Intrinsic Failure Rate**.

Finally, an individual reaches his/her retirement age, the failure rate begins to increase because of old age. This is the **Wearout Failure Period**.

It is also sometimes useful to define an average failure rate over any interval (T_1, T_2) that "averages" the failure rate over that interval. This rate, denoted by average failure rate, $AFR(T_1, T_2)$, is a single number that can be used as a specification or target for the population failure rate over that interval.

The formulas for calculating AFR's are:

$$AFR(t_1, t_2) = \frac{\left(\int_{t_1}^{t_2} h(t) dt \right)}{t_2 - t_1} = \frac{H(t_2) - H(t_1)}{t_2 - t_1} = \frac{ln\ S(t_1) - ln\ S(t_2)}{t_2 - t_1}$$

$$AFR(0, t) = AFR(t) = \frac{H(t)}{t} = \frac{-ln\ S(t)}{t}.$$

Bivariate and Multivariate Survival Function

The bivariate survival function of the lifetimes (T_1, T_2) is given by

$$S(t_1, t_2) = P[T_1 > t_1, T_2 > t_2] = \exp[-H(t_1, t_2)],$$

where $H(t_1, t_2)$ is the bivariate integrated hazard function of (T_1, T_2) which can be written in term of bivariate survival function as

$$H(t_1, t_2) = -\ln S(t_1, t_2).$$

The multivariate survival function of the lifetimes $(T_1, \ldots, T_k)$

$$S(t_1, \ldots, t_k) = P[T_1 > t_1, \ldots, T_k > t_k] = \exp[-H(t_1, \ldots, t_k)],$$

where $H(t_1, \ldots, t_k)$ is the multivariate integrated hazard function of $(T_1, \ldots, T_k)$ which can be written in term of multivariate survival function as

$$H(t_1, \ldots, t_k) = -\ln S(t_1, \ldots, t_k).$$

The multivariate hazard rate of $(T_1, \ldots, T_k)$ is defined by

$$h(t_1, \ldots, t_k) = \frac{f(t_1, \ldots, t_k)}{S(t_1, \ldots, t_k)}$$
$$= \frac{(-1)^k \frac{\partial^k S(t_1, \ldots, t_k)}{\partial t_1, \ldots, \partial t_k}}{S(t_1, \ldots, t_k)}.$$

1.12 Censoring

One peculiar feature, often present in time to event data, is known as censoring, which, broadly speaking, occurs when some events are known to occur at some point of time or within certain intervals. The meaning of censoring is already discussed in the introduction of this chapter. For example, n patients under some specific disease (cancer or AIDS) are chosen for the treatment, some of them die and the remaining will be survived from the disease at the end of the study period. The patients who survived are censored at that particular time or end of the study period.

When fitting models and estimating failure rates from survival data, the precision of the estimates (as measured by the width of the confidence intervals) tends to vary inversely with the square root of the number of failures observed—not the number of individuals on the test or the length of the test. In other words, a test where 5 fail out of a total of 10 on a test gives more information than a test with 1000 units but only 2 failures.

Since the number of failures r is critical, and not the sample size n on a test, it becomes increasingly difficult to assess the failure rates of highly censored data.

1.12.1   Censored Type I Data

Consider a situation in which we have n cancer patients taken from a population. In the typical scenario, we have a fixed time T to observe patients whether they survive or fail. The data obtained are called **censored type I** data.

Suppose we observe r deaths (where r can be any number from 0 to n) out of n patients admitted in a hospital under some specific disease. Let T (in days) be the time when the treatment is terminated. The (exact) death times are $t_1, t_2, \ldots, t_r$ and there are $(n - r)$ individuals that survived the entire T-days without failing. Note that T is fixed in advance and r is random, since we don't know how many deaths will occur until T days. Note also that we assume the exact times of failure are recorded when there are failures.

This type of censoring is also called "right censored" data since the times of failure to the right (i.e., larger than T) are missing.

1.12.2   Censored Type II Data

Another (much less common) way to test is to decide in advance that you want to see exactly r failure times and then test until they occur. For example, you might put 100 patients on the test and decide you want to see at least half of them fail. Then $r = 50$, but T is unknown until the 50th fail occurs. This is called **censored type II** data.

We observe $t_1, t_2, \ldots, t_r$, where r is specified in advance. The test ends at time $T = t_r$, and $(n - r)$ units have survived. Again we assume it is possible to observe the exact time of death for dead individuals.

Type II censoring has the significant advantage that you know in advance how many failure times your test will yield—this helps enormously when planning adequate tests. However, an open-ended random test time is generally impractical from a management point of view and this type of testing are rarely seen.

1.12.3   Current Status Data or Interval Censored Data

Sometimes exact times of failure are not known; only an interval of time in which the failure occurred is recorded. This kind of data is called **Current status data** or **interval censored** data and the situation is shown in the Fig. 1.2. Let $T_i - T_{i-1}$, $i = 1, 2, \ldots, k$, $T_0 = 0$ are the k time intervals and r_i be the number of deaths in the time interval $T_i - T_{i-1}$ and $n - \sum r_i$ patients are survived (censored) at time T_k out of n patients exposed to some particular disease. Here we do not know the exact time of deaths of patients but we know the patient died during the time interval. Figure 1.2 clearly shows the during each time interval how many patients died.

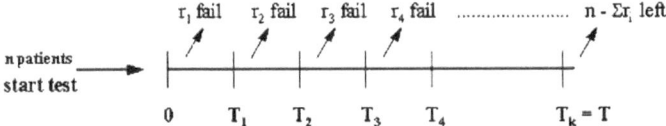

Fig. 1.2 Current status data or interval censored data diagram

1.12.4 Multicensored Data

In the most general case, every individual observed yields exactly one of the following three types of information:

- a run-time if an individual did not fail while under observation
- an exact failure time
- an interval of time during which an individual failed.

The individual may all have different run-times and/or readout intervals. Many statistical methods can be used to fit models and estimate failure rates, even with censored data. In later chapters, we will discuss the Kaplan–Meier approach, Probability Plotting, Hazard Plotting, Graphical Estimation, and Maximum Likelihood Estimation.

1.12.5 Separating Out Failure Modes

Note that when a data set consists of failure times that can be sorted into several different failure modes, it is possible (and often necessary) to analyze and model each mode separately. Consider all failures due to modes other than the one being analyzed as censoring times, with the censored run-time equal to the time it failed due to the different (independent) failure modes.

References

Avalos, B.R., Klein, J.L., Kapoor, N., Tutschka, P.J., Klein, J.P., Copelan, E.A.: Preparation of bone marrow transplantation in Hodgkin's and non-Hodgkin's lymphoma using Bu/Cy. Bone Marrow Transplant. **13**, 133–138 (1993)

Batchelor, J.R., Hackett, M.: HLA Matching in the treatment of burned patients with skin allographs. Lancet **2**, 581–583 (1970)

Duffy, D.L., Martin, N.G., Mathews, J.D.: Appendectomy in Australian twins. Aust. J. Hum. Genet. **47**(3), 590–592 (1990)

Freireich, E.J., Gehan, E., Frei, E., Schroeder, L.R., Wolman, I.J., Anbari, R., Burgert, E.O., Mills, S.D., Pinkel, D., Selawry, O.S., Moon, J.H., Gendel, B.R., Spurr, C.L., Storrs, R., Haurani, F., Hoogstraten, B., Lee, S.: The effect of 6-Mercaptopurine on the duration of steroid-induced remissions in acute Leukemia: a model for evaluation of other potential useful therapy. Blood **21**, 699–716 (1963)

Huster, W.J., Brookmeyer, R., Self, S.G.: Modelling paired survival data with covariates. Biometrics **45**, 145–156 (1989)

Klein, J.P., Moeschberger, M.L.: Survival Analysis, 2nd edn. Springer, New York (2003)

Krall, J.M., Uthoff, V.A., Harley, J.B.: A step-up procedure for selecting variables associated with survival. Biometrics **31**, 49–57 (1975)

McGilchrist, C.A., Aisbett, C.W.: Regression with frailty in survival analysis. Biometrics **47**, 461–466 (1991)

Nahman, N.S., Middendorf, D.F., Bay, W.H., McElligot, R., Powell, S., Anderson, J.: Modification of percutaneous approach to peritoneal dialysis catheter placement under peritoneoscopic visualization: clinical results in 78 patients. J. Am. Soc. Nephrol. **3**, 103–107 (1992)

Therneau, T.M., Grambsch, P.M.: Modeling Survival Data: Extending the Cox Model. Springer, New York (2000)

Chapter 2
Some Parametric Models

2.1 Introduction

There are a handful of parametric models that have successfully served as population models for failure times. Sometimes there are probabilistic arguments based on the physics of the failure mode that tend to justify the choice of model. Sometimes the model is used solely because of its empirical success in fitting actual failure data.

Six parametric models will be described in this section:

1. Exponential,
2. Weibull,
3. Extreme Value,
4. Lognormal,
5. Gamma, and
6. Log-logistic.

2.2 Exponential Distribution

The exponential model, with only one unknown parameter, is the simplest of all life distribution models. The key equations for the exponential distribution are shown below:

CDF: $F(t) = 1 - e^{-\lambda t}$, $0 < t < \infty$,

SURVIVAL: $S(t) = e^{-\lambda t}$,

PDF: $f(t) = \lambda e^{-\lambda t}$,

MEAN: $\frac{1}{\lambda}$,

MEDIAN: $\frac{\ln 2}{\lambda} \simeq \frac{.693}{\lambda}$,

VARIANCE: $\frac{1}{\lambda^2}$, and

HAZARD RATE: $h(t) = \lambda$.

© Springer Nature Singapore Pte Ltd. 2019
D. D. Hanagal, *Modeling Survival Data Using Frailty Models*,
Industrial and Applied Mathematics, https://doi.org/10.1007/978-981-15-1181-3_2

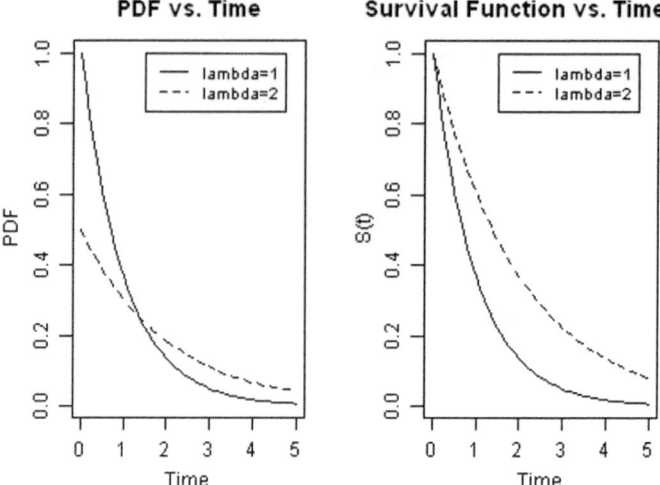

Fig. 2.1 PDF and survival function graphs of exponential distribution

Note that the failure rate reduces to the constant λ for any given time. The exponential distribution is the only distribution to have a constant failure rate. Also, another name for the exponential mean is the **mean time to fail** or **MTTF** and we have MTTF = $1/\lambda$. It has one most important property, that is, loss of memory property (LMP). Exponential is the only continuous distribution which has LMP.

The cumulative hazard function for the exponential is just the integral of the failure rate or $H(t) = \lambda t$.

Figure 2.1 presents the probability density function and survival function of the exponential distribution with parameter λ taking values 1 and 0.5.

2.3   Weibull Distribution

The Weibull is a very flexible life distribution model with two parameters. The CDF, survival, PDF, and other key formulas of Weibull distribution are, respectively, given by

CDF: $F(t) = 1 - e^{-\left(\frac{t}{\lambda}\right)^{\gamma}}, 0 < t < \infty,$

SURVIVAL: $S(t) = e^{-\left(\frac{t}{\lambda}\right)^{\gamma}},$

PDF: $f(t) = \frac{\gamma}{t}\left(\frac{t}{\lambda}\right)^{\gamma} e^{-\left(\frac{t}{\lambda}\right)^{\gamma}},$

HAZARD RATE: $\frac{\gamma}{\lambda}\left(\frac{t}{\lambda}\right)^{\gamma-1},$

MEAN: $\lambda\Gamma\left(1 + \frac{1}{\gamma}\right),$

MEDIAN: $\lambda(\ln 2)^{1/\gamma},$ and

VARIANCE: $\lambda^2\Gamma\left(1 + \frac{2}{\gamma}\right) - \left[\lambda\Gamma\left(1 + \frac{1}{\gamma}\right)\right]^2.$

with λ as the scale parameter (the **Characteristic Life**), γ, the **Shape Parameter**, and Γ, the Gamma function with $\Gamma(N) = (N-1)!$ for integer N.

The cumulative hazard function for the Weibull is the integral of the failure rate or

$$H(t) = \left(\frac{t}{\lambda}\right)^{\gamma}.$$

A more general three-parameter form of the Weibull includes an additional **waiting time** parameter μ (sometimes called a **shift** or **location** parameter). The formulas for the three-parameter Weibull are easily obtained from the above formulas by replacing t by $(t-\mu)$ wherever t appears. No failure can occur before μ hours, so the timescale starts at μ, and not 0. If a shift parameter μ is known (based, perhaps, on the physics of the failure mode), then all you have to do is subtract μ from all the observed failure times and/or readout times and analyze the resulting shifted data with a two-parameter Weibull.

Special Case: When $\gamma = 1$, the Weibull reduces to the exponential model, with $1/\lambda =$ the **mean time to fail (MTTF)**.

Depending on the value of the shape parameter γ, the Weibull model can empirically fit a wide range of data histogram shapes. Figure 2.2 gives the Weibull density with scale parameter $\lambda = 1$ and several different values of the shape parameter γ.

From a failure rate model viewpoint, the Weibull is a natural extension of the constant failure rate exponential model since the Weibull has a polynomial failure rate with exponent $\{\gamma - 1\}$. This makes all the failure rate curves shown in the following Fig. 2.3 when $\lambda = 1$. When $\gamma = 1$, the failure rate remains constant as time increases; this is the exponential case. The failure rate increases when $\gamma > 1$ and decreases when $\gamma < 1$ as time increases. Thus, the Weibull distribution is used to model the survival distribution of a population with increasing, decreasing, or

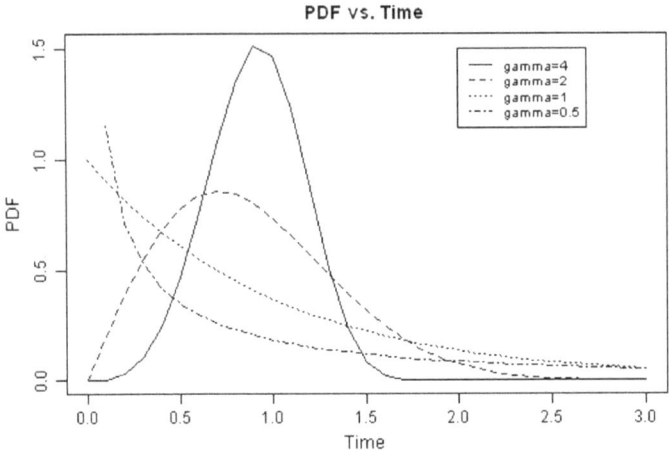

Fig. 2.2 Graphs of PDF of Weibull distribution with $\lambda = 1$

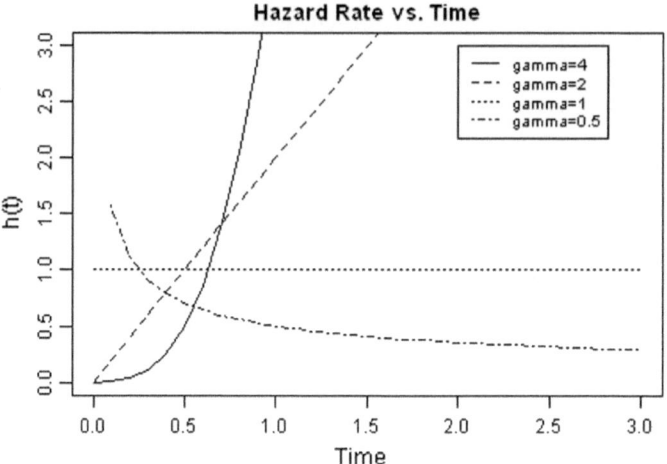

Fig. 2.3 Failure rate curves of Weibull distribution with $\lambda = 1$

constant risk. Examples of increasing and decreasing failure rates are, respectively, patients with lung cancer and patients who undergo successful major surgery.

For the survival curve, it is simple to plot the logarithm of $S(t)$,

$$\ln S(t) = -(\frac{t}{\lambda})^{\gamma}.$$

Figure 2.4 gives $\ln S(t)$ for $\lambda = 1$ and $\gamma = 1, > 1, < 1$, where $\gamma = 1$ is a straight line with a negative slope. When $\gamma < 1$, negative aging, $\ln S(t)$ decreases very slowly from 0 and then approaches a constant value. When $\gamma > 1$, positive aging, $\ln S(t)$ decreases sharply from 0 as time increases. The above equation can also be written as

$$\ln(-\ln S(t)) = -\gamma \ln \lambda + \gamma \ln t.$$

2.4 Extreme Value Distributions

The Weibull distribution and extreme value distribution have a useful mathematical relationship. If $t_1, t_2, \ldots, t_n$ are a sample of random times of fail from a Weibull distribution, then $ln\ t_1, ln\ t_2, \ldots,\ ln\ t_n$ are random observations from the extreme value distribution. In other words, the natural log of a Weibull random time is an extreme value random observation.

If the Weibull has shape parameter γ and characteristic life λ, then the extreme value distribution (after taking natural logarithms) has $\mu = ln\ \lambda$, $\beta = 1/\gamma$.

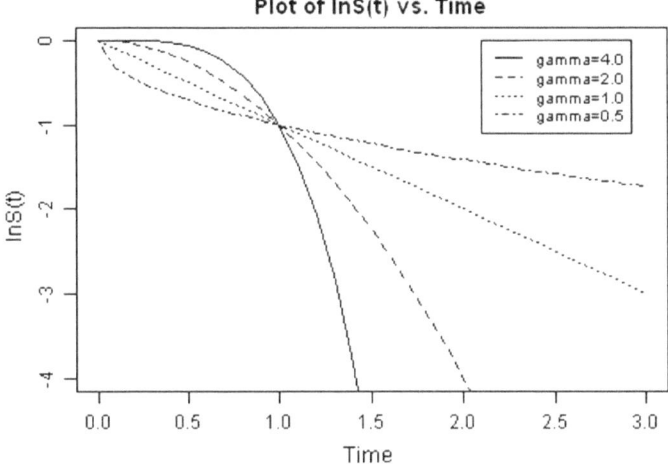

Fig. 2.4   Weibull distribution: $\ln S(t)$ versus time with $\lambda = 1$

Because of this relationship, computer programs designed for the extreme value distribution can be used to analyze Weibull data. The situation exactly parallels using normal distribution programs to analyze lognormal data, after first taking natural logarithms of the data points.

Extreme value distributions are the limiting distributions for the minimum or the maximum of a very large collection of random observations from the same arbitrary distribution. For any well-behaved initial distribution (i.e., $F(t)$ is continuous and has an inverse), only a few models are needed, depending on whether you are interested in the maximum or the minimum, and also if the observations are bounded above or below.

The distribution often referred to as the Extreme Value Distribution (type I) is the limiting distribution of the minimum of a large number of unbounded identically distributed random variables. The PDF and CDF are given by

$$f(t) = \frac{1}{\beta} e^{\frac{t-\mu}{\beta}} e^{-e^{\frac{t-\mu}{\beta}}}, \quad -\infty < t < \infty, \quad \beta > 0$$

$$F(t) = 1 - e^{-e^{\frac{t-\mu}{\beta}}}, \quad -\infty < t < \infty, \quad \beta > 0.$$

In any modeling application for which the variable of interest is the minimum of many random factors, all of which can take positive or negative values, try the extreme value distribution as a likely candidate model. For lifetime distribution modeling, since failure times are bounded below by zero, the Weibull distribution is a better choice.

2.5 Lognormal

The lognormal life distribution, like the Weibull, is a very flexible model that can empirically fit many types of failure data. The two-parameter form has parameters σ = the **shape** parameter and T_{50} = the **median** (a **scale** parameter).

NOTE: If time to failure, t_f, has a lognormal distribution, then the (natural) logarithm of time to failure has a normal distribution with mean $\mu = \ln T_{50}$ and standard deviation σ. This makes lognormal data convenient to work with just take natural logarithms of all the failure times and censoring times and to analyze the resulting normal data. Later on, convert back to real time and lognormal parameters using σ as the lognormal shape and $T_{50} = e^{\mu}$ as the (median) scale parameter. The density, cumulative density, survival, hazard, mean, and variance of lognormal distribution are, respectively,

$$\text{PDF: } f(t) = \frac{1}{\sigma t \sqrt{2\pi}} e^{-\left(\frac{1}{2\sigma^2}\right)(\ln f - \ln T_{50})^2}, \ 0 < t < \infty,$$

$$\text{CDF: } F(t) = \int_0^t \frac{1}{\sigma x \sqrt{2\pi}} e^{-\left(\frac{1}{2\sigma^2}\right)(\ln x - \ln T_{50})^2} \, dx = \Phi\left(\frac{\ln t - \ln T_{50}}{\sigma}\right)$$

with $\Phi(z)$ denoting the standard normal CDF,

SURVIVAL: $S(T) = 1 - F(t)$,

FAILURE RATE: $h(t) = \frac{f(t)}{S(t)} = \frac{(1/t\sigma\sqrt{2\pi}) \exp[-(\ln t - \ln T_{50})^2/2\sigma^2]}{1 - G[(\ln t - \ln T_{50})/\sigma]}$,

MEAN: $T_{50}e^{\sigma^2/2}$,

MEDIAN: T_{50}, and

VARIANCE: $T_{50}^2 e^{\sigma^2}\left(e^{\sigma^2} - 1\right)$.

NOTE: A more general three-parameter form of the lognormal includes an additional **waiting** time parameter θ (sometimes called a **shift** or **location** parameter). The formulas for the three-parameter lognormal are easily obtained from the above formulas by replacing t by $(t - \theta)$ wherever t appears. No failure can occur before θ hours, so the timescale starts at θ and not 0. If a shift parameter θ is known, then all you have to do is subtract θ from all the observed failure times and/or readout times and analyze the resulting shifted data with a two-parameter lognormal.

Examples of lognormal density curves are shown in Figs. 2.5 and 2.6. Figure 2.5 gives the lognormal frequency curves for $\mu = 0$, $\sigma = 0.5, 1, 2$, from which the idea of the flexibility of the distribution may be obtained. It is obvious that the distribution is positively skewed and that the greater the value of σ^2, the greater the skewness. Figure 2.6 shows the frequency curves for $\sigma = 1$, $\mu = 0, 0.5, 1.5$. Note that lognormal shapes for small sigma values are very similar to Weibull shapes when the shape parameter γ is large and large sigma values give plots similar to small Weibull γ's. Both distributions are very flexible and it is often difficult to choose which to use based on empirical fits to small samples of (possibly censored) data.

The failure (hazard) rate functions of lognormal distribution for different combinations of μ and σ are plotted in Fig. 2.7. The three hazard curves in Fig. 2.7 are corresponding to the parameters $\mu = 0.4$, $\sigma = 0.4$, $\mu = 0.6$, $\sigma = 0.6$, and $\mu = 1$, $\sigma = 1$, respectively.

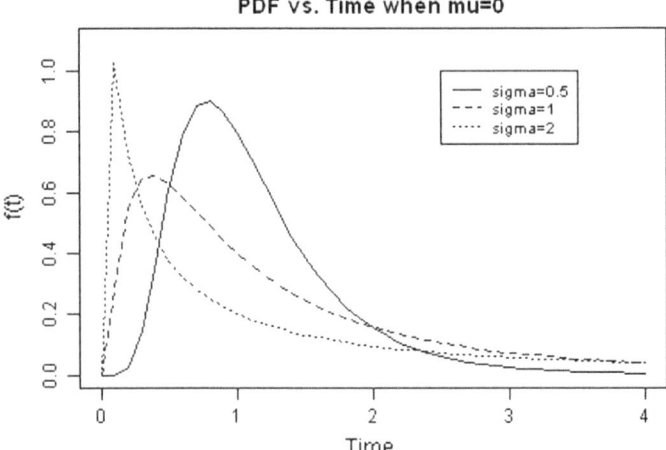

Fig. 2.5 Lognormal density curves with $\mu = 0$

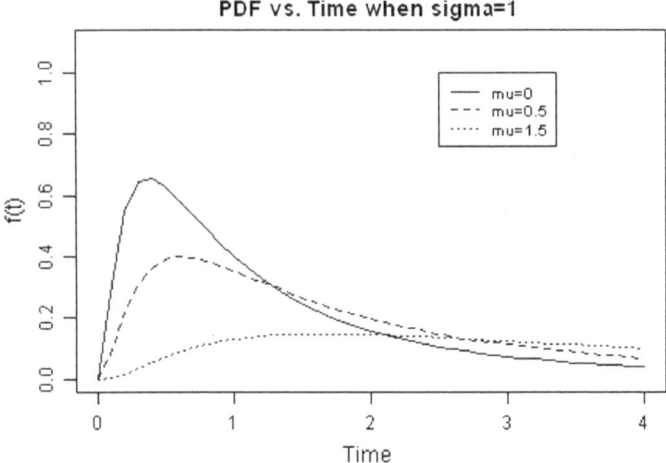

Fig. 2.6 PDF curves of the lognormal distribution with $\sigma = 1$

As shown in the preceding plots, the lognormal PDF and failure rate shapes are flexible enough to make the lognormal a very useful empirical model. Taking logarithmic transformation to all the data and time points makes it easy to work with mathematically, with many good software analysis programs available to treat normal data.

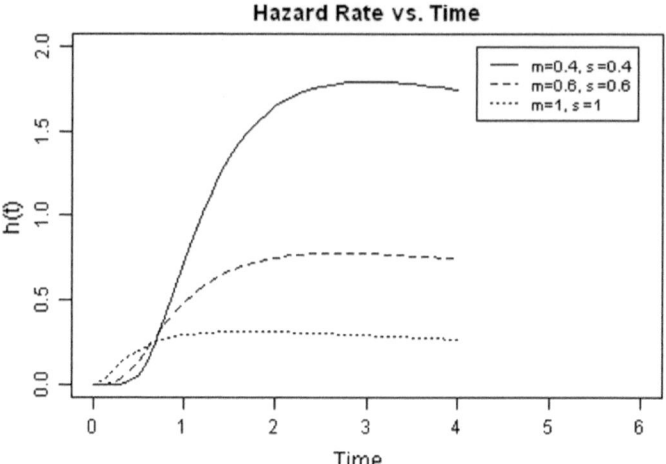

Fig. 2.7 Hazard rate of the lognormal with different parameters

2.6 Gamma

There are different ways of writing (parameterizing) the gamma distribution that are common in the literature. In addition, different authors use different symbols for the shape and scale parameters. Below, we define the gamma, with γ, the "shape" parameter, and λ, the "scale" parameter. This choice of parameters (γ, λ) will be the most convenient for later applications of the gamma. The density, cumulative density, survival, hazard, mean, and variance of gamma distribution are, respectively,

PDF: $f(t, \gamma, \lambda) = \frac{\lambda^{\gamma}}{\Gamma(\gamma)} t^{\gamma-1} e^{-\lambda t}, \quad 0 < t < \infty,$

CDF: $F(t) = \int_0^t f(t) dt,$

SURVIVAL: $S(t) = 1 - F(t),$

HAZARD RATE: $h(t) = \frac{f(t)}{S(t)},$

MEAN: $\frac{\gamma}{\lambda},$ and

VARIANCE: $\frac{\gamma}{\lambda^2}.$

NOTE: When $\gamma = 1$, the gamma reduces to an exponential distribution with λ.

Another well-known statistical distribution, the chi-square, is also a special case of the gamma. A chi-square distribution with n degrees of freedom is the same as a gamma with $\gamma = n/2$ and $\lambda = .5$.

Figures 2.8 and 2.9 give examples of gamma density functions with various values of γ and λ, respectively. It is seen that varying γ changes the shape of the distribution while varying λ changes only the scaling. Consequently, γ and λ are shape and scale parameters, respectively. When $\gamma > 1$, there is a single peak at $t = (\gamma - 1)/\lambda$.

When $0 < \gamma < 1$, there is negative aging and the failure rate decreases monotonically from infinity to λ as time increases from 0 to infinity. When $\gamma > 1$, there is positive aging and the failure rate increases monotonically from 0 to λ as time

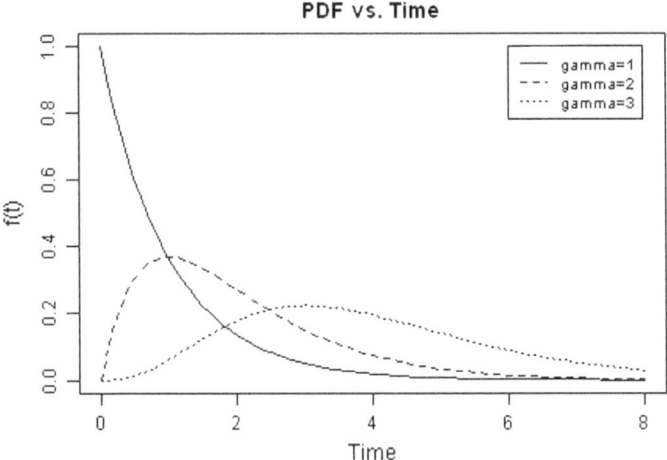

Fig. 2.8 Gamma density functions with $\lambda = 1$

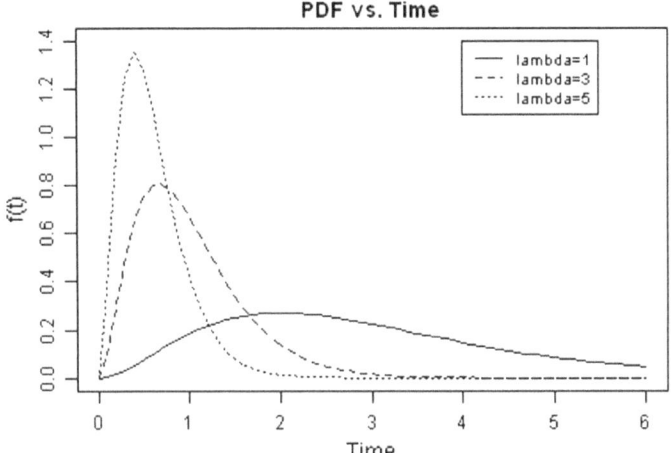

Fig. 2.9 Gamma density functions with $\gamma = 3$

increases from 0 to infinity. When $\gamma = 1$, the failure rate equals λ, a constant, as in the exponential case. Figure 2.10 shows the gamma failure rate function for $\lambda = 1$ and $\gamma = 0.5, 1, 2, 4$. Thus, the gamma distribution describes a different type of survival pattern where the failure rate is decreasing or increasing to a constant value as the time approaches infinity.

The gamma is a flexible life distribution model that may offer a good fit for some sets of failure data. It is not, however, widely used as a life distribution model for common failure mechanisms.

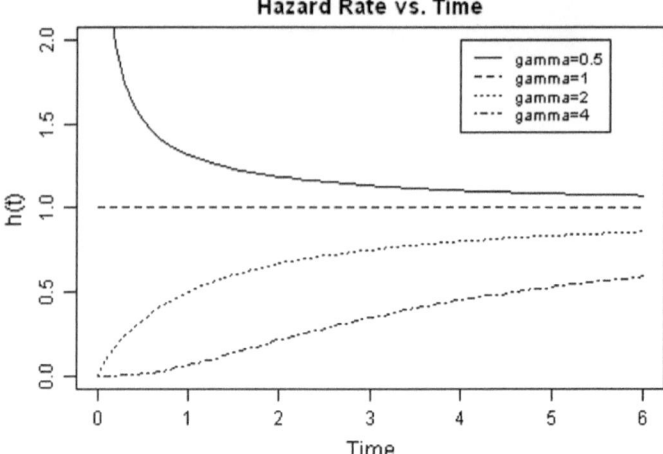

Fig. 2.10 Gamma failure rate functions with $\lambda = 1$

NOTE: When γ is a positive integer, the gamma is sometimes called an **Erlang distribution**. The Erlang distribution is used frequently in queuing theory applications.

A common use of the gamma model occurs in Bayesian reliability applications. When a system follows an HPP (exponential) model with a constant repair rate λ, and it is desired to make use of prior information about possible values of λ, a gamma Bayesian prior to λ is a convenient and popular choice.

2.7 Log-Logistic

The survival time T has a log-logistic distribution if $\ln(T)$ has a logistic distribution. The density, survival, hazard, and cumulative hazard functions of the log-logistic distribution are, respectively,

PDF: $f(t, a, b) = \frac{\alpha\gamma t^{\gamma-1}}{(1+\alpha t^{\gamma})^2}$, $0 < t < \infty$,

CDF: $F(t) = \frac{\alpha t^{\gamma}}{1+\alpha t^{\gamma}}$,

SURVIVAL: $S(t) = \frac{1}{1+\alpha t^{\gamma}}$,

HAZARD RATE: $h(t) = \frac{\alpha\gamma t^{\gamma-1}}{1+\alpha t^{\gamma}}$, and

CUMULATIVE HAZARD: $\ln(1 + \alpha t^{\gamma})$

$t \geq 0$, $\alpha > 0$, $\gamma > 0$.

The log-logistic distribution is characterized by two parameters α, and γ. The median of the log-logistic distribution is $\alpha^{-1/\gamma}$. Figures 2.11, 2.12, and 2.13 show the log-logistic density, hazard, and survival functions with $\alpha = 1$ and various values of $\gamma = 2.0$, 1 and 0.67, respectively.

When $\gamma > 1$, the log-logistic hazard has the value 0 at time 0, and it increases to a peak at $t = (\gamma - 1)^{1/\gamma}/\alpha^{1/\gamma}$, and then declines, which is similar to the lognormal

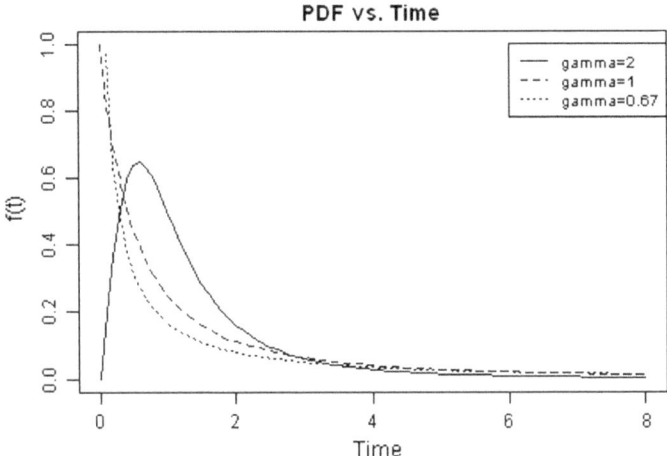

Fig. 2.11 Density function of log-logistic distribution with $\alpha = 1$

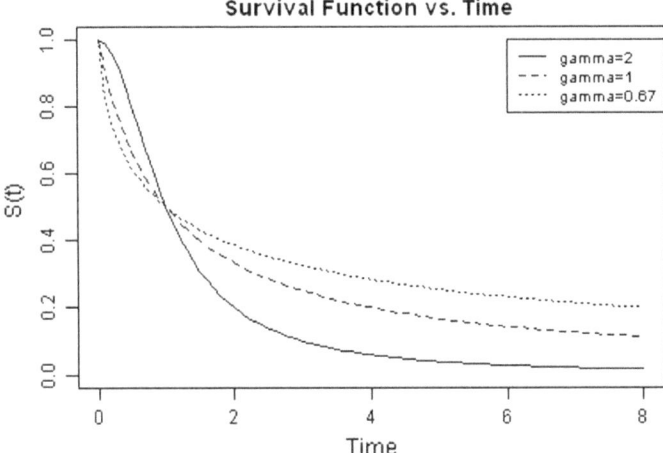

Fig. 2.12 Survival function of log-logistic distribution with $\alpha = 1$

hazard. When $\gamma = 1$, the hazard starts at $\alpha^{1/\gamma}$ and then declines monotonically. When $\gamma < 1$, the hazard starts at infinity and then declines toward 0 as t approaches infinity. Thus, the log-logistic distribution may be used to describe first, an increasing and then a decreasing hazard or a monotonically decreasing hazard.

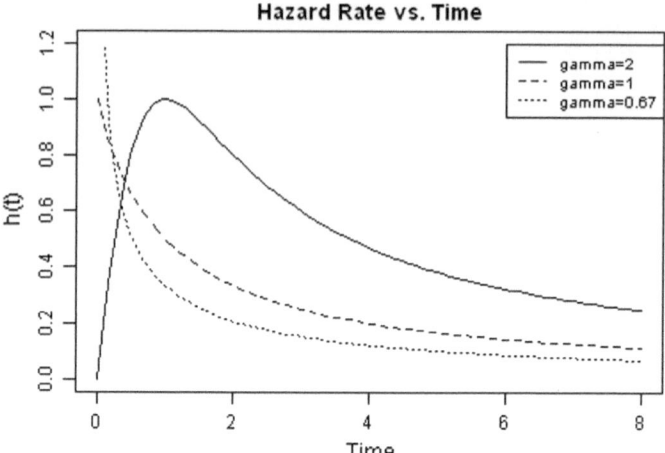

Fig. 2.13 Failure rate function of log-logistic distribution with $\alpha = 1$

2.8 Maximum Likelihood Estimation

Maximum likelihood estimation begins with writing a mathematical expression known as the **Likelihood Function** of the sample data. Loosely speaking, the likelihood of a set of data is the probability of obtaining that particular set of data, given the chosen probability distribution model. This expression contains the unknown model parameters. The values of these parameters that maximize the sample likelihood are known as the **Maximum Likelihood Estimates** or **MLE's**.

Maximum likelihood estimation is a maximization procedure. It applies to every form of censored or multicensored data, and it is even possible to use the technique across several stress cells and estimate acceleration model parameters at the same time as life distribution parameters. Moreover, MLE's and likelihood functions generally have very desirable large sample properties:

- They become unbiased minimum variance estimators as the sample size increases.
- They have approximate normal distributions and approximate sample variances that can be calculated and used to generate confidence bounds.
- Likelihood functions can be used to test hypotheses about models and parameters.

There are only two drawbacks to MLE's, but they are important ones:

- With small numbers of failures (less than 5, and sometimes less than 10 is small), MLE's can be heavily biased and the large sample optimality properties do not apply.
- Calculating MLE's often requires specialized software for solving complex nonlinear equations. This is less of a problem as time goes by, as more statistical packages are upgrading to contain MLE analysis capability every year.

Likelihood Function Examples for Survival Data

Let $f(t)$ be the PDF and $F(t)$ the CDF for the chosen life distribution model. Note that these are functions of t and the unknown parameters of the model. Assuming the independence between censoring and failure time distributions, the likelihood function for censored data is

$$L = C \prod_{i=1}^{n} [f(t_i)]^{\delta_i} [1 - F(t_i)]^{1-\delta_i} ,$$

where $\delta_i = 1$, if ith observation is failed, and 0, otherwise (censored). C denotes a constant that plays no role when solving for the MLE's. Note that with no censoring, the likelihood reduces to just the product of the densities, each evaluated at a failure time. The likelihood function for type I censored data is

$$L = C \left(\prod_{i=1}^{r} f(t_i) \right) (1 - F(T))^{n-r} .$$

For type II censored data, just replace T above by the random end of test time t_r.

The likelihood function for readout data is

$$L = C \left(\prod_{i=1}^{k} [F(T_i) - F(T_{i-1})]^{r_i} \right) (1 - F(T_k))^{n - \sum_{i=1}^{k} r_i} ,$$

with $F(T_0)$ defined to be 0.

In general, for any multi-censored data set the likelihood will be a constant times a product of terms, one for each unit in the sample, that look like either $f(t_i)$, $[F(T_i) - F(T_{i-1})]$, or $[1 - F(t_i)]$, depending on whether the unit was an exact time failure at time t_i, failed between two readouts T_{i-1} and T_i, or survived to time t_i and was not observed any longer.

The general mathematical technique for solving for the MLE's involves setting partial derivatives of $\ln L$ (the derivatives are taken with respect to the unknown parameters) equal to zero and solving the resulting (usually nonlinear) equations. The equation for the exponential model can easily be solved.

MLE's for the Exponential Model (Type I Censoring)

$$L = C \lambda^r e^{-\lambda \sum_{i=1}^{r} t_i} (e^{-\lambda(n-r)T})$$

$$\ln L = \ln C + r \ln \lambda - \lambda \sum_{i=1}^{r} t_i - \lambda(n - r)T$$

$$\frac{\partial \ln L}{\partial \lambda} = \frac{r}{\lambda} - \sum_{i=1}^{r} t_i - (n - r)T = 0$$

$$\hat{\lambda} = \frac{r}{\sum_{i=1}^{r} t_i + (n-r)T}.$$

NOTE: The MLE of the failure rate in the exponential case turns out to be the total number of failures observed divided by the total time on the test. For the MLE of the MTBF, take the reciprocal of this or use the total unit test hours divided by the total observed failures.

Conclusions

MLE analysis is an accurate and easy way to estimate life distribution parameters, provided that a good software analysis package is available. The package should also calculate confidence bounds and loglikelihood values. SAS has this capability, as do several other commercial statistical packages.

2.9 Parametric Regression Models

Before discussing parametric regression models for survival data, let us introduce the accelerated failure time (AFT) model. Denote the survival functions of two populations by $S_1(t)$ and $S_2(t)$, respectively. The AFT model is given by

$$S_1(t) = S_2(ct), \quad \text{for all } t \geq 0, \tag{2.1}$$

where c is a constant. This model implies that the aging rate of population 1 is c times as much as that of population 2. For example, if $S_1(t)$ is the survival function of rat population (in most of the clinical trials, rats are used before doing drug experiments on human beings) and $S_2(t)$ is the survival function for the human population, then by convention a year for a rat is equivalent to 20 years for a human implies $c = 20$, and $S_1(t) = S_2(20t)$. So the probability that a rat can survive for 3 years or beyond is the same as the probability that a human subject can survive for 60 years or beyond.

Let μ_i be the mean survival time for the population i and φ_i be the population quantile such that $S_i(\varphi_i) = \theta$ for some $\theta \in (0, 1)$. Then

$$\mu_2 = \int_0^\infty S_2(t)dt$$
$$= c \int_0^\infty S_2(cu)du \quad (t = cu)$$
$$= c \int_0^\infty S_1(u)du$$
$$= c\mu_1$$

and

$$S_2(\varphi_2) = \theta = S_1(\varphi_1) = S_2(c\varphi_1).$$

Then we have

$$\varphi_2 = c\varphi_1.$$

Under AFT model (2.1) and the above equations, one can note that the expected survival time, median survival time of population 2 all are C times as much as those of population 1.

Suppose, we have a sample of size n from a target population. For subject i ($i = 1, 2, \ldots, n$), we have observed values of covariates $y_{i1}, y_{i2}, \ldots, y_{ip}$ and possibly censored survival time T_i. The procedure Proc Lifereg in SAS fits models to data specified by the following equations:

$$\ln(T_i) = \beta_0 + \beta_1 y_{i1} + \cdots + \beta_p y_{ip} + \sigma\epsilon_i, \tag{2.2}$$

where $\beta_0, \ldots, \beta_p$ are the regression coefficients of interest, σ is a scale parameter, and ϵ_i are the random errors terms, usually assumed to be independent and identically distributed (i.i.d.) with some density function $F(\epsilon)$. Equation (2.2) is similar to a linear regression model for the log-transformed response variable $\ln(T_i)$ with ϵ_i are i.i.d. from N(0,1).

Let us increase the covariate y_k to $y_k + 1$ and denote by T_1 and T_2 the corresponding survival times for the two populations with covariate values y_k and $y_k + 1$ (with other covariate values fixed). Then T_1 and T_2 can be expressed as

$$T_1 = e^{\beta_0 + \beta_1 y_{i1} + \cdots + \beta_k y_k + \cdots + \beta_p y_{ip} + \sigma\epsilon_1} = c_1 e^{\sigma\epsilon_1}$$

$$T_2 = e^{\beta_0 + \beta_1 y_{i1} + \cdots + \beta_k (y_k + 1) + \cdots + \beta_p y_{ip} + \sigma\epsilon_2} = c_2 e^{\sigma\epsilon_2}$$

where c_1 and c_2 are related by $c_2 = c_1 e^{\beta_k}$. The corresponding survival functions are

$$S_1(t) = P[T_1 \geq t] = P[c_1 e^{\sigma\epsilon_1} \geq t] = P[e^{\sigma\epsilon_1} \geq c_1^{-1} t],$$

$$S_2(t) = P[T_2 \geq t] = P[c_2 e^{\sigma\epsilon_2} \geq t] = P[e^{\sigma\epsilon_2} \geq c_2^{-1} t],$$

Since ϵ_1 and ϵ_2 have the same distribution, and $c_2 = c_1 e^{\beta_k}$, we have

$$S_2(e^{\beta_k} t) = P[e^{\sigma\epsilon_2} \geq c_2^{-1} e^{\beta_k} t] = P[e^{\sigma\epsilon_2} \geq c_1^{-1} e^{-\beta_k} e^{\beta_k} t]$$

$$= P[c_1 e^{\sigma\epsilon_2} \geq t] = P[c_1 e^{\sigma\epsilon_1} \geq t] = S_1(t).$$

Therefore, we have accelerated failure time model between populations 1 (covariate value $= y_k$) and 2 (covariate value $= y_k + 1$) with $c = e^{\beta_k}$. So if we increase the covariate value of y_k by one unit while holding other covariate values unchanged, the corresponding average survival time μ_2 and μ_1 will be related by

$$\mu_2 = e^{\beta_k} \mu_1.$$

If β_k is small, then

$$\frac{\mu_2 - \mu_1}{\mu_1} = e^{\beta_k} - 1 \approx \beta_k.$$

Similarly, we have for the population quantile φ_i

$$\frac{\varphi_2 - \varphi_1}{\varphi_1} = e^{\beta_k} - 1 \approx \beta_k.$$

Therefore, when β_k is small, it can be interpreted as the percentage increase if $\beta_k > 0$ or percentage decrease if $\beta_k < 0$ in the average survival time and/or median survival time when we increase the covariate value of y_k by one unit. Thus, the greater the value of the covariate with positive β_k, the more it is beneficial in improving survival time for the target population. This interpretation of β_k is very similar to that in a linear regression.

We can assume different distributions for the error term ϵ_i in the model (2.2). For example, we can assume ϵ_i follows i.i.d. N(0,1). This assumption is equivalent to assuming that T_i has lognormal distribution (conditional on the covariates y's). In this section, we introduce exponential, Weibull, and lognormal parametric regression models for T_i (equivalently for ϵ_i) and the remaining accelerated parametric regression models can be done in a similar way.

Exponential Model

The simplest model is the exponential model where T at $y = 0$ (usually referred as baseline) has exponential distribution with constant hazard $\exp(-\beta_0)$. This is equivalent to assuming that $\sigma = 1$ and ϵ has a standard extreme value distribution given by

$$f(\epsilon) = \exp(\epsilon - e^{\epsilon}).$$

From this argument, it is easy to see that the distribution of T at any covariate vector y is exponential with constant hazard (independent of t)

$$h(t|y) = \exp(-\beta_0 - \beta_1 y_1 - \cdots - \beta_p y_p).$$

If we increase the value of covariate y_k ($k = 1, \ldots, p$) by one unit from y_k to $y_k + 1$ while holding other covariate values fixed, then the ratio of the corresponding hazards is equal to

$$\frac{\lambda(t|y_k + 1)}{\lambda(t|y_k)} = e^{-\beta_k}.$$

Thus, $e^{-\beta_k}$ can be interpreted as the hazard ratio corresponding to one unit increase in the covariate y_k, or equivalently, β_k can be interpreted as the decrease in log-hazard as the value of covariate y_k increases by one unit (while other covariate values being held fixed).

Weibull Model

In this case, the distribution of $\sigma\epsilon$ is an extreme value distribution with scale parameter σ. The survival function of T at covariate value $y = (1, y_1, \ldots, y_p)'$ is

$$S(t|y) = \exp\left\{-\left[te^{-y'\beta}\right]^{\frac{1}{\sigma}}\right\},$$

where $\beta = (\beta_0, \ldots, \beta_p)'$ is a vector of regression coefficients. Equivalently, in terms of log-hazard function:

$$\ln h(t|y) = \left(\frac{1}{\sigma} - 1\right)\ln t - \ln \sigma - y'\beta/\sigma,$$

the above expression can be written as

$$\ln h(t|y) = (\alpha - 1)\ln t + \beta_0^* + y_1\beta_1^* + \cdots + y_p\beta_p^*,$$

where $\alpha = 1/\sigma$, $\beta_0^* = -\ln\sigma - \beta_0/\sigma$, and $\beta_j^* = -\beta_j/\sigma$ for $j = 1, \ldots, p$. We also get proportional hazards model and the coefficient β_k^* ($k = 1, \ldots, p$) also has the interpretation that it is the increase in log-hazard when the value of covariate y_k increases by one unit while other covariate values are being held fixed. The function

$$\lambda_0(t) = t^{\alpha-1}e^{\beta_0^*} = \alpha t^{\alpha-1}e^{-\alpha\beta_0}$$

is the baseline hazard (i.e., when $\mathbf{y} = 0$).

Lognormal Model

The lognormal model assumes that ϵ follows $N(0,1)$. Let $h_0(t)$ be the hazard function of T when $\beta = 0$. Then $h_0(t)$ can be written as

$$h_0(t) = \frac{\phi(\frac{\ln t}{\sigma})}{\left[1 - \Phi(\frac{\ln t}{\sigma})\right]\sigma t},$$

$$\ln h_0(t) = \ln\phi(\frac{\ln t}{\sigma}) - \ln\left[1 - \Phi(\frac{\ln t}{\sigma})\right] - \ln\sigma - \ln t,$$

where $\phi(t)$ is the pdf and $\Phi(t)$ is the CDF of the standard normal distribution. Then log-hazard function of T at any covariate value y can be expressed as

$$\ln h(t|y) = \ln h_0(te^{y'\beta}) - y'\beta$$
$$= \ln \phi \left(\frac{\ln t + y'\beta}{\sigma} \right) - \ln \left[1 - \Phi(\frac{\ln t + y'\beta}{\sigma}) \right] - \ln \sigma - \ln t - y'\beta.$$

It is clear from the above expression that the above model is not a proportional hazards model. The survival function

$$\phi^{-1} \left[S(t|y) \right] = \beta_0^* + \beta_1^* y_1 + \cdots + \beta_p^* y_p - \alpha \ln(t),$$

or equivalently

$$S(t|y) = \Phi[\beta_0^* + \beta_1^* y_1 + \cdots + \beta_p^* y_p - \alpha \ln(t)],$$

where $\alpha = 1/\sigma$ and β_i/σ for $i = 0, 1, \ldots, p$. This is a probit regression model with intercept depending on t.

Log-logistic Model

The log-logistic model assumes that the error term ϵ has a standard logistic distribution

$$f(\epsilon) = \frac{e^\epsilon}{(1 + e^\epsilon)^2}.$$

The hazard function of T at any covariate value y has a closed form

$$\lambda(t|y) = \frac{\alpha t^{\alpha-1} e^{-y'\beta/\sigma}}{1 + t^\alpha e^{-y'\beta/\sigma}},$$

where $\alpha = 1/\sigma$.

The random variable T has survival function at covariate value y,

$$S(t|y) = \frac{1}{1 + (te^{-y'\beta})^{1/\sigma}}.$$

After some algebra, the above equation leads to

$$\ln \left[\frac{S(t|y)}{1 - S(t|y)} \right] = \beta_0^* + \beta_1^* y_1 + \cdots + \beta_p^* y_p - \alpha \ln(t),$$

where $\alpha = 1/\sigma$ and β_i/σ for $i = 0, 1, \ldots, p$. This is nothing but a logistic regression model with the intercept depending on t. Since $S(|y)$ is the probability of surviving to time t for any given time t, the ratio $S(t|y)/(1 - S(t|y))$ is often called the **odds** of surviving to time t. Therefore, with one unit increase in y_k while other covariate are fixed, the **odds ratio** is given by

$$\frac{S(t|y+1)/(1 - S(t|y+1))}{S(t|y)/(1 - S(t|y))} = e^{\beta_k^*} \quad \text{for all} \ \ t \geq 0,$$

which is constant over time. Therefore, we have a proportional odds model. Hence, β_k^* can be interpreted as the log odds ratio (for surviving) with one unit increase in $\mathbf{y}_k$ and $-\beta^*$ is the log odds ratio of dying before time t with one unit increase in $\mathbf{y}_k$. At times when the event of failure is rare (such as the early phase of a study), $-\beta_k^*$ can also be approximately interpreted as the log relative risk of dying. The log-logistic model is the only one that is both AFT model and a proportional odds model.

Obviously, ϵ has the following cumulative distribution:

$$F(u) = \frac{e^u}{1 + e^u}, \quad u \in (-\infty, \infty),$$

whose inverse function

$$logit(\pi) = ln\left(\frac{\pi}{1 - \pi}\right), \quad \pi \in (0, 1)$$

is often called the logit function.

Gamma Model

For a given set of covariates $(y_1, y_2, \ldots y_p)$, let $\lambda = e^{\beta_0 + y_1\beta_1 + \cdots + y_k\beta_k} = e^{\mathbf{y}'\beta}$. Then $\log(T) = \mathbf{y}'\beta + \sigma\epsilon$ implies $T = r^{\mathbf{y}'\beta}[e^\epsilon]^\sigma = \lambda T_0^\sigma$. T_0 is distributed as standard gamma and $\log T_0$ is distributed as standard log gamma.

Example 2.1

The myeloma data discussed in Sect. 1.9 are revisited here in this example. We obtain a parametric Weibull regression model for assessing the nine covariates on the survival time using the R program.

```
myeloma=read.table(file="myeloma.txt",header=T)
library(survival)
fit=survreg(Surv(T,S)~LBUN+HGB+P+Age+LW+F+LPBM+Pr+SC,myeloma,
dist="weibull")
summary(fit)
```

The output of the R program is

```
Call:
survreg(formula = Surv(T, S) ~ LBUN + HGB + P + Age + LW + F +
    LPBM + Pr + SC, data = myeloma, dist = "weibull")
            Value Std. Error     z       p
(Intercept)  7.12248   2.7422  2.597 0.00939
LBUN        -1.53251   0.5412 -2.832 0.00463
HGB          0.09698   0.0621  1.561 0.11855
P            0.26546   0.4557  0.583 0.56017
Age          0.01032   0.0169  0.611 0.54106
```

```
LW              -0.40081     0.5989 -0.669 0.50331
F               -0.33236     0.3526 -0.943 0.34589
LPBM            -0.38709     0.4290 -0.902 0.36695
Pr              -0.00923     0.0228 -0.404 0.68617
SC              -0.09985     0.0898 -1.112 0.26611
Log(scale)      -0.14255     0.1070 -1.333 0.18261


Scale= 0.867


Weibull distribution
Loglik(model)= -206.1    Loglik(intercept only)= -215.1
          Chisq= 17.95 on 9 degrees of freedom, p= 0.036
Number of Newton-Raphson Iterations: 5
n= 65
```

From the output of the R program, it is observed that the test for the regression parameters equal to zero is rejected with chi-square value 17.95 for 9 df and p-value is 0.036. log(BUN) is the most effective variable which is related to the survival of patients. Similar analysis can be done using other baseline distributions like lognormal, and log-logistic. The maximum of loglik (intercept only) among these distribution gives the best fit for the parametric model. The loglikelihood for Weibull baseline is -215.1, for lognormal baseline is -215.3, and for log-logistic baseline is -216. Weibull baseline has the maximum loglikelihood.

The SAS program commands which can be written to analyze this data are as follows. We will not give the output of SAS because of large output and similar results.

```
data Myeloma;
infile'myeloma.txt';
input LBUN HGB P Age LW FLPBM Pr SC;
label Time='Survival Time'
Status='0=Alive 1=Dead';
run;
proc phreg data=Myeloma;
model Time*Status(0)=LBUN HGB P Age LW FLPBM Pr
SC/dist=log-normal;
run;
```

Example 2.2

The data on times of infection of kidney dialysis discussed in Sect. 1.4 are revisited here in this example. We obtain a parametric Weibull regression model for assessing the catheter placement on the survival time using the R program.

```
> dialysis=read.table(file="C:/David/Book2/Data/dialysis.txt",
  header=T)
> fit1=survreg(Surv(time,ind)~place,data=dialysis,
  dist='weibull')
> summary(fit1)

Call:
survreg(formula = Surv(time, ind) ~ place, data = dialysis,
     dist = "weibull")

            Value Std. Error    z        p
(Intercept) 2.974      0.682 4.36 1.28e-05
place       0.623      0.469 1.33 1.84e-01
Log(scale)  0.129      0.167 0.77 4.41e-01

Scale= 1.14

Weibull distribution
Loglik(model)= -122   Loglik(intercept only)= -122.9
        Chisq= 1.93 on 1 degrees of freedom, p= 0.16
Number of Newton-Raphson Iterations: 7
n= 119
```

From the output of the R program, it is observed that the test for the regression parameters equal to zero is not rejected with a chi-square value 1.93 for 1 df and p-value is 0.16. Catheter placement is not a significant covariate related to the survival of patients. A similar analysis can be done using other baseline distributions like lognormal, and log-logistic. The maximum of loglik (intercept only) among these distribution gives the best fit for the parametric model. The loglikelihood for the Weibull baseline is -122.9, for lognormal baseline is -123.6, and for log-logistic baseline is -123.3. Weibull baseline has the maximum loglikelihood.

2.10 Bayesian Estimation Strategies

In classical approaches such as maximum likelihood, the inference is based on the likelihood of the data alone. In the Bayesian framework, the parameters of the model are viewed as random variables with some distribution known as a prior distribution, $p(\zeta)$. To apply Bayesian methods, we assume that, conditional on explanatory variables and on the entire set of parameters, observations are independent and prior distributions for all parameters are mutually independent. We use Bayesian estimation methods in Chaps. 9, 10, 13, and 14 and here we give idea on the Bayesian methodology.

The distribution of a parameter can be updated by combining its prior distribution and the likelihood function, called posterior density of a parameter. Thus the likelihood of the observed data y given parameters ζ, denoting $f(y|\zeta)$ or equivalently $L(y|\zeta)$, is used to modify the prior beliefs $p(\zeta)$, with the updated knowledge summarized in a posterior density, $\pi(\zeta|y)$. The relationship between these densities follows from standard probability equations. Thus, the posterior density can be written as

$$\pi(\zeta|y) \propto L(y|\zeta)p(\zeta).$$

Thus, updated beliefs are a function of prior knowledge and sample data evidence. From the Bayesian perspective, the likelihood is viewed as a function of ζ given fixed data y.

Bayesian statistics have made great strides in recent years, developing a class of methods for estimation and inference via stochastic simulation known as Markov Chain Monte Carlo (MCMC) methods. By sampling rather than optimizing, MCMC can make estimation and inference simpler for both Bayesians and frequentists. In the Bayesian framework, inference involves communicating features of the posterior distribution of ζ. For example, a Bayesian might report the mean or the mode of a posterior density, along with some measure of dispersion (perhaps quantiles or highest density regions), or perhaps even a graphical summary of the posterior (a histogram or density estimate). MCMC techniques tend to inherit this property of Bayesian analysis. Whereas procedures for conventional statistical inference focus attention on point estimates of parameters and their standard errors, MCMC methods seek to characterize a posterior distribution for parameters. Of course, sometimes, it will be convenient to summarize a posterior in terms of its mean and standard deviation. In Markov Chain Monte Carlo (MCMC) methods, each of the parameters in the model is iteratively resampled using its conditional density given the current values of other parameters. Sometimes, the MCMC approach to Bayesian inference is the only feasible method for solving the problem, particularly when the parameter space is high dimensional. Sahu et al. (1997), Bolstad and Manda (2001), Ibrahim et al. (2001), and Santos et al. (2010) used Markov Chain Monte Carlo (MCMC) methods to obtain summary statistics of the posterior distribution. For a more thorough discussion on this topic, readers are advised to refer to books such as Gamerman (1997), Gelman et al. (2003), Congdon (2006), Carlin et al. (2009), and Bolstad (2010).

2.10.1 Markov Chain Monte Carlo Methods

The Markov Chain Monte Carlo (MCMC) method is a general simulation method for sampling from posterior distributions and computing posterior quantities of interest. MCMC methods sample successively from a target distribution. Each sample depends on the previous one, hence the notion of the Markov chain. Markov Chain Monte Carlo (MCMC) methods consist of generating a set of Markov chains that has the posterior distribution of the model as its limiting distribution.

In MCMC methods, the posterior distribution of each of the parameters is approximated by the empirical distribution of the values of the corresponding Markov chain and empirical summary statistics calculated along each chain can be used to make inferences about the true value of the corresponding parameter. The Metropolis–Hastings algorithm, Gibbs sampler, etc., are the methods of doing this. Metropolis and Ulam (1949) and Metropolis et al. (1953) describe what is known as the Metropolis algorithm (see the section, Metropolis–Hastings Algorithms). The algorithm can be used to generate sequences of samples from the joint distribution of multiple variables, and it is the foundation of MCMC. Hastings (1970) generalized their work, resulting in the Metropolis–Hastings algorithm. Geman and Geman (1984) analyzed image data by using what is now called Gibbs sampling (see the section, Gibbs Sampler). These MCMC methods first appeared in the mainstream statistical literature in Tanner and Wong (1987).

A Markov chain is a sequence of random variables ζ^1, ζ^2, ... for which the random variable ζ^t depends on all previous ζ's only through its immediate predecessor ζ^{t-1}. We let the Markov chain run a long time until it has approached the limiting distribution. After the chain has run for a large number of iterations called as burn-in period, any value from the chain approximates a random draw from the posterior distribution. However, a sequence of draws after the burn-in period may have autocorrelation. Because of autocorrelation, consecutive draws may not be random, but values at widely separated time points are approximately independent. So a pseudorandom sample from the posterior distribution can be found by taking values from a single run of the Markov chain at widely spaced time points (autocorrelation lag) after the burn-in period. Alternatively, it can be obtained by taking values from independent runs of the Markov chain that runs long enough to approach stationary distribution.

With the MCMC method, it is possible to generate samples from an arbitrary posterior density $\pi(\zeta|y)$ and to use these samples to approximate expectations of quantities of interest. Several other aspects of the Markov chain method also contributed to its success. Most importantly, if the simulation algorithm is implemented correctly, the Markov chain is guaranteed to converge to the target distribution $\pi(\zeta|y)$ under rather broad conditions, regardless of where the chain was initialized. In other words, a Markov chain is able to improve its approximation to the true distribution at each step in the simulation.

Here, we use Metropolis–Hastings algorithm and Gibbs sampler to estimate the parameters of the models. The algorithm consists of successively obtaining a sample from the conditional distribution of each of the parameters given all other parameters of the models. These distributions are known as full conditional distributions. The process eventually provides samples from the joint posterior distribution of the unknown parameters. In our case, full conditional distributions are not easy to integrate out. So, full conditional distributions are obtained by considering that they are proportional to the joint distribution of the parameters of the model.

2.10.2 Metropolis–Hastings Algorithm

The Metropolis algorithm is named after its inventor, the American Physicist and computer scientist Nicholas C. Metropolis. A more general form, the Metropolis–Hastings (MH) algorithm, was proposed by Hastings (1970). Hence the algorithm is referred to as Metropolis–Hastings algorithm. The algorithm is simple but practical, and it can be used to obtain random samples from any arbitrarily complicated target distribution of any dimension that is known up to a normalizing constant. The Metropolis–Hastings (M–H) algorithm is the baseline for MCMC schemes that simulate a Markov chain ζ^t with $\pi(\zeta|y)$ as its stationary distribution. We simulate a Markov chain defined by iteratively scanning overall parameters. Replace each parameter by simulating a Metropolis step. The Metropolis–Hastings (M–H) algorithm can be summarized by the following steps:

1. Starting with initial values for the parameter vector $\zeta^0 = (\lambda_1^0, \lambda_2^0, \gamma_1^0, \gamma_2^0, \theta^0, \beta^0)$. This can be an arbitrary point as long as $\pi(\zeta|y) > 0$.
2. Set iteration counter $t = 1$.
3. Generate a candidate value for ζ say $\zeta_{new} = \zeta^*$ from transition kernel $q(\zeta^*|\zeta^{t-1})$. Mostly we use normal transition kernel such that $\zeta^* \sim N(\zeta^{t-1}, \sigma^2)$.
4. Calculate the acceptance probability a,

$$a(\zeta^*|\zeta^t) = min\left(1, \frac{\pi(\zeta^* \mid y)q(\zeta^{t-1} \mid \zeta^*)}{\pi(\zeta^{t-1} \mid y)q(\zeta^* \mid \zeta^{t-1})}\right).$$

5. Sample r from uniform distribution $U(0, 1)$.
6. Set $\zeta^t = \zeta^*$ if $r < a$; otherwise $\zeta^t = \zeta^{t-1}$.
7. Change the iteration counter from t to $t + 1$ and return to step 3 until convergence is reached.

This algorithm defines a chain of random variates whose distribution will converge to the desired distribution $\pi(\zeta|y)$ and so from some point forward, the chain of samples is a sample from the distribution of interest. In Markov chain terminology, this distribution is called the stationary distribution of the chain, and in Bayesian statistics, it is the posterior distribution of the model parameters. The random walk Metropolis algorithm is used in the MCMC procedure.

2.10.3 Gibbs Sampling Method

The Gibbs sampler is the most basic MCMC method used in Bayesian statistics. The Gibbs sampler, named by Geman and Geman (1984) after the American Physicist Josiah W. Gibbs, is a special case of the more general Metropolis–Hastings algorithm in which the proposal distributions exactly match the posterior conditional distributions and proposals are accepted 100% of the time. Although Gibbs sampling was developed and used in physics prior to 1990, its widespread use in Bayesian statistics originated in 1990 with its introduction by Gelfand and Smith (1990).

Gibbs sampling involves ordering the parameters and sampling from the full conditional distribution for each parameter given the current value of all the other parameters and repeatedly cycling through this updating process. Each "loop" through these steps is called an "iteration" of the Gibbs sampler, and when a new sampled value of a parameter is obtained, it is called an "updated" value. The sampler can be efficient when the parameters are not highly dependent on each other and the full conditional distributions are easy to sample from. Some researchers favor this algorithm because it does not require an instrumental proposal distribution as Metropolis methods do. However, while deriving, the conditional distributions can be relatively easy; it is not always possible to find an efficient way to sample from these conditional distributions. For Gibbs sampling, the full conditional density for a parameter needs only to be known up to a normalizing constant. The full posterior conditional distribution of is proportional to the joint posterior density; that is,

a generic Gibbs sampler follows the following iterative process:

1. Set $t = 0$ and choose arbitrary initial values for the parameter vector $\zeta^0 = (\lambda_1^0, \lambda_2^0, \gamma_1^0, \gamma_2^0, \theta^0, \beta^0)$. Relabel the parameter vector as $\zeta = (\zeta_1, \ldots, \zeta_p)$ (i.e., write ζ_1 for λ_1, ζ_2 for λ_2, etc.).
2. Generate each component of ζ as follows:

   - draw ζ_1^{t+1} from $\pi(\zeta_1 | \zeta_2^t, \zeta_3^t, \ldots, \zeta_p^t, y)$,

   - draw ζ_2^{t+1} from $\pi(\zeta_2 | \zeta_1^{t+1}, \zeta_3^t, \ldots, \zeta_p^t, y)$, $\vdots$
   - draw ζ_p^{t+1} from $\pi(\zeta_p | \zeta_1^{t+1}, \zeta_2^{t+1}, \ldots, \zeta_{p-1}^{t+1}, y)$.

3. Change the iteration counter from t to $t + 1$ and return to step 3 until convergence is reached.

2.10.4 Convergence Diagnostics

Operationally, effective convergence of Markov chain simulation has been reached when inferences for quantities of interest do not depend on the starting point of the simulations. This suggests monitoring convergence by comparing inferences made from several independently sampled sequences with different starting points. One way to see if our chain has converged is to see how well our chain is mixing, or moving around the parameter space. If our chain is taking a long time to move around the parameter space, then it will take longer to converge. We can see how well our chain is mixing through visual inspection. We need to do the inspections for every parameter. The convergence of Markov chain to a stationary distribution can be monitored by trace plots, coupling from past plots, running mean plot, Gelman–Rubin convergence statistic, and Geweke test.

- **Trace Plots** monitor the behavior of the chain. Trace plots of samples versus the simulation index can be very useful in assessing convergence. A trace plot is a graphical visualization of the iteration number against the value of the draw of the parameter at each iteration. It is obtained by joining the points by taking the iteration number on the horizontal axis and generated parameter values on the vertical axis. The trace plot tells us if the chain has not yet converged to its stationary distribution that is, if it needs a longer burn-in period. A trace can also tell us whether the chain is mixing well. The wavy pattern typically indicates strong autocorrelation within the chain while a zigzag pattern suggests the parameter is moving freely. A chain might have reached stationarity if the distribution of points is not changing as the chain progresses. We can see whether our chain gets stuck in certain areas of the parameter space, which indicates bad mixing. The aspects of stationarity that are most recognizable from a trace plot are a relatively constant mean and variance.
- **Burn-in Period** refers to the practice of discarding an initial portion of a Markov chain sample so that the effect of initial values on the posterior inference is minimized and the chain converges to a unique stationary distribution. If the Markov chain is run for an infinite amount of time, the effect of the initial values decreases to zero. We assume that after t iterations, the chain has reached its target distribution and we can throw away the early portion by considering iterations as sample from the posterior distribution. and use the good samples for posterior inference. The value of t is the burn-in number. The most obvious approach for determining the burn-in period is time series plot of all m parallel chains. One such plot developed by Prop and Wilson (1996) is coupling from the past plots.
- **Coupling from Past Plots** can be used to decide the burn-in period. It is actually a plot that represents the graphical view of all the generated chains on the same graph paper. To plot a chain, join the points corresponding to an iteration number of the horizontal axis and generated parameter value of the vertical axis. To diminish the effect of the starting distribution, we generally discard the early iterations (burn-in) of each sequence and focus attention on the remaining. A point at which all the m parallel chains overlap each other can be taken as burn-in value.
- **Running Mean Plots** can also be used to check how well our chains are mixing. A running mean plot is a plot of the iterations against the mean of the draws up to each iteration. In fact, running mean plots display a time series of the running mean for each parameter in each chain. These plots should be converging to a value. Running mean plot for each parameter converges to the posterior mean of the parameter, thus, representing a good mixing of the chain.

- **Autocorrelation** assessment between the draws of our Markov chain is another way to assess convergence. The lag k autocorrelation k is the correlation between every draw and its kth lag

$$\rho_k = \frac{\sum_{i=1}^{n-k}(y_i - \bar{y})(y_{i+k} - \bar{y})}{\sum_{i=1}^{n}(y_i - \bar{y})^2}. \tag{2.3}$$

However, a sequence of draws after the burn-in period may have autocorrelation. Because of autocorrelation, consecutive draws may not be random, but values at widely separated time points are approximately independent. So, a pseudorandom sample from the posterior distribution can be found by taking values from a single run of the Markov chain at widely spaced time points (autocorrelation lag) after burn-in period. Sample autocorrelation plots can also be used to decide autocorrelation lag.

- **Gelman and Rubin Diagnostics** (Gelman and Rubin 1992; Brooks and Gelman 1998) use parallel chains with dispersed initial values to test whether they all converge to the same target distribution. This diagnostic is based on analyzing multiple simulated MCMC chains by comparing the variances within each chain and the variance between chains for each variable. The large deviation between these two variances indicates non-convergence and the presence of a multimode posterior distribution (different chains converge to different local modes) or the need to run a longer chain (burn-in is yet to be completed). This diagnostic is an estimate of the potential scale reduction factor. When values of this diagnostic are approximately equal to one, then the sample can be considered to have arisen from the stationary distribution. In this case, descriptive statistics or posterior summary can be seen as valid estimates of unknown parameters.

Consider a scalar summary, that is, a random variable ζ, that has mean μ and variance σ^2 under the target distribution. Suppose that we have some unbiased estimator $\hat{\mu}$ for μ. Assume that we have m independently parallel MCMC generated chains. After obtaining suitable starting points, the chains are run for $2n$ iterations, of which the first n are discarded as the burn-in period. Define $\{\zeta_t\}, t = 1, \ldots, n$ to be the collection of a single Markov chain output. The parameter ζ_t is the tth sample of the Markov chain. For each ζ_t, the simulations are labeled as ζ_{tj}, $t = 1, \ldots, n$ and $j = 1, \ldots, m$. The variance between chains (B) and variance within chain (W) are given by

$$B = \frac{m}{n-1} \sum_{j=1}^{m}(\bar{\zeta}_{.j} - \bar{\zeta}_{..})^2,$$

and

$$W = \frac{1}{m(n-1)} \sum_{j=1}^{m}\sum_{t=1}^{n}(\zeta_{tj} - \bar{\zeta}_{.j})^2, \tag{2.4}$$

where

$$\bar{\zeta}_{.j} = \frac{1}{n} \sum_{t=1}^{n} \zeta_{tj} \quad \text{and} \quad \bar{\zeta}_{..} = \frac{1}{m} \sum_{j=1}^{m} \bar{\zeta}_{.j}.$$

Having observed these estimates, we can estimate σ^2 by a weighted average of B and W

$$\sigma^2 = \frac{n-1}{n} W + \frac{B}{n} \tag{2.5}$$

which would be an unbiased estimate of the true variance σ^2 if the starting points of the sequences were drawn from the target distribution, but overestimates σ^2 if the starting distribution is appropriately overdispersed. On the other hand, before convergence, W will tend to underestimate σ^2 because the individual chains have not had time to range over all of the target distribution and as a result will have less variability. Thus as $n \to \infty$, both $\hat{\sigma}^2$ and W approaches to $var(\zeta)$, but from the opposite direction. An indicator of convergence can be formed by the estimator of potential scale reduction factor (PSRF) given by $\hat{R} = \sqrt{\frac{\hat{\sigma}^2}{W}}$. As the chain converges, the PSRF decreases to one, meaning that the parallel chains are essentially overlapping. Alternatively, if the PSRF is close to 1, we can conclude that each of the m sets of n simulated observations is close to the target distribution. In general, if $\hat{R}$ is not near one, it is probably a good idea to continue the iterations. In practice, values of $\hat{R}$ less than 1.1 or 1.2 are sufficient for convergence diagnosis.

- **Geweke test** examines the convergence of a Markov chain based on the subparts of a chain at the end and at the beginning of the convergence period. The large standardized difference between ergodic averages at the beginning and at the end of the convergence period indicates non-convergence. This tests whether the mean estimates have converged by comparing means from the early and latter part of the Markov chain.
  Consider two subsequences $\{\zeta_t^a\}, t = 1, \ldots, n_1$ and $\{\zeta_t^b\}, t = n', \ldots, n; 1 < n_1 < n' < n$ of the Markov chain $\{\zeta_t\}, t = 1, \ldots, n$.
  Let $n_2 = n - n' + 1$ and define

$$\bar{\zeta}^a = \frac{1}{n_1} \sum_{t=1}^{n_1} \zeta_t \quad \text{and} \quad \bar{\zeta}^b = \frac{1}{n_2} \sum_{t=n'}^{n} \zeta_t.$$

Let $\hat{s}_1(0)$ and $\hat{s}_2(0)$ denote consistent spectral density estimates at zero frequency for the two MCMC chains, respectively. If the ratios n_1/n and n_2/n are fixed, $(n_1 + n_2)/n < 1$, and the chain is stationary, then the following statistic converges to a standard normal distribution as $n \to \infty$:

$$Z_n = \frac{\bar{\zeta}^a - \bar{\zeta}^b}{\sqrt{\frac{\hat{s}_1(0)}{n_1} + \frac{\hat{s}_2(0)}{n_2}}}. \tag{2.6}$$

This is a two-sided test, and large absolute Z-scores indicate rejection. The standardized difference Z_n between the ergodic averages at the beginning and at the end of the convergence period should not be large if convergence has been achieved. One can calculate p-value based on standard normal distribution of the Geweke test statistic Z_n for testing convergence of chains.

References

Bolstad, W.M.: Understanding Computational Bayesian Statistics. Wiley, New York (2010)

Bolstad, W.M., Manda, S.O.: Investigating child mortality in Malawi using family and community random effects: a Bayesian analysis. J. Am. Stat. Assoc. **96**, 12 (2001)

Brooks, S.P., Gelman, A.: Alternative methods for monitoring convergence of iterative simulations. J. Comput. Graph. Stat. **7**, 434–55 (1998)

Carlin, B.P., Louis, T.A.: Bayesian methods for data analysis. 3rd edn. CRC press, chapman and Hall, Boca Raton (2009)

Congdon, P.: Bayesian Statistical Modelling, 2nd edn. Wiley, New York (2006)

Gamerman, D.: Markov Chain Monte Carlo: Stochastic Simulation for Bayesian Inference. Chapman and Hall, London (1997)

Gelfand, A.E., Smith, A.F.M.: Sampling-based approaches to calculating marginal densities. J. Am. Stat. Assoc. **85**, 398–409 (1990)

Gelman, A., Rubin, D.B.: A single series from the Gibbs sampler provides a false sense of security. In: Bernardo, J.M., Berger, J.O., Dawid, A.P., Smith, A.F.M., (eds.), Bayesian Statistics, vol. 4, pp. 625–632. Oxford University Press, Oxford (1992)

Gelman, A., Carlin, J.B., Stern, H.S., Rubin, D.B.: Bayesian data analysis, 2nd edn. Chapman and Hill, NewYork (2003)

Geman, S., Geman, D.: Stochastic relaxation, gibbs distributions and the bayesian restoration of images. IEEE Trans. Pattern Anal. Mach. Intell. **6**, 721–41 (1984)

Hastings, W.K.: Monte Carlo sampling methods using Markov chains and their applications. Biometrika **57**, 97–109 (1970)

Ibrahim, J.G., Chen, M.H., Sinha, D.: Bayesian Survival Analysis. Springer Inc, New York (2001)

Metropolis, N., Ulam, S.: The Monte Carlo method. J. Am. Stat. Assoc. **44**(247), 335–41 (1949)

Metropolis, N., Rosenbluth, A.W., Rosenbluth, M.N., Teller, A.H., Teller, E.: Equations of state calculations by fast computing machine. J. Chem. Phys. **21**, 1087–91 (1953)

Prop, J.G., Wilson, D.B.: Exact sampling with coupled markov chains and applications to statistical mechanics. Random Struct. Algorithms **9**, 223–52 (1996)

Sahu, S.K., Dey, D.K., Aslanidou, H., Sinha, D.: A Weibull regression model with gamma frailties for multivariate survival data. Life Time Data Anal. **3**, 123–137 (1997)

Santos, C.A., Achcar, J.A.: A Bayesian analysis for multivariate survival data in the presence of covariates. Jr. Stat. Theor. Appl. **9**, 233–253 (2010)

Tanner, M.A., Wong, W.H.: The calculation of posterior distributions by data augmentation. J. Am. Stat. Assoc. **82**, 528–49 (1987)

Chapter 3
Nonparametric and Semiparametric Models

Survival data are conveniently summarized through estimates of the survival function and hazard function. Methods of estimating these functions from a sample of survival data are said to be *nonparametric* or *distribution-free*, since they do not require specific assumptions to be made about the underlying distribution of the survival times. An initial step in the analysis of survival data is to present numerical or graphical summaries of the survival times for individuals in a particular group. Such summaries may be of interest in their own right, or as a precursor to a more detailed analysis of the data. Once the estimated survival function has been found, the median and other percentiles of the distribution of survival times can be estimated. When the survival times of two groups of patients are being compared, an informal comparison of the survival experience of each group of individuals can be made using the estimated survival functions. However, there are more formal procedures that enable two groups of survival data to be compared. Nonparametric procedure for comparing two or more groups of survival times is the *logrank test* which is the most powerful test against the alternatives that the hazard functions are proportional.

3.1 Empirical Survival Function

Suppose, we have a single sample of survival times, where none of the observations are censored. The survivor function $S(t)$ is the probability that an individual survives for a time greater than or equal to t. This function can be estimated by the **empirical survival function**, given by

$$\hat{S}(t) = \frac{\text{Number of individuals with survival times} \geq t}{\text{Number of individuals in the data set}}.$$

© Springer Nature Singapore Pte Ltd. 2019   49
D. D. Hanagal, *Modeling Survival Data Using Frailty Models*,
Industrial and Applied Mathematics, https://doi.org/10.1007/978-981-15-1181-3_3

Note that the empirical survival function is equal to unity for values of t before the first death time, and zero after the final death time. The estimated survival function $\hat{S}(t)$ is assumed to be constant between two adjacent times, and so a plot of $\hat{S}(t)$ against t is a step function. The function decreases immediately after each observed survival time.

3.2 Graphical Plotting

Graphical plots of survival data are quick, useful visual tests of whether a particular model is consistent with the observed data. The basic idea behind virtually all graphical plotting techniques is the following:

If the survival data consist of (possibly multicensored) failure data from a population, then the models are life distribution models such as the exponential, Weibull, or lognormal.

The kinds of plots we will consider for failure data are

- Probability (CDF) plots,
- Hazard and Cum Hazard plots.

NOTE: Many of the plots discussed in this chapter can also be used to obtain quick estimates of model parameters. This will be covered in later sections. While there may be other, more accurate ways of estimating parameters, simple graphical estimates can be very handy, especially when other techniques require software programs that are also readily available.

3.2.1 Probability Plotting

Probability plots are simple visual ways of summarizing survival data by plotting CDF estimates versus time.

Plotting Positions: Censored Data (Type I or Type II)

At the time t_i of the ith failure, we need an estimate of the cumulative population percent failure (CDF). The simplest and most obvious estimate is just $100 \times i/n$ (with a total of n units on test). This, however, is generally an overestimate (i.e., biased). Various texts recommend corrections such as $100 \times (i - .5)/n$ or $100 \times i/(n + 1)$. Here, we recommend what are known as (approximate) **median rank** estimates.

Corresponding to the time t_i of the ith failure, use a CDF or Percentile estimate of $100 \times (i - .3)/(n + .4)$.

Plotting Positions: Readout Data

Let the readout times be $T_1, T_2, \ldots, T_k$ and let the corresponding new failures recorded at each readout be $r_1, r_2, \ldots, r_k$. Again, there are n individuals on test.

Corresponding to the readout time T_j, use a CDF or percentile estimate of

$$100 \times \frac{\sum_{i=1}^{j} r_i}{n}.$$

Plotting Positions: Multicensored Data

The calculations are more complicated for multicensored data. K–M estimates (described in Sect. 3.4) can be used to obtain plotting positions at every failure time. The more precise modified K–M estimates are recommended. They reduce to the censored type I or the censored type II median rank estimates when the data consist of only failures, without any removals except possibly at the end of the study period.

The general idea is to take the model CDF equation and write it in such a way that a function of $F(t)$ is a linear equation of a function of t. This will be clear after a few examples. In the formulas that follow, "*ln*" always means "natural logarithm", while "log" always means "base 10 logarithm".

(a) **Exponential Model**: Take the exponential survival function and rewrite it as

$$- \ln S(t) = \lambda t \quad \text{or, equivalently.}$$

If $- \ln S(t)$ is linear in t with slope λ, then exponential model is a good fit.

(b) **Weibull Model**: Take the Weibull survival function and rewrite it as

$$+ \ln (- \ln S(t)) = \gamma \, ln \, t - \gamma \, ln \, \alpha.$$

If $\ln(- \ln S(t))$ is linear in $\ln t$ with slope γ and intercept $-\gamma \ln \alpha$, then Weibull model is a good fit.

(c) **Lognormal Model**: Take the lognormal survival function and rewrite it as

$$ln \, t = \sigma \Phi^{-1}\{1 - S(t)\} + ln \, T_{50},$$

where Φ^{-1} denotes the inverse function for the standard normal distribution. If $\ln t$ is linear in $\Phi^{-1}\{1 - S(t)\}$ with slope σ and intercept $\ln T_{50}$, then lognormal model is a good fit.

(d) **Extreme Value Distribution (Type I—for minimum)**: Take the survival function of extreme value distribution and rewrite it as

$$\ln \{- \ln S(t)\} = (t - \mu)/\beta.$$

If $\ln \{- \ln S(t)\}$ is linear in t with slope $1/\beta$ and intercept $-\mu/\beta$, then extreme value model is a good fit.

Example 3.1 To generate Weibull random failure times, we generate 20 Weibull failure times with a shape parameter of $\gamma = 1.5$ and $\alpha = 500$. Assuming a test time of $T = 500\,\text{h}$, only ten of these failure times would have been observed. They are to the nearest hour: 54, 187, 216, 240, 244, 335, 361, 373, 375, and 386. First, we will compute plotting position survival function estimates based on these failure times, and then a probability plot is plotted. Table 3.1 gives the empirical CDF and $-\ln S(t)$ for this data.

Figure 3.1 shows Weibull plot of $\ln \ln(1/(1 - F(t)))$ versus $\ln t$ for the data given in Example 3.1.

Note that the configuration of points appears to have some curvature. This is mostly due to the very first point on the plot (the earliest time of failure). The first

Table 3.1 Empirical CDF calculations

(1)	(2)	(3)	(4)
Fail $\# = i$	Time of fail	$F(t_i)$ estimate	$\ln\{1/(1 - F(t_i)\}$
	(x)	$(i - 0.3)/20.4$	(y)
1	54	0.034	0.035
2	187	0.083	0.087
3	216	0.132	0.142
4	240	0.181	0.200
5	244	0.230	0.262
6	335	0.279	0.328
7	361	0.328	0.398
8	373	0.377	0.474
9	375	0.426	0.556
10	386	0.475	0.645

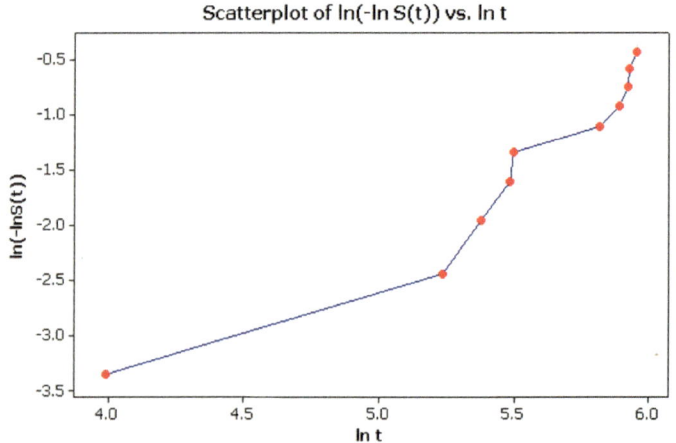

Fig. 3.1 Graphical Weibull fitting plot

few points on a probability plot have more variability than points in the central range and less attention should be paid to them when visually testing for "straightness".

This would give a slope estimate of 1.46, which is close to the 1.5 value used in the simulation.

The intercept is -4.114 and setting this equal to $-\gamma log\alpha$, we estimate $\alpha = 657$ (the "true" value used in the simulation was 500).

3.2.2   Hazard and Cumulative Hazard Plotting

Since probability plots are generally more useful, we will only give a brief description of hazard plotting. We describe how to make cumulative probability plots in the following steps.

1. Order the failure times and running times for each of the n units on test in ascending order from 1 to n. The order is called the rank of an individual. Calculate the reverse rank for each individual (reverse rank $= n-$ rank $+1$).
2. Calculate a hazard "value" for every failed individual (do this only for the failed individuals). The Hazard value for the failed individual with reverse rank k is just $1/k$.
3. Calculate the cumulative hazard values for each failed individual. The cumulative hazard value corresponding to a particular failed individual is the sum of all the hazard values for failed individuals with ranks up to and including that failed individual.
4. Plot the time of fail versus the cumulative hazard value as covered below for the exponential and the Weibull model.

Example 3.2   Ten cancer patients in a clinical trial were under observation up to 250 days. Six patients dead at 37, 73, 132, 195, 222, and 248 days. Four patients discontinued the treatment and got admitted to another hospital at the following times: 50, 100, 200, and 250 days. Cumulative hazard values were computed in Table 3.2.

Next, ignore the rows with no cumulative hazard value and plot column (1) versus column (6) of Table 3.2.

3.2.3   Exponential and Weibull Hazard Plots

The cumulative hazard for the exponential is just $H(t) = \lambda t$, which is linear in t with a 0 intercept. So a simple linear graph paper plot of $y = $ col (6) versus $x = $ col (1) should line up as approximately a straight line going through the origin with slope λ if the exponential model is appropriate. Figure 3.2 gives the plot of $H(t)$ versus t for the data given in Example 3.2.

Table 3.2 Empirical cumulative hazard calculations

(1) Time of event	(2) 1=Failure 0 = Censored	(3) Rank	(4) Reverse rank	(5) Hazard value (2)/(4)	(6) Cum. hazard value
37	1	1	10	1/10	0.10
50	0	2	9		
73	1	3	8	1/8	0.225
100	0	4	7		
132	1	5	6	1/6	0.391
195	1	6	5	1/5	0.591
200	0	7	4		
222	1	8	3	1/3	0.924
248	1	9	2	1/2	1.424
250	0	10	1		

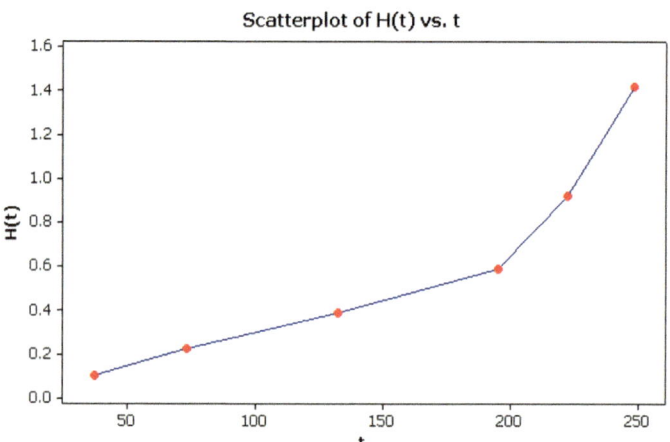

Fig. 3.2 Graphical exponential fitting of the data

The cumulative hazard for the Weibull is $H(t) = (t/\alpha)^{\gamma}$, so a plot of $\ln H(t) = \ln\ col(6)$ versus $\ln t = \ln\ col(1)$ resembles a straight line with slope γ if the Weibull model is appropriate. Figure 3.3 gives the probability plot for Weibull distribution for the data given in Example 3.2.

The Weibull fit looks better, although the slope estimate is 1.27, which is not far from an exponential model slope of 1. Of course, with a sample of just ten, and only six failures, it is difficult to pick a model from the data alone.

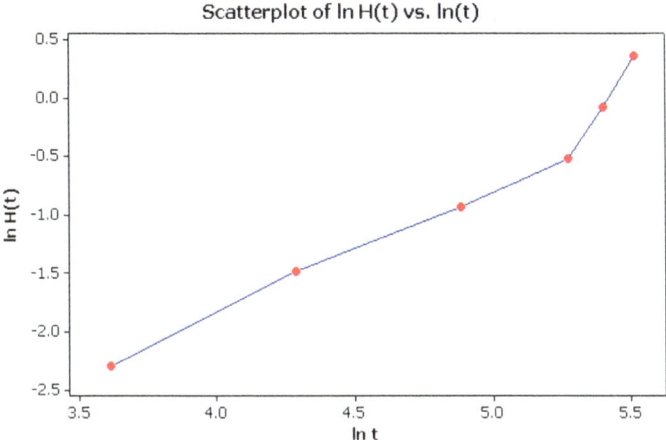

Fig. 3.3 Graphical Weibull fitting of the data

3.3   Graphical Estimation

Once you have calculated the plotting positions from your failure data and put the points on the appropriate graph paper for your chosen model, parameter estimation follows easily. But along with the mechanics of graphical estimation, be aware of both the advantages and the disadvantages of graphical estimation methods.

Graphical Estimation Mechanics

If you draw a line through the points, and the paper is a commercially designed probability paper, there are usually simple rules to find estimates of the slope (or shape parameter) and the scale parameter. On a lognormal paper with time on the x-axis and cumulative percent on the y-axis, draw horizontal lines from the 34th and the 50th percentiles across to the line, and drop vertical lines to the time axis from these intersection points. The time corresponding to the 50th percentile is the T_{50} estimate. Divide T_{50} by the time corresponding to the 34th percentile (this is called T_{34}). The natural logarithm of that ratio is the estimate of sigma or the slope of the line ($\sigma = ln(T_{50}/T_{34})$).

On commercial Weibull probability paper, there is often a horizontal line through the 62.3 percentile point. That estimation line intersects the line through the points at a time that is the estimate of the characteristic life parameter α. In order to estimate the line slope (or the shape parameter γ), some papers have a special point on them called an estimation point. You drop a line from the estimation point perpendicular to the fitted line and look where it passes through a special **estimation scale**. The estimate of γ is read off the estimation scale where the line crosses it.

Other papers may have variations on the methods described above. To remove the subjectivity of drawing a line through the points, a least squares (regression) fit can be performed.

Advantages of Graphical Methods of Estimation

- Graphical methods are quick and easy to use and make visual sense.
- Calculations can be done with little or no special software needed.
- Visual test of the model (i.e., how well the points line up) is an additional benefit.

Disadvantages of Graphical Methods of Estimation

The statistical properties of graphical estimates (i.e., how precise they are on the average) are not good due to the following:

- They are biased.
- Even with large samples, they do not become minimum variance (i.e., most precise) estimates.
- Graphical methods do not give confidence intervals for the parameters (intervals generated by a regression program for this kind of data are incorrect).
- Formal statistical tests about model fit or parameter values cannot be performed with graphical methods.

As we have seen in the last chapter, maximum likelihood estimates overcome all these disadvantages—at least for survival data sets with a reasonably large number of failures—at a cost of losing all the advantages listed above for graphical estimation.

3.4 Empirical Model Fitting: Distribution Free (Kaplan–Meier) Approach

Kaplan and Meier (1958) proposed an estimator called as Kaplan–Meier (K–M) Product Limit estimator which provides quick, simple estimates of the survival function or the CDF based on failure data that may even be multicensored. No underlying model (such as Weibull or lognormal) is assumed; K–M estimation is an empirical (nonparametric) procedure. Exact times of failure are required.

Calculating Kaplan–Meier Estimates

The steps for calculating K–M estimates are the following:

1. Order the actual failure times from t_1 through t_r, where there are r failures.
2. Corresponding to each t_i, associate the number n_i, with $n_i =$ the number of operating units just before the ith failure occurred at time t_i.
3. Estimate $S(t_1)$ by $(n_1 - 1)/n_1$.
4. Estimate $S(t_i)$ by $S(t_{i-1})(n_i - 1)/n_i$.
5. Estimate the CDF $F(t_i)$ by $1 - S(t_i)$.

Note that unfailed individuals taken off the test (i.e., censored) only count up to the last actual failure time before they were censored. They are included in the n_i counts up to and including that failure time, but not after.

Example 3.3 A simple example will illustrate the K–M procedure. Assume that 20 patients with some disease in a clinical study are on life test and six deaths occur at the following times: 10, 32, 56, 98, 122, and 181 days. There were four patients who discontinued from the clinical study at the following times: 50, 100, 125, and 150 days. The remaining ten patients were survived at the end of the clinical study, i.e., on the 200th day. The K–M estimates for this life test are

$$S(10) = 19/20$$
$$S(32) = 19/20 \times 18/19$$
$$S(56) = 19/20 \times 18/19 \times 16/17$$
$$S(98) = 19/20 \times 18/19 \times 16/17 \times 15/16$$
$$S(122) = 19/20 \times 18/19 \times 16/17 \times 15/16 \times 13/14$$
$$S(181) = 19/20 \times 18/19 \times 16/17 \times 15/16 \times 13/14 \times 10/11.$$

A General Expression for K–M Estimates

A general expression for the K–M estimates can be written. Assume that we have n individuals on the test and order the observed lifetimes for these n individuals from t_1 to t_n. Some of these are actual failure times and some are running times for individuals taken off test before they die. Suppose, there are r deaths that have occurred, and the ordered death times are $t_{(1)}, \ldots, t_{(r)}$, where $r \leq n$. The number individuals who are alive just before time $t_{(j)}$, including those who are about to die at this time, will be denoted by n_j, $j = 1, 2, \ldots, r$, and d_j will denote the number who die at this time. The probability that an individual dies during the interval from $t_{(j)} - \delta$ to $t_{(j)}$ is estimated by d_j/n_j where δ is an infinitesimal time interval. The corresponding estimated probability of survival through that interval is then $(n_j - d_j)/n_j$. The probability of surviving through the interval from $t_{(k)}$ to $t_{(k+1)}$ and all preceding intervals leads to the Kaplan–Meier estimate of the survival function, which is given by

$$\hat{S}(t) = \prod_{j=1}^{k} \left(\frac{n_j - d_j}{n_j} \right),$$

for $t_{(k)} \leq t < t_{(k+1)}$, $k = 1, 2, \ldots, r$. A plot of Kaplan–Meier estimate of the survival function is a step function, in which the estimated survival probabilities are constant between adjacent death times and decrease at each death time.

The estimated variance of the estimate of $S(t)$ and is given by

$$var\{\hat{S}(t)\} \approx [\hat{S}(t)]^2 \sum_{j=1}^{k} \frac{d_j}{n_j(n_j - d_j)}.$$

The standard error of the K–M estimate of survival function is

$$se(\hat{S}(t)) \approx \hat{S}(t) \left\{ \sum_{j=1}^{k} \frac{d_j}{n_j(n_j - d_j)} \right\}^{\frac{1}{2}},$$

for $t_{(k)} \leq t < t_{(k+1)}$.

Nelson–Aalen Estimator

The most common estimate of integrated hazard is the Nelson–Aalen estimate which was first introduced by Nelson (1969) based on counting process and is given by

$$\hat{H}(t) = \sum_{i:t_i \leq t} \frac{\overline{N}(t_i) - \overline{N}(t_i-)}{\overline{Y}(t_i)},$$

where $\overline{Y}(t_i) = \sum_j Y_j(t_i)$, $\overline{N}(t_i) = \sum_j N_j(t_i)$.

The $N_j(t)$ is the counting process, that is, the number of observed events in $[0, t]$ for the unit j, and $Y(t)$ is a predictable process—a process whose value at time t is known infinitesimally before t. The Nelson–Aalen estimator is essentially a method of moment estimator. Its variance is estimated consistently by

$$var[\hat{H}(t)] = \sum_{i:t_i \leq t} \frac{\overline{N}(t_i) - \overline{N}(t_i-)}{\overline{Y}^2(t_i)}.$$

Breslow (1972) suggested a nonparametric estimate for survival function and is given by $\hat{S}_B(t) = \exp[-\hat{H}(t)]$. Fleming and Harrington (1984) showed the close relationship between the Breslow and Kaplan–Meier estimators, and compared them numerically for several sample sizes and censoring percentages. Let $d\hat{H}(t_i) = [\overline{N}(t_i) - \overline{N}(t_i-)]/\overline{Y}(t_i)$, the increment in the Nelson–Aalen (N–A) estimator at the ith failure. Then Breslow estimator can be written as

$$\hat{S}_B(t) = \prod_{j:t_j \leq t} e^{-d\hat{H}(t_j)}$$

and the Kaplan–Meier estimate is

$$\hat{S}_{KM}(t) = \prod_{j:t_j \leq t} [1 - d\hat{H}(t_j)].$$

Since $e^{-x} \approx 1 - x$ for small x, the two estimators are quite similar when the increments $d\hat{H}$ are small, that is, when there are many subjects still at risk. The two estimates are asymptotically equivalent since, as $n \to \infty$, the individual increments get arbitrarily small. Since $e^{-x} \geq 1 - x$, $\hat{S}_B(t) \geq \hat{S}_{KM}(t)$ in finite samples. If the largest time T in a data set is a death, $\hat{S}_{KM}(t) = 0$, but $\hat{S}_B(t)$ is positive.

Example 3.4 The data on kidney infection is presented in Sect. 1.5 in Chap. 1. We plot survival function for the time to first infection or censoring at the point of insertion of the catheter-based K–M estimate and Breslow (or N–A) estimate. We also obtain 95% confidence intervals for K–M estimates. We can very easily observe from the survival function of the graph that Breslow (or N–A) estimates are larger than the K–M estimates. The R program commands to draw this graph are as follows.

```
jpeg(file="D:/David/Book2/surv01.jpg",height=5,width=6.5,
units="in",quality=100,bg="white",par(mfrow=c(1,1)),res=72)
kidney=read.table(file="D:/David/Book2/kidney.txt",header=T)
afit=survfit(Surv(T1,I1)~1,kidney,type="fleming-harrington")
kfit=survfit(Surv(T1,I1)~1,kidney,type="kaplan-meier")
plot(kfit,mark.time=F,main="Survival Function vs Time",
xlim=c(0,600),ylim=c(0,1),xlab="Survival Time(days)",
ylab="Survival Function",pch=" ")
lines(afit$time,afit$surv,type="s",lty=2)
legend(0,0.3,c("K-M","N-A"),lty=c(1,2),cex=0.8)
dev.off()
```

The graph of survival functions based on K–M and Breslow(or N–A) estimates are displayed in Fig. 3.4 and it is observed from the graph that Breslow estimates are slightly larger than the K–M estimates.

Example 3.5 The data on bone marrow transplantation (BMT) is presented in Sect. 1.2 of Chap. 1. The patient's age, sex, and disease group (1-ALL, 2-AML low risk, 3-AML high risk) were considered as covariates. We compare the graph of survival function based on K–M and Breslow (or N–A) estimates in three different groups (1-ALL, 2-AML low risk, 3-AML high risk) using the R program. The R program commands are as follows.

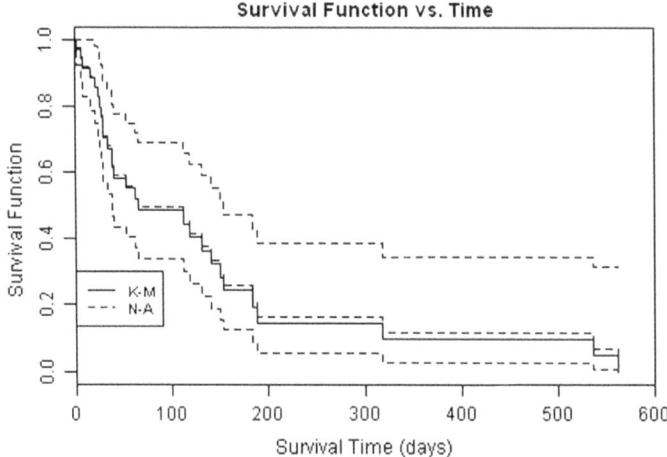

Fig. 3.4 K–M and Breslow (or N–A) estimates for kidney infection data set with 95% CI for K–M

```
jpeg(file="surv0.jpg",height=5,width=6.5,units="in",quality=100,
bg="white",par(mfrow=c(1,1)),res=72)
bone1=read.table(file="D:/David/SurvivalAnalysis/BMT1.txt",
header=T)
fit=survfit(Surv(T2,I2)~g,conf.type=c("plain"),bone1)
fit1=fit[g=1]
fit2=fit[g=2]
fit3=fit[g=3]
plot(0,0,main="Survival Function vs Time",xlim=c(0,600),
ylim=c(0,1),xlab="Survival Time(days)",
ylab="Survival Function",pch=" ")
lines(fit1$time,fit1$surv,type="s",lty=1)
lines(fit2$time,fit2$surv,type="s",lty=2)
lines(fit3$time,fit3$surv,type="s",lty=3)
legend(0,0.3,c("Group1=ALL","Group2=Low-AML","Group3=High-AML"),
lty=c(1,2,3),cex=0.8)
dev.off()
```

The graph of K–M survival function for three groups are displayed in Fig. 3.5.
We obtain the graph of $-lnS(t)$ versus t for the three groups (1-ALL, 2-AML
low risk, 3-AML high risk) using the R program. The R program commands are as
follows.

```
jpeg(file="surv1.jpg",height=5,width=6.5,units="in",quality=100,
bg="white",par(mfrow=c(1,1)),res=72)
bone1=read.table(file="D:/David/SurvivalAnalysis/BMT1.txt",
header=T)
fit=survfit(Surv(T2,I2)~g,conf.type=c("plain"),bone1)
fit1=fit[g=1]
fit2=fit[g=2]
fit3=fit[g=3]
plot(0,0,main="-Log(S(t)) vs Time",xlim=c(0,600),ylim=c(0,1),
```

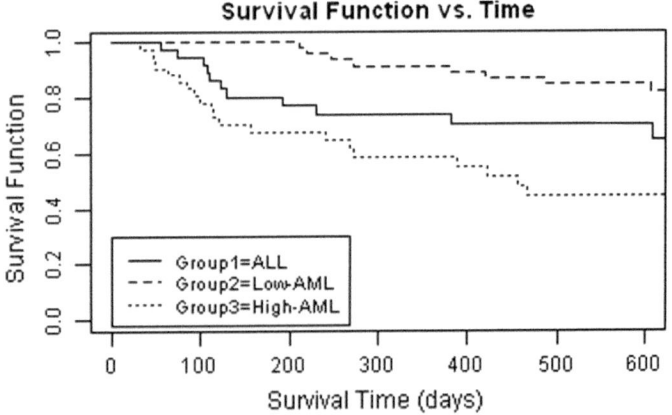

Fig. 3.5 Graph of the survival function of three groups for BMT data set

```
xlab="Survival Time(days)",ylab="-Log(S(t))",pch=" ")
lines(fit1$time,-log(fit1$surv),type="s",lty=1)
lines(fit2$time,-log(fit2$surv),type="s",lty=2)
lines(fit3$time,-log(fit3$surv),type="s",lty=3)
legend(1,1,c("Group1=ALL","Group2=Low-AML",
"Group3=High-AML"),lty=c(1,2,3),cex=0.8)
dev.off()
```

The graph of $-\ln S(t)$ versus t for three groups are displayed in Fig. 3.6.

We obtain a graph of $\ln[-\ln S(t)]$ versus $\ln t$ for the three groups (1-ALL, 2-AML low risk, 3-AML high risk) using the R program. The R program commands are as follows.

```
jpeg(file="surv2.jpg",height=5,width=6.5,units="in",quality=100,
bg="white",par(mfrow=c(1,1)),res=72)
bone1=read.table(file="D:/David/SurvivalAnalysis/BMT1.txt",
header=T)
fit=survfit(Surv(T2,I2)~g,conf.type=c("plain"),bone1)
fit1=fit[g=1]
fit2=fit[g=2]
fit3=fit[g=3]
plot(0,0,main="Log(-Log(S(t))) vs log of Time",xlim=c(3.5,7),
ylim=c(-4,0.5),xlab="Log of Survival Time(days)",
ylab="Log(-Log(S(t)))",pch=" ")
lines(log(fit1$time),log(-log(fit1$surv)),type="s",lty=1)
lines(log(fit2$time),log(-log(fit2$surv)),type="s",lty=2)
lines(log(fit3$time),log(-log(fit3$surv)),type="s",lty=3)
legend(3.5,0.5,c("Group1=ALL","Group2=Low-AML","Group3=High-AML"),
lty=c(1,2,3),cex=0.8)
dev.off()
```

The graph of $\ln[-\ln S(t)]$ versus $\ln t$ for three groups are displayed in Fig. 3.7.

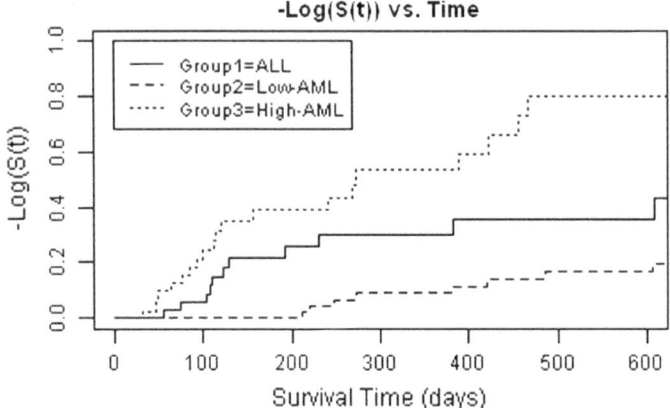

Fig. 3.6 Graph of the $-\ln S(t)$ versus t of three groups for BMT data set

One can compare the nonparametric K–M estimate of survival curves with survival curves of parametric models, say, exponential and Weibull distributions. Figure 3.8 gives the graph of K–M survival curve and 95% confidence intervals of K–M estimate with exponential and Weibull survival curves using R program and SAS program together. The exponential survival curve is very close to K–M survival curve. The R program is as follows.

```
plot(0,0,xlim=c(0,600),ylim=c(0,1),xlab="Survival time(days)",
ylab="Survival probability",pch=" ")
bone=read.table(file="BMT1.txt",header=T)
fit=survfit(Surv(T2,I2),conf.type=c("plain"),bone)
lines(fit,lty=1)
x=seq(0,600, by=5)
lam=exp(-7.163) # value 7.163 is obtained from SAS program
# using proc lifereg
sf=exp(-lam*x)
lines(x,sf,lty=2)
gam=1/1.72     # value 1.72 is obtained from SAS program
# using proc lifereg
lamb=exp(-7.294/1.72)
sf1=exp(-lamb*x^gam)
lines(x,sf1,lty=3)
legend(400,1,c("KM estimate","Exponential fit","Weibull fit"),
lty=c(1,2,3),cex=0.8)
```

The SAS program is used to calculate $\lambda = \exp(-intercept)$ in the exponential distribution. In the same way, the SAS program is used to calculate $\lambda = \exp(-intercept/scale)$ and $\gamma = 1/scale$ in the Weibull distribution. The following are the SAS commands.

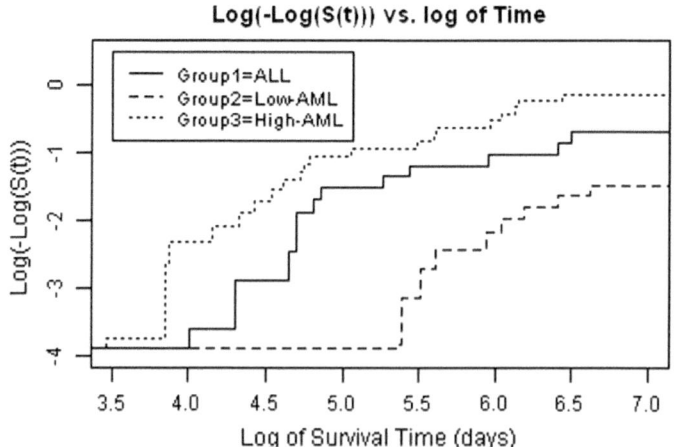

Fig. 3.7 Graph of the $\ln[-\ln S(t)]$ versus $\ln t$ of three groups for BMT data set

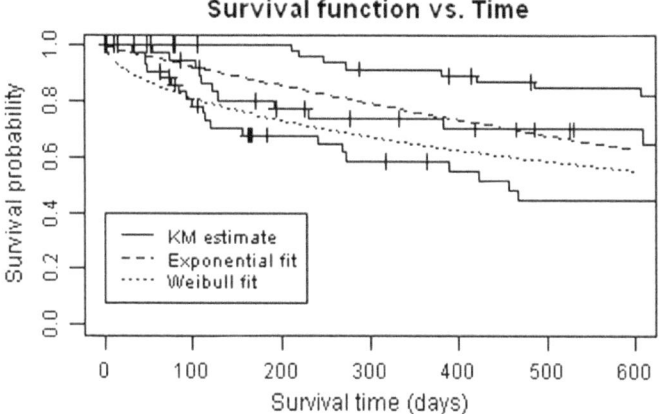

Fig. 3.8 Graph of the $\ln[-\ln S(t)]$ versus $\ln t$ of three groups for BMT data set

```
proc lifereg data=BMT1;
model T2*I2(0)=/dist=exponential;
run;
proc lifereg data=BMT1;
model T2*I2(0)=/dist=weibull;
run;
```

3.5 Comparison Between Two Survival Functions

Let us consider the comparison between two survival functions $S_1(t)$ and $S_2(T)$. The test is developed for the hypothesis

$$H_0 : S_1(t) = S_2(t)$$

that the two survival functions are the same. Treating the observations from both distributions as coming from a single population and by defining a dummy regressor, variable y takes on the value 0 or 1 based on whether an observation comes from the first or second distribution. The hazard functions for the two survival functions are $h_1(t) = h_0(t)$ and $h_2(t) = h_0(t)e^{\beta}$, and the two distributions are identical if and only if $\beta = 0$, i.e.,

$$S_2(t) = S_1(t)^{\exp(\beta)}$$

so that by testing $\beta = 0$, one is testing the hypothesis

$$H_0 : S_2(t) = S_1(t) \quad \text{versus} \quad H_1 : S_2(t) = S_1(t)^{\delta}, \quad \delta \neq 1$$

where $\delta = \exp(\beta)$.

Logrank Test:

Let n_1 and n_2 be the number on individuals in group 1 and 2, respectively, and $n = n_1 + n_2$. Let n_{1i} and n_{2i} be the number of individuals at risk just prior to $t_{(i)}$ from the treatments 1 and 2, and d_{1i} and d_{2i} be the number of deaths at $t_{(i)}$ among the individuals in group 1 and group 2 and $d_{1i} + d_{2i} = d_i$, $n_{1i} + n_{2i} = n_i$. The logrank statistic is given by

$$X_{LR} = \frac{\left[\sum_{i=1}^{r}(d_{1i} - e_{1i})\right]^2}{\sum_{i=1}^{r} V_{1i}},$$

where

$$e_{1i} = n_{1i}d_i/n_i, \quad V_{1i} = \frac{n_{1i}n_{2i}d_i(n_i - d_i)}{n_i^2(n_i - 1)}, \quad i = 1, \ldots, r,$$

X_{LR} is the logrank statistic which is the distributed approximately central chi-square distribution with one degree of freedom when the null hypothesis is true and the sample size is moderate.

Wilcoxon Test:

The Wilcoxon test, sometimes known as the **Breslow test**, is also used to test the null hypothesis that there is no difference in the survival functions for two groups of survival data. The Wilcoxon test is based on the test statistic

$$X_W = \frac{\left[\sum_{i=1}^{r} n_i(d_{1i} - e_{1i})\right]^2}{\sum_{i=1}^{r} n_i^2 V_{1i}}$$

which has a central chi-square distribution with one degree of freedom when the null hypothesis is true. The Wilcoxon test is conducted in the same manner as the logrank test.

The difference between logrank and Wilcoxon tests is that in the Wilcoxon test, each difference $(d_{1i} - e_{1i})$ is weighted by n_i, the total number of individuals at risk at time $t_{(i)}$. The effect of this is to give less weight to differences between d_{1i} and e_{1i} at those times when the total number of individuals who are still alive is small, that is, at the longest survival times. This statistic is, therefore, less sensitive than the logrank statistic to deviations of d_{1i} from e_{1i} in the tail of the distribution of the survival times.

The logrank test is more suitable to test the null hypothesis of no difference between two groups of survival times when the alternative hypothesis is the hazard of death at any given time for an individual in one group is proportional to the hazard at that time for a similar individual in the other group. This is the assumption of proportional hazards, which underlies a number of methods for analyzing survival data. For other types of departure from the null hypothesis, the Wilcoxon test is more appropriate than the logrank test for comparing the two survival functions. When the hazard functions are proportional, the survival functions for the two groups of survival data do not cross one another.

Example 3.6 The data on bone marrow transplantation is presented in Sect. 1.4 of Chap. 1 and also in Example 3.6 of this chapter. Patient's age, sex, and disease group (1-ALL, 2-AML low risk, 3-AML high risk) were considered as covariates. We obtain the test for testing equality of survival functions for the three groups (1-ALL, 2-AML low risk, 3-AML high risk) using an R program based on logrank and Wilcoxon tests. We also obtain estimates and 95% confidence intervals of the estimates of survival functions. The R program commands are as follows.

```
bone=read.table(file="BMT1.txt",header=T)
fit=survfit(Surv(T2,I2),conf.type=c("plain"),bone)
summary(fit)
survdiff(Surv(T2,I2)~g,bone,rho=0)
survdiff(Surv(T2,I2)~g,bone,rho=1)
```

The output of these R program commands is as follows.

```
Call: survfit(formula=Surv(T2, I2),data=bone,
      conf.type = c("plain"))
```

time	n.risk	n.event	survival	std.err	lower 95% CI	upper 95% CI
32	133	1	0.992	0.00749	0.978	1.000
47	131	2	0.977	0.01294	0.952	1.000
48	129	1	0.970	0.01489	0.941	0.999
55	126	1	0.962	0.01665	0.929	0.995
64	124	1	0.954	0.01823	0.919	0.990
. . . .						
609	62	1	0.658	0.04523	0.569	0.747
625	61	1	0.647	0.04576	0.558	0.737
662	59	1	0.636	0.04628	0.546	0.727
748	56	1	0.625	0.04683	0.533	0.717

```
Call:
survdiff(formula = Surv(T2, I2) ~ g, data = bone, rho = 0)
```

	N	Observed	Expected	(O-E)^2/E	(O-E)^2/V
g=1	38	12	11.2	0.0625	0.0854
g=2	54	9	20.2	6.1851	12.0778
g=3	45	21	10.7	10.0122	13.5301

Chisq= 16.5 on 2 degrees of freedom, p= 0.000263

```
Call:
survdiff(formula = Surv(T2, I2) ~ g, data = bone, rho = 1)
```

	N	Observed	Expected	(O-E)^2/E	(O-E)^2/V
g=1	38	10.08	9.36	0.0555	0.0896
g=2	54	6.72	16.47	5.7688	13.1752
g=3	45	18.04	9.02	9.0355	14.4025

Chisq= 17.8 on 2 degrees of freedom, p= 0.000138

This output shows that there is a difference in the observed and expected observations in group 2 and 3, i.e., AML low risk and AML high risk. Both logrank test and the Wilcoxon test are rejected for testing the hypothesis of the equality survival functions in three groups. The chi-square with 2 df is 17.8 and p-value is 0.000138. There is a very high significant difference between the survival curves of the three groups.

3.6   Cox's Proportional Hazards Model

The proportional hazards model, proposed by Cox (1972, 1975), has been used primarily in medical testing analysis, to model the effect of secondary variables on survival. Its strength lies in its ability to model and test many inferences about survival without making any specific assumptions about the form of the life distribution model.

This section will give only a brief description of the proportional hazards model. It has wide applications in medicine and biology.

Proportional Hazards Model Assumption

Let $y = \{y_1, y_2, \ldots y_k\}$ be a vector of one or more **explanatory** variables believed to affect lifetime. These variables may be continuous (dosage level of a particular drug in medical studies) or they may be indicator variables with the value 1 if a given factor or condition is present, and 0 otherwise.

Let the hazard rate for a nominal (or baseline) set $y^0 = (y_1^0, y_2^0, \ldots, y_k^0)$ of these variables be given by $h_0(t)$, with $h_0(t)$ denoting legitimate hazard function (failure rate) for some unspecified life distribution model.

The proportional hazards model assumes that we can write the changed hazard function for a new value of y as

$$h_y(t) = g(y)h_0(t).$$

In other words, changing y, the explanatory variable vector results in a new hazard function that is proportional to the nominal hazard function, and the proportionality constant is a function of y, $g(y)$, independent of the time variable t.

A common and useful form for $g(y)$ is the equation: $g(y) = e^{\beta y}$ for one variable, $g(y_1, y_2) = e^{\beta_1 y_1 + \beta_2 y_2}$ for two variables, etc.

Properties and Applications of the Proportional Hazards Model

1. The proportional hazards model is equivalent to the acceleration factor concept if and only if the life distribution model is a Weibull (which includes the exponential model, as a special case). For a Weibull with shape parameter γ, and an acceleration factor AF between nominal use fail time t_0 and high stress fail time t_s (with $t_0 = AF t_s$), we have $g(y) = AF^\gamma$. In other words, $h_s(t) = AF^\gamma h_0(t)$.

2. Under a log-linear model assumption for $g(y)$, without any further assumptions about the life distribution model, it is possible to analyze experimental data and compute maximum likelihood estimates and use likelihood ratio tests to determine which explanatory variables are highly significant.

The general proportional hazards model for the ith individual is

$$h_i(t) = h_0(t) \exp(\beta_1 y_{1i} + \beta_2 y_{2i} + \cdots + \beta_p y_{pi}).$$

This model can be reexpressed in the following form

$$\ln\left\{\frac{h_i(t)}{h_0(t)}\right\} = \beta_1 y_{1i} + \beta_2 y_{2i} + \cdots + \beta_p y_{pi}.$$

Notice that there is no constant term in the linear component of the proportional hazards model.

There are two unknown components in the proportional hazards model, one is the regression parameter and the second, the baseline hazard function $h_0(t)$. One can write the baseline survival function as

$$S_0(t) = \exp\left(-\int_0^t h_0(u)du\right) = \exp[-H_0(t)],$$

where $H_0(t)$ is the baseline cumulative hazard function. The survival function of T given $\mathbf{y}$ is

$$S(t|\mathbf{y}) = \exp\left(-\int_0^t h_0(u|\mathbf{y})du\right) = [S_0(t)]^{\exp(\beta'\mathbf{y})}.$$

We wish to estimate β and $S_0(t)$, or $h_0(t)$, from data that are possibly censored. One approach would be to attempt to maximize the likelihood function for the observed data simultaneously with respect to β and $h_0(t)$. A more attractive approach is that given by Cox (1972), in which a likelihood that does not depend upon $h_0(t)$ is obtained for β. This can be maximized to give an estimate β and to provide tests for β in the absence of knowledge of $h_0(t)$. Once β has been estimated, $h_0(t)$ (or $S_0(t)$) can be estimated by the K–M product limit estimate. This approach is taken here.

Suppose that data are available for n individuals, among whom there are r distinct death times and $n - r$ right-censored survival times. We will, for the moment, assume that only one individual dies at each death time so that there are no ties in the data. The r ordered death times will be denoted by $t_{(1)} < t_{(2)} < \cdots < t_{(r)}$. The β coefficients in the proportional hazards model can be estimated using the *method of maximum likelihood*. To operate this method, we first obtain the likelihood of the sample data.

Cox (1972) showed the partial likelihood function for the proportional hazards model which is given by

$$L(\beta) = \prod_{j=1}^{r} \frac{\exp(\beta' y_{(j)})}{\sum_{l \in R(t_{(j)})} \exp(\beta' y_l)},$$

where $y_{(j)}$ is the vector of covariates for the individual who dies at the jth ordered death time, $t_{(j)}$. The summation in the denominator of this likelihood function is the sum of the $\exp(\beta'y)$ over all individuals who are at risk at time $t_{(j)}$. Notice that the product is taken over by the individuals for whom death times have been recorded. Individuals for whom the survival times are censored do not contribute to the numerator of the loglikelihood function, but they do enter into the simulation over the risk sets at death that occur before a censored time. Moreover, the likelihood function depends only on the ranking of the death times since this determines the risk set at each death time. When there are more than one deaths at each time, Peto (1972) and Breslow (1974) obtained the partial likelihood function $L(\beta)$ which is given by

$$L(\beta) = \prod_{j=1}^{r} \frac{\exp(\beta'S_j)}{\left(\sum_{l\in R(t_{(j)})} \exp(\beta'y_l)\right)^{d_j}},$$

where d_j is the number of lifetimes equal to $t_{(j)}$ and S_j is the sum of the regression vectors y for these d_j individuals. That is, if D_j represents the set of individuals who die at $t_{(j)}$, then $d_j = |D_j|$ and $S_j = \sum_{l\in D_j} y_l$. When there are no ties, all $d_j = 1$. The loglikelihood is

$$\ln L(\beta) = \sum_{j=1}^{r} S_j\beta - \sum_{j=1}^{r} d_j \ln\left(\sum_{l\in R(t_{(j)})} e^{\beta'y_l}\right)$$

and the first derivatives of $\log L(\beta)$ are

$$\frac{\partial \ln L}{\partial \beta_m} = \sum_{j=1}^{r}\left(S_{jm} - \frac{d_j \sum_{l\in R(t_{(j)})} y_{lm}e^{\beta'y_l}}{\sum_{l\in R(t_{(j)})} e^{\beta'y_l}}\right), \quad m = 1, \ldots, p,$$

where S_{jm} is the mth component of $S_j = (S_{j1}, \ldots, S_{jp})$. The matrix I containing minus the second order partial derivatives of $\log L(\beta)$ has entries

$$I_{mn} = \frac{-\partial^2 \ln L(\beta)}{\partial \beta_m \partial \beta_n}, \quad m, n = 1, \ldots, p.$$

$$= \sum_{j=1}^{r} d_j \left[\sum_{l\in R(t_{(j)})} y_{lm}y_{ln}e^{\beta'y_l} \Big/ \sum_{l\in R(t_{(j)})} e^{\beta'y_l} \right.$$
$$\left. - \left(\sum_{l\in R(t_{(j)})} y_{lm}e^{\beta'y_j}\right)\left(\sum_{l\in R(t_{(j)})} y_{ln}e^{\beta'y_l}\right) \Big/ \left(\sum_{l\in R(t_{(j)})} e^{\beta'y_l}\right)^2 \right].$$

The inverse of matrix I is the variance–covariance matrix and it is used in the Newton–Raphson procedure to obtain the maximum likelihood estimates of β.

Example 3.7 The myeloma data discussed in Sect. 1.9 of Chap. 1 is revisited here
in this example. We take Cox's proportional hazards model for assessing the nine
covariates on the survival time using R program commands.

```
> myeloma=read.table(file="myeloma.txt",header=T)
> library(survival)
> fit <- coxph(Surv(T,S)~LBUN+HGB+P+Age+LW+F+LPBM+Pr+SC,myeloma)
> plot( survfit( fit),xlab="Time (in months)",
+ ylab="Survival Function")
> summary(fit)
```

The output of the R program is as follows.

```
Call:
coxph(formula = Surv(T, S) ~ LBUN + HGB + P + Age + LW + F +
    LPBM + Pr + SC, data = myeloma)

  n= 65
          coef exp(coef) se(coef)      z      p
LBUN   1.8556      6.395    0.6563  2.827 0.0047
HGB   -0.1263      0.881    0.0721 -1.751 0.0800
P     -0.2549      0.775    0.5119 -0.498 0.6200
Age   -0.0131      0.987    0.0196 -0.668 0.5000
LW     0.3539      1.425    0.7158  0.494 0.6200
F      0.3423      1.408    0.4072  0.841 0.4000
LPBM   0.3816      1.465    0.4874  0.783 0.4300
Pr     0.0130      1.013    0.0261  0.498 0.6200
SC     0.1298      1.139    0.1050  1.236 0.2200

       exp(coef) exp(-coef) lower .95 upper .95
LBUN       6.395      0.156     1.767     23.15
HGB        0.881      1.135     0.765      1.02
P          0.775      1.290     0.284      2.11
Age        0.987      1.013     0.950      1.03
LW         1.425      0.702     0.350      5.79
F          1.408      0.710     0.634      3.13
LPBM       1.465      0.683     0.563      3.81
Pr         1.013      0.987     0.963      1.07
SC         1.139      0.878     0.927      1.40

Rsquare= 0.237    (max possible= 0.991 )
Likelihood ratio test= 17.6   on 9 df,    p=0.0399
Wald test             = 17.9   on 9 df,    p=0.0361
Score (logrank) test = 19.0   on 9 df,    p=0.0255
```

Here also, LBUN is the most effective variable which is related to the survival of
patients as we have seen in the parametric regression model in Chap. 2. The global
test for testing all the regression parameters equal to zero is rejected at a 5% level of
significance. 95% confidence interval for $\exp(-\beta_i)$, $i = 1, \ldots 9$ are displayed in the
output of the R program.

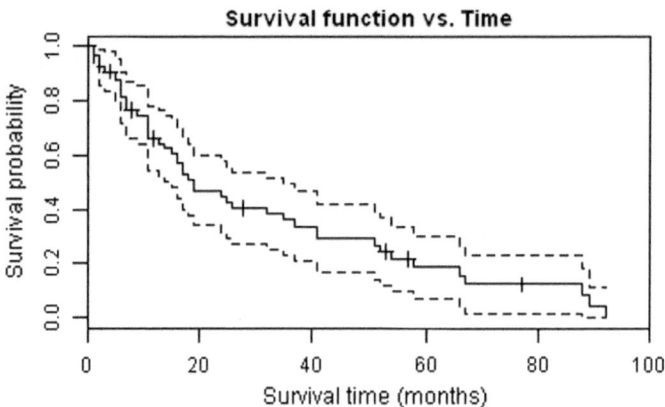

Fig. 3.9 K–M curve with 95% CI for Myeloma data

Figure 3.9 shows the graph of survival function versus time (in days) for the myeloma data along with 95% confidence interval.

References

Breslow, N.E.: Discussion of professor Cox's paper. J. R. Stat. Soc. B **34**, 216–217 (1972)

Breslow, N.E.: Covariate analysis of censored survival data. Biometrics **30**, 89–100 (1974)

Cox, D.R.: Regression models and life tables (with discussions). J. R. Stat. Soc. B **34**, 187–220 (1972)

Cox, D.R.: Partial likelihood. Biometrika **62**, 269–276 (1975)

Fleming, T.R., Harrington, D.P.: Nonparametric estimation of survival distribution in censored data. Commun. Stat. Theory Methods **13**, 2469–2486 (1984)

Kaplan, E.L., Meier, P.: Nonparametric estimation from incomplete observations. J. Am. Stat. Assoc. **53**, 457–481 (1958)

Nelson, W.: Hazard plotting for incomplete failure data. J. Qual. Technol. **1**, 27–52 (1969)

Peto, R.: Contribution to the discussion of paper by D.R. Cox. J. R. Stat. Soc. B **34**, 205–207 (1972)

Part II
Shared Frailty Models for Survival Data

Chapter 4
The Frailty Concept

4.1 Introduction

An individual said to be frail if he or she is much more susceptible (exposed or infected) to adverse events than others. Clayton (1978) introduced the term frailty to indicate that different individuals are at risk even though on the surface they may appear to be quite similar with respect to measurable attributes such as age, gender, weight, etc. He used the term frailty to represent an unobservable random effect shared by subjects with similar (unmeasured) risks in the analysis of mortality rates. A random effect describes excess risk or frailty for distinct categories, such as individuals or families, over and above any measured covariates. Thus, random effect or frailty models have been introduced into the statistical literature in an attempt to account for the existence of unmeasured attributes such as genotype that do introduce heterogeneity into a study population. It is recognized that individuals in the same family are more similar than the individuals in different families because they share similar genes and similar environment. Thus, frailty or random effect models try to account for correlations within groups. Such groups arise naturally in those studies involving two or more failure times on the same individual subject. These failure times may be times to the recurrence of the same event or times to the occurrence of different types of events. Examples include the time sequences of asthmatic attacks, infection episodes, tumor diagnosis, tumor recurrences or bleeding incidents in individual subjects (Prentice et al. 1981).

Frailties are useful in modeling correlations in multivariate survival and event history data. Examples include recurrent events such as epileptic seizures or depressive episodes, where an individual's frailty influences the occurrence of events, and community trials, where the different events within each community share a common frailty (or shared frailty), shared by each individual within the community, each unit belongs to precisely one category, and frailties of different categories are independent. More complex models are possible. Frailties can be nested; individuals within a family may share common frailty, while families within communities share another common frailty. Frailties can be correlated, as in studies of pedigrees.

© Springer Nature Singapore Pte Ltd. 2019
D. D. Hanagal, *Modeling Survival Data Using Frailty Models*,
Industrial and Applied Mathematics, https://doi.org/10.1007/978-981-15-1181-3_4

A common approach to the analysis of survival data is to assume a homogeneous population of individuals with the same covariate structure. However, it is clear that individuals identical in many respects such as age, sex, and treatment may differ in unmeasured ways, if only because of genotypical differences.

It is easy to see that it is important to consider the effect of ignoring frailty in any study where the existence of such heterogeneity may be present. Consider the study of survival times for a population consisting of one high-risk subgroup and one low-risk subgroup. Early in the study, one would estimate the population hazard to be high as the high-risk individuals start to die off rather quickly; after a period of time the remaining population consists primarily of low-risk individuals and this would give rise to a low hazard rate. Thus, the population hazard function would appear to decrease over time, even if the individuals in the same subpopulation had the same hazard. More formally, if the high and low-risk subpopulation was of the same size and had exponentially distributed failure times with hazards of 3 and 1, respectively, the population hazard at time t would be

$$
\begin{aligned}
h(t) &= \frac{f(t)}{S(t)} \\
&= \frac{3\exp(-3t) + \exp(-t)}{\exp(-3t) + \exp(-t)} \\
&= 1 + \frac{2}{1 + \exp(2t)}
\end{aligned}
$$

with hazard decreasing from 2 to 1 over time.

Hougaard (1995) and Aalen (1988) provide illuminating discussions of more complex scenarios. In one example where the relative risk of failure is high in one group, the population relative risk could even drop below over time due to selection pressures.

Keyfitz and Littman (1979) developed a procedure to estimate life expectancy in a heterogeneous population and showed that ignoring heterogeneity results in overestimates of life expectancy. When Lancaster (1990) modeled the unemployment rate, he found an underestimation of the covariate effects when frailty was ignored in the model. In their view, Pickles and Crouchley (1995) suggests that ignoring such heterogeneity generally attenuates parameter estimates towards zero.

If one's experimental material involves grouped or clustered data at either the individual or population level, one should consider the use of frailty (random effect) models. Examples would include situations where students are nested within the classroom, animals are nested within the litter, individuals related by family membership or shared exposure to unmeasured environmental exposures, multiple measurements on the same individual, etc. Sometimes frailty effects are modeled in a hope to account for measurement error.

More formally, a heterogeneous population can be sometimes be modeled as a mixture problem with an underlying random variable called frailty. For example, suppose T is the failure time of a subject (for example, the time to infection for a kidney patient using portable dialysis), then the probability density of T might be modeled conditional on Z, an unobserved nonmeasurable random variable, called frailty, which is intended to allow for individual variation. This representation can be symbolized by $f(t; y, z)$. The additional variable Y represents measurable covariates which are thought to be related to the failure time. Under this representation, the failure time distribution can be considered to be continuous mixture induced by the frailty Z.

Recent research has addressed the problem of heterogeneity. Hougaard (1986a, b) suggested the power variance function (PVF) distribution which includes gamma, inverse gaussian, positive stable distributions as frailty model. Hedeker et al. (1996) discussed a frailty regression model for the analysis of correlated grouped time survival data. Frailty models have been applied to the analysis of event history data, including the study of age at the time of death for individuals in terms of population (Zelterman 1992), unemployment duration (McCall 1994), pregnancy in women (Aalen 1987), and migration (Lindstorm 1996).

4.2   The Definition of Shared Frailty

In a frailty model, it is assumed that the hazard function can be separated into multiplicative components: frailty, the baseline hazard function and the linear predictor. For data classified by genotype group, the hazard function for individual j in the group i would be $z_i h_0(t) \exp(y'_{ij}\beta)$, where z_i is the common frailty of each individual in the group i which is shared by all the individuals in the group i and we call it as shared frailty, $h_0(t)$ gives the baseline hazard function and $\exp(y'_{ij}\beta)$ is the exponential of the linear predictor. The variability of z_i determines the degree of heterogeneity among the groups and its distribution is described by the probability density function $g(z)$, where $g(z)$ is interpreted as the distribution of genotypic frailty in the population. In empirical applications, the observed survival data are used to estimate the parameters of the distribution of frailty $g(z)$ and to actually predict the individual frailties.

Frailty is a measure of relative risk because the greater an individual's frailty, with regard to some cause of death, the greater the individual's susceptibility to the cause of death. For example, if an individual with frailty 1 is called a "standard" individual, then an individual with frailty 2 is having double hazard as compared to a standard individual for any given time t and covariates. This definition of frailty assumes that each individual is born at certain level of relative frailty and stays at this level all its life (Vaupel et al. 1979). Individuals in the same cluster usually share the same unobserved frailty (Shih and Louis 1995).

Extensive research has been devoted to the frailty issue in survival analysis and generalized linear model (GLIM). Recently, investigators have recognized that ignoring individual heterogeneity may lead to inaccurate conclusions. Models for heterogeneity have been proposed by Vaupel et al. (1979), who introduced frailty as an unobserved quantity in population mortality. Oakes (1989) proposed frailty models for bivariate survival times and introduced several possible frailty models. Flinn and Heckman (1982) also introduced heterogeneity into their model for analyzing individual event histories. They believed that improper modeling of heterogeneity will result in biased estimates since the covariates in the model fail to explain the true effect of the covariates on a response variable. Keyfitz and Littman (1979) showed that ignoring heterogeneity will lead to an incorrect calculation of the life expectancy from known death rates. A similar conclusion was reached by Vaupel et al. (1979) using a continuous mixture model in which an unobserved nonnegative random frailty represents all individual differences in endowment for longevity.

For reasons of convenience, analysts often choose parametric representations of frailty models that are mathematically tractable. Hougaard (1986a) used several distributions for frailty including gamma, inverse gaussian, positive stable distributions and claimed that these two distributions are relevant and mathematically tractable as a frailty distribution for heterogeneous populations. Flinn and Heckman (1982) used a log-normal distribution for frailty, whereas Vaupel et al. (1979) assumed that frailty is distributed across individuals as a gamma distribution. Frailty models have been used by demographers, economists, epidemiologists, and biostatisticians to denote proneness to disease, accidents, and other events because there are persistent differences in susceptibility among individuals.

4.3   The Implications of Frailty

In hazard rate analysis, it is assumed that any differences in failure rates among individuals are picked up by the covariate structure which typically is assumed to act multiplicatively on a baseline hazard. This assumption can be relaxed by allowing for different baseline hazards in different strata and by allowing for time-dependent covariates. Even this structure assumes that individuals with the same covariate strata value have the same hazard rate. It is useful and important to examine this assumption that all heterogeneity has been picked up by the statistical model (Trussel and Richards 1985). The issue of ignoring heterogeneity as a result of omitting important (possibly unmeasurable) variables in the model, was investigated in a real-world application by Flinn and Heckman (1982). When they incorporated frailty into the analysis of event history data, they found that there was no effect of the covariates on the response variable (duration). On the other hand, when frailty was omitted from the model, some covariates had an effect. Thus, ignoring such heterogeneity may have a drastic effect on the fitted statistical model with obvious consequences in its application in real-world settings. Another example of the consequences of ignoring frailty is an underestimation of the covariate effects on the risk of bladder cancer (Babikar and Cuzick 1994).

The shared gamma frailty models were suggested by Clayton (1978) for the analysis of the correlation between clustered survival times in genetic epidemiology. An advantage is that without covariates its mathematical properties are convenient for estimation (See Oakes 1982, 1986). However, when adjusting for environmental risk factors the analysis of the clustering is more difficult (See Parner 1998). Until recently, a lack of theory and reliable software had prevented widespread use of the model.

In a frailty model, it is absolutely necessary to be able to include explanatory variables. The reason is that frailty describes the influence of common unknown factors. If some common covariates are included in the model, the variation owing to unknown covariates should be reduced. Common covariates are common for all members of the group.

For monozygotic twins, examples are sex and any other genetically based covariate. Both monozygotic and dizygotic twins share date of birth and common pre-birth environment. By measuring some potentially important covariates, we can examine the influence of the covariates and we can examine, whether they explain the dependence, that is, whether the frailty has no effect (or more correctly, no variation), when the covariate is included in the model.

It is not possible in practice to include all relevant covariates. For example, we might know that some given factor is important, but if we do not know the value of the factor for each individual, we cannot include the variable in the analysis. For example, it is known that the excretion of small amounts of albumin in the urine is a diagnostic marker for increased mortality, not only for diabetic patients but also for the general population. However, we are unable to include this variable unless we actually obtain urine and analyze samples for each individual understudy. It is furthermore possible that we are not aware that there exist variables that we ought to include. For example, this could be a genetic factor, as we do not know all possible genes having an influence on survival. This consideration is true for all regression models, not only survival models. If it is known that some factor is important, it makes sense to try to obtain the individual values, but if it is not possible, the standard is to ignore the presence of such variables. In general terms, we let the heterogeneity go into the error term. This will, of course, lead to an increase in the variability of the response compared to the case, when the variables are included. In the survival data case, however, the increased variability implies a change in the form of the hazard function, as this will be illustrated by some more detailed calculations.

In statistics, one is frequently interested in extracting information about unobserved quantities from observed quantities. The relationship between the two is given by a statistical model. A typical multilevel model buildup consists of a specification of a *measurement model* (i.e., the distribution of the observed quantities given the unobserved) and some description of the unobserved quantities, sometimes called *random effects*. In the context of survival studies of related individuals examples of such unobserved quantities may be genotypes, susceptibility to some disease or condition (i.e., the age-specific relative risk of death), genetic transmission pattern in a family tree, whereas the outcome is typically a survival time.

A class of random effect models is particularly useful in survival studies of related individuals is a class of *frailty* models which are based on the proportional hazards property.

4.4   Shared Frailty

Let T be a survival time with an absolutely continuous distribution. A nonnegative random variable Z is called *frailty* (Vaupel et al. 1979) if the conditional hazard function given Z has the form:

$$H(t|Z) = ZH(t)$$

where $H(t)$ is called *hazard* function. The conditional survival function is in this case is given by

$$S(t|Z) = e^{-ZH(t)}$$

where $H(t) = \int_0^t h_0(u)du$ is the cumulative baseline hazard. The marginal survival function $S(t)$ may be obtained by taking the expectation

$$S(t) = E[S(t|Z)] = E[e^{-ZH(t)}] = L_Z(H(t)).$$

where L is the Laplace transform of the frailty variable Z. In a similar way, conditionally on Z, the bivariate survival function is

$$S(t_1, t_2|Z) = \exp[-Z\{H_1(t_1) + H_2(t_2)\}],$$

where $H_i(t_i) = \int_0^{t_i} h_i(u)du, i = 1, 2$ are the integrated hazards of T_i. Here conditionally T_1 and T_2 are independent. We can derive unconditional bivariate survival function by integrating Z out

$$S(t_1, t_2) = E\left[\exp[-Z\{H_1(t_1) + H_2(t_2)\}]\right] = L[H_1(t_1) + H_2(t_2)]$$

When T_1 and T_2 are dependent, conditionally on Z, the bivariate survival function is

$$S(t_1, t_2|Z) = \exp[-ZH(t_1, t_2)],$$

where $H(t_1, t_2)$ is the bivariate integrated hazard of (T_1, T_2). The corresponding unconditional bivariate survival function is derived by integrating Z out

$$S(t_1, t_2) = = L[H(t_1, t_2)].$$

For the multivariate set up, the unconditional multivariate survival function is

$$S(t_1, ..., t_k) = L[H(t_1, ..., t_k)].$$

When $(T_1, \ldots, T_k)$ are independent the unconditional multivariate survival function is

$$S(t_1, \ldots, t_k) = L\left[\sum_{i=1}^{k} H_i(t_i)\right].$$

4.5 Frailty as a Model for Omitted Covariates

One explanation for including hidden heterogeneity effects on survival in the model is to account for the effects of omitted covariates (Hougaard et al. 1994; Keiding et al. 1997) in a Cox regression model (Cox 1972). Let $Y_0, \ldots, Y_n$ be some covariates with associated regression coefficients $\beta_0, \ldots, \beta_n$. In a Cox regression model the conditional survival function given the covariates is given by

$$S(t|Y_0, \ldots, Y_n) = \exp(-e^{\beta_0 Y_0 + \cdots + \beta_n Y_n} H(t)).$$

If the covariate Y_0 is not observed and Y_0 is independent of $Y_1, \ldots, Y_n$, the respective survival function is given by:

$$S(t|Y_1, \ldots, Y_n) = L(e^{\beta_1 Y_1 + \cdots + \beta_n Y_n} H(t))$$

where $L(s)$ is the Laplace transform of frailty random variable, $Z = \exp(\beta_0 Y_0)$. In this case, frailty is used to describe deviations from the proportional hazards assumption. This model is identifiable when the frailty Z has a finite mean (Elbers and Rider 1982).

4.6 Frailty as a Model of Stochastic Hazard

Another way of introducing frailty is through the modeling of biological processes within the organism. The basic idea is that genes and environment influence the lifespan through individual age-specific hazard rates. The health history of the organism is described by a random process $(Z_t)_{t\geq 0}$ which also incorporates the individual environment and genetic expression history. At each time t the survival chances are related to deviations of the health status from *homeostasis* (Yashin et al. 2000) which are described by the following conditional age-specific hazard rate:

$$\mu(t|\{Z_s, 0 \leq s \leq t\} = \lim_{\Delta t \to 0} \frac{1}{\Delta t} P(t \leq T < t + \Delta t | T \geq t, \{Z_s, 0 \leq s \leq t\})$$

where we assume that the limit on the right-hand side exists.

In general, many components of Z_t are not observed, although recent developments in DNA microarray techniques may facilitate studies of individual gene expression histories. Therefore, some simplification steps are necessary in order to make the problem of studying the above model analytically tractable.

Simplification 1 : The hazard rate at age t depends only on Z_t and not on the whole past history $\{Z_s | 0 \leq s \leq t\}$, i.e.,

$$h(t|\{Z_s, 0 \leq s \leq t\}) = h(t|Z_t).$$

Simplification 2 : Genetic and environmental factors described by Z_t do not change with age, i.e., $Z_t = Z, t \geq 0$ and consequently:

$$h(t|Z_t) = h(t|Z).$$

Simplification 3 : First order Taylor approximation of $h(t|Z)$ assuming that Z is one-dimensional and $h(t|0) = 0$, i.e., proportional hazards model holds:

$$h(t|Z) = Zh_0(t).$$

In the latter case all inter-individual differences in susceptibility to death at age t can be described by the nonnegative random variable Z which is called *frailty* (Vaupel et al. 1979).

4.7 Identifiability of Frailty Models

Identifiability is an important property of a statistical model, determining whether the model parameters maybe recovered from the observed data (MacLachlan and Basford 1998). A successful parameter estimation procedure or proof of consistency of the parameter estimates require that a model is identifiable to begin with. The study of identifiability property is especially important when dealing with semiparametric latent variable models (e.g., frailty models), since in these cases it is easy to specify a latent structure which is too complex to be identified from the data and also because in these models the relationship between the latent quantities and observed model characteristics is often not transparent (Iachine 2006).

Frailty models (Vaupel et al. 1979) are used in survival analysis to account for unobserved heterogeneity in individual risks to disease and death. In a univariate frailty model the observed survival time T and unobserved frailty variable Z are related by the proportional hazards assumption:

$$h(t|Z) = Zh_0(t). \tag{4.1}$$

This model is determined by the distribution of the frailty variable Z and the underlying baseline hazard $h_0(t)$ or equivalently the cumulative baseline hazard function $H(t) = \int_0^t h_0(u)du$ (determined up to a multiplicative constant). This model is not identifiable from data on T alone unless additional parametric assumptions are made about the cumulative baseline hazard $H(t)$ (Heckman and Singer 1984).

In applications, data on observed covariates $\mathbf{Y}$ are often available together with survival information. In this case, the frailty model (4.1) may be extended to include the effects of the observed covariates:

$$h(t|Z, \mathbf{Y}) = Zr(\mathbf{Y})h_0(t), \tag{4.2}$$

where $r(\mathbf{Y})$ is an unknown risk function. In fact, when $r(\mathbf{Y}) = \exp(\beta^T \mathbf{Y})$ (i.e., the risk function in the regression model of Cox (1972)) the frailty variable in model ((4.2)) may be viewed as describing the effects of unobserved covariates $\mathbf{Y}_u$, i.e., $Z = \exp(\beta^T \mathbf{Y}_u)$.

The identifiability properties of the univariate frailty model (4.2) with unspecified functional forms of the frailty distribution, baseline hazard, and risk function have been studied in detail. These properties are largely determined by the existence of a finite mean of the frailty distribution. Elbers and Rider (1982) have shown the identifiability of model (4.2) using information on T and $\mathbf{Y}$ when $EZ < \infty$ (alternative conditions of identifiability were considered by Heckman and Singer (1984)). However, this model is not identifiable when frailty has an infinite mean (Hougaard 1986a, b).

Ridder (1990) extended the result of Elbers and Rider (1982) to generalized accelerated failure time (GAFT) models and showed that the frailty model (4.2) is a GAFT model. In essence, he proved the over identifiability property of the univariate frailty models with finite mean, a fact which was also noted by Melino and Sueyoshi (1990). In the GAFT framework the frailty model (4.2) corresponds to a particular error term distribution structure of the GAFT regression model. Ridder (1990) shows that the GAFT model is identifiable without this additional structural assumption about the noise term.

To analyze bivariate data on pairs of related survival times (T_1, T_2) (e.g., matched pairs experiments, twin or family data), bivariate frailty models were suggested. Initially, such models exploited the data of shared frailty (Holt and Prentice 1974; Clayton 1978; Vaupel 1988). The bivariate model was derived by extending (4.1) to the two-dimensional case under the assumption of conditional independence of T_1, T_2 given the shared frailty Z, resulting is the following bivariate survival function:

$$S(t_1, t_2|Z) = e^{-ZH(t_1)}e^{-ZH(t_2)}.$$

The identifiability property of this model using data on T_1, T_2 was shown to hold by Honore (1993) without the assumption of finite mean of frailty.

It turns out that univariate frailty models without observed covariates and without any additional parametrical assumptions about $h_0(x)$ are not identifiable from univariate survival data. Moreover, even in the presence of observed covariates there exist frailty models that cannot be identified (e.g. the positive stable distribution, Hougaard 1986b) from univariate data alone. Bivariate survival data present a unique opportunity to identify the frailty distribution and the underlying hazards. For example, all *shared frailty* models (e.g., the positive stable) are identifiable from bivariate survival data without observed covariates (Iachine and Yashin 1998).

References

Aalen, O.O.: Two examples of modelling heterogeneity in survival analysis. Scand. J. Stat. **14**, 19–25 (1987)

Aalen, O.O.: Heterogeneity in survival analysis. Stat. Med. **7**, 1121–1137 (1988)

Babikar, A., Cuzick, J.: A simple frailty model for family studies with covariates. Stat. Med. **13**, 1679–1692 (1994)

Clayton, D.G.: A model for association in bivariate life tables and its application in epidemiological studies of familial tendency in chronic disease incidence. Biometrika **65**, 141–151 (1978)

Cox, D.R.: Regression models and life tables (with discussions). J. R. Stat. Soc., B **34**, 187–220 (1972)

Elbers, C., Rider, G.: True and spurious duration dependence: the identifibility of the proportional hazard model. Rev. Econ. Stud. **49**, 403–409 (1982)

Flinn, C.J., Heckman, J.J.: New methods for analyzing individual event histories. Social. Methodol. pp. 99–140 (1982)

Heckman, J., Singer, B.: The identifiability of the proportional hazard model. Rev. Econ. Stud. **51**(2), 231–241 (1984)

Hedeker, D., Siddiqui, O., Hu, F.B.: Random effects regression analysis of correlated group time survival data. School of Public Health and Prevention Research Cancer. University of Illinois, Chicago (1996)

Holt, J.D., Prentice, R.L.: Survival analysis in twin studies and matched pair experiments. Biometrika **61**(1), 17–30 (1974)

Honore, B.E.: Identification results for duration models with multiple spells. Rev. Econ. Stud. **60**, 241–246 (1993)

Hougaard, P., Muglogaard., Borch-Johnsen, K.: Heterogeneity models of disease susceptibility with application to diabetic nephropathy. Biometrics **50**(4), 1178–1188 (1994)

Hougaard, P.: Frailty models for survival data. Lifetime Data Analysis, **1**, 255–274 (1995)

Hougaard, P.: A class of multivariate failure time distributions. Biometrika **73**, 671–678 (1986a)

Hougaard, P.: Survival models for hetrogeneous populations derived from stable distributions. Biometrika **73**, 387–396 (1986b)

Iachine, I.A., Yashin, A.I.: Identifiability of bivariate frailty models based on additive independent components. Research Report 8, Department of Statistics and Demography, Odense University, Denmark (1998)

Iachine, I.A.: . Identifiability of bivariate frailty models. Working Paper, Department of Statistics and Demography, University of Southern Denmark, Denmark (2006)

Keiding, N., Andersen, P.K., Klein, J.P.: The role of frailty models and accelerated failure time models in describing heterogeneity due to omitted covariates. Stat. Med. **16**(1–3), 215–224 (1997)

Keyfitz, N., Littman, G.: Mortality in a heterogeneous population. Popul. Stud. **33**, 333–342 (1979)

Lancaster, T.: The Economic Analysis of Transition Data. University Press Cambridge, London (1990)

Lindstorm, D.P.: Economic opportunities in Mexico and return to the United States. Demography **33**, 357–374 (1996)

MacLachlan, G.J., Basford, K.E.: Mixture models: Inference and applications to clustering. Statistics:Textbooks and monographs, Vol. 84. Marcel Dekker, New York (1998)

McCall, B.P.: Testing the proportional hazard assumptions in the presence of unmeasured hetero-geneity: an application to the unemployment durations of displaced workers. J. Appl. Econ., B **44**, 226–233 (1994)

Melino, A., Sueyoshi, G.T.: A simple approach to the identifiability of the proportional hazard model. Econ. Lett. **33**, 63–68 (1990)

Oakes, D.: Bivariate survival models induced by frailties. J. Am. Stat. Assoc. **84**, 487–493 (1989)

Oakes, D.: A model for association in bivariate survival data. J. R. Stat. Soc., B **44**, 414–493 (1982)

Oakes, D.: Semiparametric inference in bivariate survival data. Biometrika **73**, 353–361 (1986)

Parner, E.: Asymptotic theory for the correlated gamma-frailty model. Ann. Stat. **26**(1), 183–214 (1998)

Pickles, A., Crouchley, R.: A comparison of frailty models for multivariate survival data. Stat. Med. **14**, 1447–1461 (1995)

Prentice, R.L., Williams, B.J., Peterson, A.V.: On the regression analysis of multivariate failure time data. Biometrika **68**, 373–379 (1981)

Ridder, G.: The non-parametric identification of generalized accelerated failure time models. Rev. Econ. Stud. **57**(2), 167–181 (1990)

Shih, J.H., Louis, T.A.: Inferences on the association parameter in copula models for bivariate data. Biometrics **51**(4), 1384–1399 (1995)

Trussel, J., Richards, T.: Correcting for unobserved heterogeneity in hazard models using Heckman-Singer procedure. Social. Methodol. pp. 242–276 (1985)

Vaupel, J.W.: Inherited frailty and longevity. Demography **25**(2), 139–149 (1988)

Vaupel, J.W., Manton, K.G., Stallard, E.: The impact of heterogeneity on individual frailty on the dynamic of mortality. Demography **16**(3), 439–454 (1979)

Yashin, A.I., Iachine, I.A., Begun, A.S.: Mortality modeling: a review. Math. Popul. Stud. **8**(4), 305–332 (2000)

Zelterman, D.: A statistical distribution with an unbounded hazard function and its application to a theory from demography. Biometrics **48**, 807–818 (1992)

Chapter 5
Various Frailty Models

5.1 Introduction

The shared frailty model is relevant to event time of the related individuals, similar organs, and repeated measurements. In this model individuals from a group shares common covariates. For the shared frailty model it is assumed that survival times are conditionally independent, for given shared frailty. Shared frailty means dependence between survival times is only due to unobservable covariates or frailty.

Mazroui et al. (2013) proposed multivariate frailty model that jointly analyzes two types of recurrent events with a dependent terminal event and illustrated their model with breast cancer data. Cosco et al. (2015) discussed the similarities and differences between successful aging and frailty in terms of scope and emphasis of their constituent components and functioning. Callegaro and Lacobelli (2012) introduced log-skew-normal frailty model and illustrated with a case study of multiple myeloma patients with autologous stem cells transplantation. Kau et al. (2011) applied a shared frailty model to analyze the mortgage termination risks. Preter et al. (2015) compared Cox model and shared frailty model to analyze retirement timing of dual earner couples in 11 European countries. Unkel et al. (2013) explored time-dependent frailty models, in which the frailty is modulated over time in a deterministic fashion and illustrated with paired serological survey data on a range of infections with same or different routes of transmission. Mauguen et al. (2013) proposed a dynamic prediction tool based on joint frailty models where joint modeling accounts for the dependence between recurrent events and death, by the introduction of a random effect shared by the two processes. They applied these proposed models to patients diagnosed with a primary invasive breast cancer and treated with breast-conserving surgery, followed for more than 10 years in a French comprehensive cancer center. Enky et al. (2014) proposed time-varying shared frailty model to represent changes over time in population heterogeneity, for use with bivariate current status data and illustrated with data on infectious diseases.

© Springer Nature Singapore Pte Ltd. 2019   85
D. D. Hanagal, *Modeling Survival Data Using Frailty Models*,
Industrial and Applied Mathematics, https://doi.org/10.1007/978-981-15-1181-3_5

Govindarajulu et al. (2011) analyzed using multivariate frailty models in a nonparametric hazards setting on biomedical data sets and discussed the implications of choosing to use frailty and relevance to genetic applications. Unkel and Farrington (2012) proposed a measure for assessing the temporal variation in the strength of association for shared frailty models with bivariate current status data. These methods were illustrated with bivariate serological survey data on a pair infections, where the time-varying association is likely to represent heterogeneities in activity levels and/or susceptibility to infection. Farrington et al. (2012) discussed the properties of the relative frailty variance which characterizes frailty distributions and that, suitably rescaled, it may be used to compare patterns of dependence across proposed models and data sets. The benefits of approach of methods are illustrated with two applications to bivariate current status data obtained from serological surveys. Chen et al. (2013) proposed generalized gamma frailty distribution, which can accommodate most of the popular frailty distributions. They applied the proposed modes to a data set of coronary heart disease patients. Xu and Zhang (2010) developed an estimation method for the semiparametric accelerated failure time gamma frailty model based on the EM algorithm and rank-like estimation method. They applied the proposed method to the data set of coronary heart disease patients. Molenberghs et al. (2011) proposed Weibull-Gamma frailty model, which can accommodate most of the popular frailty distributions and they illustrated the proposed models using data from survival in cancer patients.

In this chapter, we discuss some important frailty distributions which are used more often and they have a lot of applications. The main frailty distributions discussed in this chapter are gamma, inverse Gaussian, positive stable, power variance function, log-normal, Weibull, and compound Poisson, compound negative binomial, piecewise gamma, generalized exponential, generalized gamma, and Birnbaum–Saunders distributions. Frailty models can be expressed in terms of Laplace transform. Once the Laplace transform of frailty distribution is obtained, it is easy to obtain the estimates the parameters of frailty models. Now we will discuss various frailty models here one by one as follows.

5.2 Gamma Frailty

The shared gamma frailty model is more widely used frailty distribution in the literature. Gamma distributions have been used for many years to generate mixtures in exponential and Poisson models. From a computational point of view, gamma models fit very well into survival models, because it is easy to derive the formulas for any number of events. This is due to simplicity of the derivatives of the Laplace transform. This is also the reason why this distribution has been applied in most of the applications published until now. The probability density function (pdf) of gamma distribution as

$$f(z) = \theta^{\alpha} z^{\alpha-1} e^{-\theta z} / \Gamma(\alpha), \quad z > 0, \theta, \alpha > 0.$$

For many calculations and in order to solve non-identifiability problem, it makes sense to take $E(Z) = 1$ which leads to restrict the scale parameter, and the standard restriction is $\theta = \alpha$, when $\alpha \longrightarrow \infty$, the distribution becomes degenerate. The pdf and Laplace transform of gamma distribution are, respectively, as follows:

$$
f_Z(z) = \begin{cases} \frac{\frac{1}{\theta}^{\frac{1}{\theta}}}{\Gamma\frac{1}{\theta}} z^{\frac{1}{\theta}-1} e^{-\frac{z}{\theta}} & ; \; z > 0, \theta > 0 \\ 0 & ; \; \text{otherwise.} \end{cases}
$$

$$
L_Z(s) = (1 + \theta s)^{-\frac{1}{\theta}}
$$

with variance of Z as θ. Let T be a survival times and Z be the frailty variable which is distributed as gamma. The conditional survival function in this case is given by

$$
S(t|z) = \exp(-zH(t))
$$

and the unconditional survival function is given by integrating out Z from the above equation

$$
S_\theta(t) = E[S(t|z)] = L_Z[H(t)] = [1 + \theta H(t)]^{-\frac{1}{\theta}}, \quad \theta > 0.
$$

Let T_1 and T_2 be the lifetimes of two individuals or twins or paired organs, then the unconditional bivariate survival function with gamma frailty is given by

$$
S_\theta(t_1, t_2) = L_Z(H(t_1) + H_2(t_2))
$$

When Z is distributed as gamma frailty, then the bivariate survival function is

$$
= [1 + \theta(H(t_1) + H_2(t_2))]^{-\frac{1}{\theta}} . \tag{5.1}
$$

where $H_1(t_1)$ and $H_2(t_2)$ are the integrated hazard functions of the two lifetimes T_1 and T_2. The bivariate distribution when the frailty variable is degenerate is given by,

$$
S(t_1, t_2) = e^{-(H_1(t_1) + H_2(t_2))}
$$

According to different assumptions on the baseline distributions we get different shared gamma frailty models.

The various families of distributions have some theoretical advantages. If the frailty distribution is a natural exponential family, selection, that is truncation (updating when no events have happened), implies that the conditional distribution of the frailty is still within the same family. The hazard for death of individual 1 at time t_1, conditional on individual 2's being alive at time t_2, that is, conditional on the event $(T_2 > t_2)$, is $h_1(t_1)[1 + \theta(H_1(t_1) + H_2(t_2))]^{-1}$. The hazard for death of individual

1 at time t_1, conditional on death of individual 2 at time $(T_2 = t_2)$, the hazard is $h_1(t_1)(1 + \theta)[1 + \theta(H_1(t_1) + H_2(t_2))]^{-1}$. This implies that the cross-ratio function is given by (See Clayton 1978; Oakes 1989)

$$\theta^*(t_1, t_2) = \frac{\lambda(t_1 \mid T_2 = t_2)}{\lambda(t_1 \mid T_2 > t_2)}$$

$$= \frac{(\frac{\partial^2 S_\theta(t_1, t_2)}{\partial t_1 \partial t_2})(S_\theta(t_1, t_2))}{(\frac{\partial S_\theta(t_1, t_2)}{\partial t_1})(\frac{\partial S_\theta(t_1, t_2)}{\partial t_2})}$$

$$= 1 + \theta.$$

Here $\theta^*(t_1, t_2)$ is independent of the lifetimes. The expression $\theta^*(t_1, t_2)$ can be interpreted as the relative risk for an individual if the other one has experienced the event rather than being event free at a given time (See Liang 1991). Therefore, it is an association function such that $\theta^*(t_1, t_2) > 1$ represents positive association, $\theta^*(t_1, t_2) < 1$ indicates negative association and $\theta^*(t_1, t_2) = 1$ implies no association.

$F(t_1)$ and $F(t_2)$, corresponds a unique function,

$$C : [0, 1] \times [0, 1] \rightarrow [0, 1],$$

is called a copula such that

$$F(t_1, t_2) = C(F(t_1), F(t_2)) \text{ for } (t_1, t_2) \in (0, \infty) \times (0, \infty)$$

For a given copula C, there exists a unique survival copula $\overline{C}$, such that

$$\overline{C}(u, v) = u + v - 1 + C(1 - u, 1 - v)$$

and

$$S_{T_1, T_2}(t_1, t_2) = \overline{C}(S_{T_1}(t_1), S_{T_2}(t_2))$$

Here S_{T_1, T_2}, S_{T_1} and S_{T_2} are the survival functions. Conversely it is possible to construct a bivariate survival function using copula having the desired marginal survivals and a chosen dependence structure, see Nelsen (2006) for details. The joint bivariate survival function (5.1) can be expressed in terms of survival copula as

$$\overline{C}(u, v) = \left[u^{-\theta} + v^{-\theta} - 1 \right]^{-1/\theta}$$

where $u = S_{T_1}(\cdot)$ and $v = S_{T_2}(\cdot)$

The above equation is often called as Clayton Archimedean copula.

5.3 Inverse Gaussian Frailty

The gamma distribution is most commonly used frailty distribution because of its mathematical convenience. Another choice is the inverse Gaussian distribution. The inverse Gaussian makes the population homogeneous with time, whereas for gamma the relative heterogeneity is constant (Hougaard 1984). Duchateau and Janssen (2008) fit the inverse Gaussian (IG) frailty model with Weibull hazard to the udder quarter infection data. The IG distribution has a unimodal density and is a member of the exponential family. Furthermore, there are many striking similarities between the statistics derived from this distribution and those of the normal; see Chhikara and Folks (1996). These properties make it potentially attractive for modeling purposes with survival data. The models derived above are bases on the assumption that a common random effect acts multiplicatively on the hazard rate function.

Alternative to the gamma distribution, Hougaard (1984) introduced the inverse Gaussian as a frailty distribution. It provides much flexibility in modeling, when early occurrences of failures are dominant in a lifetime distribution and its failure rate is expected to be non-monotonic. In such situations, the inverse Gaussian distribution might provide a suitable choice for the lifetime model. Also inverse Gaussian is almost an increasing failure rate distribution when it is slightly skewed and hence is also applicable to describe lifetime distribution which is not dominated by early failures. The inverse Gaussian distribution has shape resembles the other skewed density functions, such as log-normal and gamma. These properties of inverse Gaussian distribution motivate us to use inverse Gaussian as frailty distribution. The inverse Gaussian distribution has a history dating back to 1915 when Schrodinger and Smoluchowski presented independent derivations of the density of the first passage time distribution of Brownian motion with positive drift. Vilmann et al. (1990) have studied the histomorphometrical analysis of the influence of soft diet on masticatory muscle development in the muscular dystrophic mouse. The muscle fiber size distributions were fitted by an inverse Gaussian law. Barndorff-Nielsen (1994) considers a finite tree whose edges are endowed with random resistances, and shows that, subject to suitable restrictions on the parameters, if the resistances are either inverse Gaussian or reciprocal inverse Gaussian random variables, then the overall resistance of the tree follows a reciprocal inverse Gaussian law. Gacula and Kubala (1975) have analyzed shelf life of several products using the IG law and found to be a good fit. For more real-life applications (see seshadri (1999)).

Let a continuous random variable Z follows inverse Gaussian distribution with parameters μ and θ then density function of Z is

$$f_Z(z) = \begin{cases} \left[\dfrac{1}{2\pi\theta} \right]^{\frac{1}{2}} z^{-\frac{3}{2}} e^{\frac{(z-\mu)^2}{2z\theta\mu^2}} & ; \ z > 0, \mu > 0, \theta > 0 \\ 0 & ; \ \text{otherwise}, \end{cases}$$

and the Laplace transform is,

$$L_Z(s) = \exp\left[\frac{1}{\mu\theta} - \left(\frac{1}{\theta^2\mu^2} + \frac{2s}{\theta}\right)^{\frac{1}{2}}\right].$$

The mean and variance of frailty variable are $E(Z) = \mu$ and $V(Z) = \mu^3\theta$. For identifiability, we assume Z has expected value equal to one i.e. $\mu = 1$. Under this restriction, the density function and the Laplace transformation of the inverse Gaussian distribution reduces to

$$f_Z(z) = \begin{cases} \left[\dfrac{1}{2\pi\theta}\right]^{\frac{1}{2}} z^{-\frac{3}{2}} e^{\frac{(z-1)^2}{2z\theta}} & ; \ z > 0, \theta > 0 \\ 0 & ; \ \text{otherwise,} \end{cases}$$

and the Laplace transform is,

$$L_Z(s) = \exp\left[\frac{1 - (1 + 2\theta s)^{\frac{1}{2}}}{\theta}\right],$$

with variance of Z as θ. The frailty variable Z is degenerate at $Z = 1$ when θ tends to zero. The unconditional bivariate distribution function of lifetimes T_1 and T_2 with inverse Gaussian frailty is

$$L_Z(H_1(t_1) + H_2(t_2)) = \exp\left[\frac{1 - (1 + 2\theta(H_1(t_1) + H_2(t_2)))^{\frac{1}{2}}}{\theta}\right]$$

$$= S(t_1, t_2) \tag{5.2}$$

where $H_1(t_1)$ and $H_2(t_2)$ are the cumulative baseline hazard functions of the lifetime T_1 and T_2, respectively. Clayton (1978) define cross-ratio function as

$$\theta^*(t_1, t_2) = \frac{\frac{\partial^2 S(t_1, t_2)}{\partial t_1 \partial t_2} S(t_1, t_2)}{\frac{\partial S(t_1, t_2)}{\partial t_1} \frac{\partial S(t_1, t_2)}{\partial t_2}}$$

The cross-ratio function of inverse Gaussian frailty is

$$\theta^*(t_1, t_2) = 1 + \frac{1}{\frac{1}{\theta} - \ln(S(t_1, t_2))}$$

The highest value is obtained at the start and equals $1 + \theta$, and goes to one as the survival function goes to zero. It is decreasing function of t_1, t_2.

The joint bivariate survival functions in (5.2) can be expressed in terms of survival copula as (see Nelsen (2006) for details)

$$\overline{C}(u, v) = \exp \left\{ \frac{1 - \left[(1 - \theta \log u)^2 + (1 - \theta \log v)^2 - 1\right]^{\frac{1}{2}}}{\theta} \right\}$$

where $u = S_{T_1}(\cdot)$ and $v = S_{T_2}(\cdot)$. This is a new copula and not appeared in the earlier literature.

5.4 Positive Stable Frailty

The shared positive stable frailty model is of special interest for two reasons. First, similar to the gamma frailty model, the simple form of the Laplace transform allows simple maximum likelihood estimation in the parametric model. Second, there exist no moments of this distribution. This was the reason why Hougaard (1986a) introduced this distribution in the shared frailty approach. Because of the infinite mean, the univariate positive stable frailty model is not identifiable. This makes sense because, in shared frailty models, the frailty parameter is interpreted as an association parameter, that should not be identifiable from univariate observations. In practice, the gamma frailty specification may not fit well (Shih 1998; Glidden 1999; Fan et al. 2000). The positive stable (PS) model (Hougaard 2000) is a useful alternative, in part because it has the attractive feature that predictive hazard ratio decrease to 1 over time (Oakes 1989). The property is observed in familial associations of the ages of onset of diseases with etiologic heterogeneity, where genetic cases occur early and long-term survivors are weakly correlated. The gamma model has predictive hazard ratios which are time invariant and may not be suitable for these patterns of failures (Fine et al. 2003). The probability density function (pdf) of positive stable distribution with two parameters α and δ is given by

$$f_Z(z) = \frac{-1}{\pi z} \sum_{k=1}^{\infty} \frac{\Gamma(k\alpha + 1)}{k!} (-z^{-\alpha} \delta/\alpha)^k \sin(\alpha k \pi); \quad z > 0, 0 < \alpha < 1$$

with the Laplace transform
$$L_Z(s) = E\left[e^{-sZ}\right] = e^{-\delta s^\alpha/\alpha}. \quad \text{(See Hougaard 2000)}.$$
In order to solve the non-identifiability, we restrict the parameter ($\alpha = \delta = \theta$) in the positive stable distribution. With this restriction, PDF is

$$f_Z(z) = \frac{1}{\pi} \sum_{k=1}^{\infty} \frac{\Gamma(k\theta + 1)}{k!} (-1)^{k+1} \left(\frac{1}{z}\right)^{\theta k + 1} \sin(\theta k \pi); \quad z > 0, 0 < \theta < 1$$

with the Laplace transform

$$L_Z(s) = E\left[e^{-sZ}\right] = e^{-s^\theta}.$$

Unconditional bivariate survival function

The unconditional bivariate survival function at time $t_1 > 0$ and $t_2 > 0$ with positive stable frailty is,

$$L_Z(H_1(t_1), H_2(t_2)) = e^{-[(H_1(t_1)+H_2(t_2))]^{\theta}},$$
$$= S(t_1, t_2) \tag{5.3}$$

where $H_1(t_1)$ and $H_2(t_2)$ are the cumulative baseline hazard functions of the lifetime random variables T_1 and T_2, respectively. When $\theta = 1$, the frailty distribution is degenerate $Z = 1$.

Cross-Ratio Function

The cross-ratio function is given by

$$\theta^*(t_1, t_2) = \frac{S(t_1, t_2) \frac{\partial^2 S(t_1, t_2)}{\partial t_1 \partial t_2}}{\frac{\partial S(t_1, t_2)}{\partial t_1} \frac{\partial S(t_1, t_2)}{\partial t_2}}$$
$$= 1 + \frac{\theta - 1}{\theta \ln S(t_1, t_2)}$$

It is a decreasing function of (t_1, t_2) and decreases from ∞ to one.

The Stable Weibull Model

The Weibull distribution is particularly well suited to the positive stable frailty model. The bivariate Weibull model is obtained by assuming $H_i(t) = \lambda_i t^{c_i}$, $i = 1, 2$. This means that conditionally on $Z = z$, the distribution of T_i's are independent Weibull (λ_i, z, c_i), $i = 1, 2$. The bivariate survival function is

$$S_\alpha(t_1, t_2) = e^{-[\lambda_1 t_1^{c_1} + \lambda_2 t_2^{c_2}]^{\theta}}.$$

The advantage of this model is that the marginal distributions are also of Weibull form. Also, the time to the first event, $T_{(1)} = \min(T_1, T_2)$, is of Weibull form when $c_1 = c_2$.

The positive stable model has the advantage that it fits proportional hazards which means that if the conditional model has proportional hazards, so does the marginal distribution. This is an advantage, when considering the model as a random effects model.

The joint bivariate survival function (5.3) can be expressed in terms of survival copula as (see Nelsen (2006) for details)

$$\overline{C}(u, v) = e^{\left[-((-\ln u)^{1/\theta} + (-\ln v)^{1/\theta})^{\theta}\right]}$$

where $u = S_{T_1}(\cdot)$ and $v = S_{T_2}(\cdot)$.

Hanagal and Bhambure (2014) and Hanagal and Kamble (2014) developed positive stable frailty models to analyze kidney infection data. Hanagal and Bhambure (2017) obtained positive stable frailty model to analyze Australian twin data.

5.5 Power Variance Function Frailty

Power variance function (PVF) distribution is a three-parameter family uniting gamma and positive stable distributions. The distribution is denoted PVF(α, δ, θ). For $\alpha = 0$, the gamma distributions are obtained, with same parametrization. Some formulas are valid, but many are others are different in this case. For $\theta = 0$, the positive stable distributions are obtained. For $\alpha = 1/2$, the inverse Gaussian distributions are obtained. For $\alpha = -1$, the noncentral gamma distribution of shape parameter zero is obtained. For $\alpha = 1$, a degenerate distribution is obtained.

The parameter set is ($\alpha \leq 1, \delta > 0$), with ($\theta \geq 0$ for $\alpha > 0$), and ($\theta > 0$ for $\alpha \leq 0$). The distribution is concentrated on the positive numbers for $\alpha \geq 0$, and is positive or zero for $\alpha < 0$. In the case $\alpha > 0$, the p.d.f. of PVF is given by (See Hougaard 2000, p. 504)

$$f(z) = e^{-\theta z + \delta \theta^\alpha / \alpha} \frac{1}{\pi} \sum_{k=1}^{\infty} \frac{\Gamma(k\alpha + 1)}{k!} (-\frac{1}{z})^{\alpha k + 1} \sin(\alpha k \pi), \quad z > 0.$$

In the case $\alpha < 0$, the Γ-term in the density is not necessarily defined, and therefore we can use the alternative expression for p.d.f. of PVF as (See Hougaard 2000, p. 504)

$$f(z) = e^{-\theta z + \delta \theta^\alpha / \alpha} \frac{1}{z} \sum_{k=1}^{\infty} \frac{(-\delta z^\alpha / \alpha)^k}{k! \Gamma(-k\alpha)}, \quad z > 0.$$

This expression is valid for all α values, except 0 and 1, with the convention that when the Γ-function in the denominator is undefined (which happens when $k\alpha$ is a positive integer), the whole term in the sum is zero. For $\alpha < 0$, there is probability $\exp(\delta \theta^\alpha / \alpha)$ of the random variable being zero. For $\alpha \geq 0$, the distribution is unimodal.

If Z_1 and Z_2 are independent, and Z_i follows PVF(α, δ_i, θ), $i = 1, 2$ the distribution of $Z_1 + Z_2$ is PVF($\alpha, \delta_1 + \delta_2, \theta$). So, PVF distribution is infinitely divisible. When $\theta > 0$, all (positive) moments exist, and the mean is $\delta \theta^{\alpha-1}$. The variance is $\delta(1 - \alpha)\theta^{\alpha-2}$.

In order to solve the non-identifiability problem, we assume $E(Z) = 1$. Thus $E(Z) = 1$ is achieved by setting $\delta = \theta^{1-\alpha}$. The pdf of PVF when $\delta = \theta^{1-\alpha}$ is given by

$$f(z) = e^{\theta z + \theta / \alpha} \frac{1}{z} \sum_{k=1}^{\infty} \frac{[z^\alpha / (\alpha \theta^{\alpha-1})]^k}{k! \Gamma(-k\alpha)}, \quad z > 0.$$

The Laplace transform of the above PVF distribution is

$$L(s) = e^{-\theta\{(1+s/\theta)^\alpha - 1\}/\alpha}.$$

The unconditional survival function of the lifetime T with PVF frailty is given by

$$S_{\alpha,\theta}(t) = L[H(t)] = \exp(-\theta\{[1 + H(t)/\theta]^\alpha - 1\}/\alpha).$$

When $\alpha = 1$ or $\theta = \infty$, Z is degenerate at $Z = 1$. The unconditional bivariate survival function of the lifetimes T_1 and T_2 with PVF frailty is given by

$$S_{\alpha,\theta}(t_1, t_2) = e^{-\theta\{[1+H_1(t_1)+H_2(t_2)/\theta]^\alpha - 1\}/\alpha}.$$

The cross-ratio function of PVF frailty distribution is given by

$$\theta^*(t_1, t_2) = 1 + \frac{\alpha - 1}{1 - \frac{\alpha}{\theta} \ln S(t_1, t_2)}$$

The cross-ratio function is decreasing function of (t_1, t_2) and decreases from α to one.

Hanagal (2007c, 2009) considered PVF frailty models with bivariate Weibull as a baseline distributions.

5.6 Compound Poisson Frailty

Aalen (1988, 1992) introduced a compound Poisson distribution as a mixing distribution in survival models which is an extension of one studied by Hougaard (1986b) The compound Poisson distribution plays a prominent role in this extension, being used here as a mixing distribution. Quite often hazard rates or intensities are raising at the start, reaching a maximum and then declining. Hence the intensity has a unimodal shape with finite mode. For example, (1) death rates for cancer patients, meaning that the longer the patient lives, beyond a certain time, the more improved are his or her chances, (2) divorce rates, the maximal rate of divorce which occurs after a few years which means most marriages are going through crisis and then improving (Aaberge et al. 1989). The population intensity starts to decline simply because of the high-risk individuals have already died or been divorced, and so forth.

An additional feature which is often seen is that the total integral under the intensity (hazard rate) is to be finite; that is, the distribution is defective. In practical terms this means that some individuals have zero susceptibility; they will 'survive forever'. For instance, some patients survive their cancer, some people never marry, some marriages are not prone to be dissolved, and so on. In medicine, there are several examples of diseases primarily attacking people with a particular susceptibility, for instance, a genetic kind, other people having virtually zero susceptibility of getting the disease. Another example is fertility. Some couples are unable to conceive children so that the distribution of times to having first childbirths for a population of couples will be defective. In unemployment data, one is also faced with the fact that some people may be completely unable to get a job. In such type of data, compound distribution having some positive mass at zero value can be a suitable choice. Compound Poisson distribution is conveniently used in the literature, since it has an explicit Laplace transform and it deals with the feature that some people may have zero susceptibility. Aalen (1992) considered a compound Poisson distribution as a mixture distribution in survival analysis. Also Aalen and Tretli (1995), Moger and Aalen (2005), Hanagal (2010a, b, c) have considered compound Poisson frailty models. Hanagal and Dabade (2012) and Hanagal and Kamble (2015) developed compound Poisson frailty models to analyze kidney infection data.

The use of the compound Poisson distribution for Z is not only mathematically convenient but might also be seen as natural in a more substantial sense. The distribution arises as a sum of a random number of independent gamma variables, where the number of terms in the sum is Poisson distributed. This might be viewed as a kind of shock model, where the vulnerability of the subject has been shaped by a random number of shocks, each of random size.

Some Definitions and Properties

Definition

A random variable Z is said to have the compound Poisson distribution if Z is such that,

$$Z = \begin{cases} X_1 + X_2 + \cdots + X_N \; ; & N > 0 \\ 0 & ; \quad N = 0. \end{cases}$$

where N is Poisson distributed with mean ρ, while $X_1, X_2, \ldots, X_N$ are independent and identically gamma distributed random variables with scale parameter ν and shape parameter γ.

The distribution of Z consists of two parts; a discrete part which corresponds to the probability of zero susceptibility, and a continuous part on the positive real line. The discrete part is

$$P(Z = 0) = e^{-\rho},$$

which decreases as ρ increases.

We know that, if $X_1, X_2, \ldots, X_N$ are independent and identically distributed gamma variates with scale parameter ν and shape parameter γ then for given N = n, $Z = \sum_{i=1}^{N} X_i$ is also gamma variate with same scale parameter ν and shape parameter $n\gamma$ having density function,

$$g(z \mid n) = \begin{cases} \frac{\nu^{n\gamma}}{\Gamma(n\gamma)} z^{n\gamma-1} e^{-\nu z} \; ; & z > 0, \nu > 0, \gamma > 0 \\ 0 & ; \text{ otherwise.} \end{cases}$$

Also N is a Poisson variable with probability mass function,

$$P(n) = \begin{cases} \frac{e^{-\rho}\rho^n}{n!} & ; \ n = 0, 1, \ldots, ; \rho > 0 \\ 0 & ; \ \text{otherwise.} \end{cases}$$

Then the distribution of the continuous part of compound Poisson distribution can be found by conditioning on N as

$$f(z) = \sum_{n=0}^{\infty} \frac{\nu^{n\gamma}}{\Gamma(n\gamma)} z^{n\gamma-1} e^{-\nu z} \cdot \frac{e^{-\rho}\rho^n}{n!}$$

$$= \exp\left[-(\rho + \nu z)\right] \frac{1}{z} \sum_{n=0}^{\infty} \frac{\rho^n (\nu z)^{n\gamma}}{\Gamma(n\gamma)n!}$$

Thus density function of compound Poisson variate Z is given by,

$$f(z; \gamma, \nu, \rho) = \begin{cases} e^{[-(\rho+\nu z)]} \frac{1}{z} \sum_{n=0}^{\infty} \frac{\rho^n(\nu z)^{n\gamma}}{\Gamma(n\gamma)n!} & ; \ z > 0, \rho > 0, \nu > 0, \gamma > 0 \\ 0 & ; \ \text{otherwise.} \end{cases} \tag{5.4}$$

The parameter set for the compound Poisson distribution is $\rho > 0, \nu > 0, \gamma > 0$.

Laplace transform

To obtain Laplace transform of compound Poisson variate we first have to obtain Laplace transform of Poisson and gamma distribution. The Laplace transform of gamma distribution is

$$L_X(s) = \left(1 + \frac{s}{\nu}\right)^{-\gamma}$$

and Laplace transform of Poisson distribution is,

$$L_N(s) = E\left(e^{-sN}\right) = \sum_{n=0}^{\infty} e^{-sn} \frac{e^{-\rho}\rho^n}{n!} = e^{-\rho+\rho e^{-s}} = e^{-\rho[1-e^{-s}]}$$

Let $L_Z(s)$ be the Laplace transform of Z then,

$$L_Z(s) = E\left\{e^{-sz}\right\}$$
$$= E_N\left\{E_{X_i}\left[e^{-s(X_1+X_2+\cdots+X_N)|N}\right]\right\}$$
$$= E_N\left\{E_{X_i}\left[\prod_{i=1}^{N} e^{-sX_i} \mid N\right]\right\}$$
$$= E_N\left\{E_X\left[e^{-sX|N}\right]^N\right\} \qquad X_i\text{'s are i.i.d.}$$
$$= E_N\left\{L_{X|N}^N(s)\right\}$$
$$= E_N\left\{e^{-[-N\ln L_X(s)]}\right\}$$
$$= L_N\left[-\ln L_X(s)\right]$$

Substituting Laplace transforms of gamma distribution and Poisson distribution in the above equation, we have

$$L_Z(s) = \exp\left\{-\rho\left[1 - \left(1 + \frac{s}{\nu}\right)^{-\gamma}\right]\right\}$$

$$= \exp\left\{-\rho\left[1 - \left(\frac{\nu}{\nu + s}\right)^{\gamma}\right]\right\} \tag{5.5}$$

Moments

Now to obtain mean and variance of Z we obtain derivatives of Laplace transform.

$$L'_Z(s) = \frac{d}{ds}\exp\left\{-\rho\left[1 - \left(\frac{\nu}{\nu + s}\right)^{\gamma}\right]\right\}$$

$$= \exp\left\{-\rho\left[1 - \left(\frac{\nu}{\nu + s}\right)^{\gamma}\right]\right\}\frac{d}{ds}\left\{-\rho\left[1 - \left(\frac{\nu}{\nu + s}\right)^{\gamma}\right]\right\}$$

$$= -\gamma\rho\nu^{\gamma}\frac{L_Z(s)}{(\nu + s)^{\gamma+1}}$$

$$L''_Z(s) = \frac{d}{ds}\left\{-\gamma\rho\nu^{\gamma}\frac{L_Z(s)}{(\nu + s)^{\gamma+1}}\right\}$$

$$= -\gamma\nu^{\gamma}\rho\left\{L_Z(s)\frac{d}{ds}\frac{1}{(\nu + s)^{\gamma+1}} + \frac{1}{(\nu + s)^{\gamma+1}}\frac{dL_Z(s)}{ds}\right\}$$

$$= \frac{\rho\gamma(\gamma + 1)\nu^{\gamma}}{(\nu + s)^{\gamma+2}}L_Z(s) - \frac{\rho\gamma\nu^{\gamma}}{(\nu + s)^{\gamma+1}}L'_Z(s)$$

Then $E(Z)$ is given by

$$E(Z) = -L'_Z(s)\mid_{s=0} = \frac{\rho\gamma}{\nu} \tag{5.6}$$

The $E(Z^2)$ is

$$E(Z^2) = L''_Z(s)\mid_{s=0} = \frac{\rho\gamma(\gamma + 1)\nu^{\gamma}}{\nu^{\gamma+2}} - \frac{\rho\gamma\nu^{\gamma}}{\nu^{\gamma+1}}\left[-\frac{\rho\gamma\nu^{\gamma}}{\nu^{\gamma+1}}\right]$$

$$= \frac{\rho\gamma(\gamma + 1)}{\nu^2} + \frac{\rho^2\gamma^2}{\nu^2}$$

therefore the variance of Z is

$$var(Z) = E(Z^2) - E(Z)^2 = \frac{\rho\gamma(\gamma + 1)}{\nu^2} \tag{5.7}$$

For identifiability of the model, we assume Z has expected value equal to one i.e. $E(Z) = 1$. Under the restriction $E(Z) = 1$ which leads to $\nu = \rho\gamma$. Under this restriction, variance of Z is given by $\sigma^2 = \frac{\gamma+1}{\rho\gamma}$. Laplace transform under the restriction is

$$L_Z(s) = \exp\left\{-\rho\left[1 - \left(1 + \frac{s}{\rho\gamma}\right)^{-\gamma}\right]\right\}$$

Unconditional Bivariate Survival Function

We obtain the unconditional bivariate survival function for at time $t_1 > 0$ and $t_2 > 0$ as,

$$S(t_{1j}, t_{2j}) = L_Z(H_1(t_1) + H_2(t_2))$$

$$= \exp\left\{-\rho\left[1 - \left(1 + \frac{(H_{01}(t_{1j}) + H_{02}(t_{2j}))\eta_j}{\rho\gamma}\right)^{-\gamma}\right]\right\}$$

where $H_1(t_1)$ and $H_2(t_2)$ are cumulative baseline hazard functions of lifetime random variables T_1 and T_2, respectively.

Cross-ratio Function

The cross-ratio function $\theta^*(t_1, t_2)$ can be written as

$$\theta^*(t_1, t_2) = 1 + \frac{\gamma + 1}{\rho\gamma}\left[1 + \frac{\ln S(t_1, t_2)}{\rho}\right]^{-1}$$

but $\sigma^2 = \frac{\gamma + 1}{\rho\gamma}$ therefore,

$$\theta^*(t_1, t_2) = 1 + \sigma^2\left[1 + \frac{\ln S(t_1, t_2)}{\rho}\right]^{-1}$$

Thus cross-ratio function is greater than one and is a function of t_1, t_2. This implies there is always positive association between the survival times t_1 and t_2. We know that as $t_1 > 0$, $t_2 > 0$ survival function $S(t_1, t_2)$ is a nonincreasing function from 1 to 0, hence log of $S(t_1, t_2)$ is decreasing function and decreases from 0 to $-\infty$. Thus cross-ratio function is an decreasing function of $t_1 > 0$, $t_2 > 0$ and decreases from $1 + \sigma^2$ to 1.

5.7 Compound Negative Binomial Frailty

To add non-susceptibility or zero susceptibility a convenient frailty distribution, compound Poisson distribution, is suggested in literature which we have considered in the previous chapter. Aalen (1992), Aalen and Tretli (1999), Moger and Aalen (2005), Hanagal (2010a, b, c) have considered compound Poisson frailty models. For example, Aalen and Tretli (1995) analyzed testis cancer data by means of a compound

Poisson frailty model. They represented X_i as size of the damage at ith occasion and N be the number of damages occurred. A man receives damages during a critical period of their fetal development which may develop testis cancer after the hormonal process of puberty has started. The damage may be a result of the mother's exposure to environmental factors, for example, an excessive estrogen burden, and may also interact with genetic factors. So Z is now cumulative effect of damages before testis cancer is observed with a man. In such situations negative binomial distribution or in particular geometric distribution is a suitable choice of distribution for variate N. In risk model also, another parallel choice to compound Poisson model is compound negative binomial model or compound geometric model. When the number of successes is equal to one, the compound negative binomial distribution reduces to compound geometric distribution. Every compound negative binomial distribution can be considered as a compound Poisson distribution. If Z_1 and Z_2 are, respectively, follows compound Poisson and compound negative binomial distribution with $Z_1 = X_1 + X_2 + \cdots X_{N_1}$ and $Z_2 = X_1 + X_2 + \cdots X_{N_2}$, where N_1 is Poisson random variate with intensity λ and N_2 is negative binomial random variate with parameters, number of successes r and probability of success p then Z_1 and Z_2 are identically distributed if $\lambda = -r \log p$. Hanagal and Dabade (2013) and Hanagal and Kamble (2016) developed compound negative binomial frailty models to analyze kidney infection data.

Some Definitions and Properties

A random variable Z is said to have the compound negative binomial distribution if Z is such that,

$$Z = \begin{cases} X_1 + X_2 + \cdots + X_N & ; \ N > 0 \\ 0 & ; \ N = 0. \end{cases}$$

where N is a negative binomial variate with parameters r and p; r and p denotes, respectively, the number of successes and the probability of success. If $N > 0$ then we can interpret Z as aggregate heterogeneity due to failures before we get first success or in general rth success. $X_1, X_2, \ldots, X_N$ are i.i.d. gamma variates with scale parameter ν and shape parameter γ.

The distribution of Z consists of two parts; a discrete part which corresponds to the probability of zero susceptibility, and a continuous part on the positive real line. The discrete part is $P(Z = 0) = p^r$ which decreases as p decreases.

We know that, if $X_1, X_2, \ldots, X_N$ are independent and identically distributed gamma variates with scale parameter ν and shape parameter γ then for given N = n, $Z = \sum_{i=1}^{N} X_i$ is also gamma variate with same scale parameter ν and shape parameter $n\gamma$ having density function,

$$g(z \mid n) = \begin{cases} \frac{\nu^{n\gamma}}{\Gamma(n\gamma)} z^{n\gamma-1} e^{-\nu z} & ; \ z > 0, \nu > 0, \gamma > 0 \\ 0 & ; \ \text{otherwise.} \end{cases}$$

Also N is a negative binomial variate with probability mass function,

$$P(n) = \begin{cases} {}^{n+r-1}C_{r-1} p^r q^n \; ; \; n = 0, 1, \ldots ; 0 < p < 1; q = 1 - p, r = 1, 2, \ldots \\ 0 \qquad\qquad\qquad ; \text{ otherwise.} \end{cases}$$

Then the distribution of the continuous part of compound negative binomial distribution can be found by conditioning on N as,

$$f(z) = \sum_{n=0}^{\infty} g(z \mid N = n) \cdot P(n)$$

$$= \sum_{n=0}^{\infty} \frac{\nu^{n\gamma}}{\Gamma(n\gamma)} z^{n\gamma-1} e^{-\nu z} \cdot {}^{n+r-1}C_{r-1} p^r q^n$$

$$= p^r \frac{1}{z} e^{-\nu z} \sum_{n=0}^{\infty} {}^{n+r-1}C_{r-1} q^n \frac{(\nu z)^{n\gamma}}{\Gamma(n\gamma)}$$

Thus density function of compound negative binomial variate Z is given by,

$$f(z) = \begin{cases} p^r \frac{1}{z} e^{-\nu z} \sum_{n=0}^{\infty} {}^{n+r-1}C_{r-1} q^n \frac{(\nu z)^{n\gamma}}{\Gamma(n\gamma)} \; ; z > 0, \nu > 0, \gamma > 0, 0 < p < 1; \\ \qquad\qquad\qquad\qquad\qquad\qquad q = 1 - p, r = 1, 2, \ldots \\ 0 \qquad\qquad\qquad\qquad\qquad ; \text{ otherwise.} \end{cases}$$

The parameter set for the compound negative binomial distribution is
  $0 < p < 1, \nu > 0$ and $\gamma > 0$.

Laplace transform

The Laplace transform of gamma distribution is given by,

$$L_X(s) = \left(1 + \frac{s}{\nu}\right)^{-\gamma}$$

and Laplace transform of negative binomial distribution is,

$$L_N(s) = E\left(e^{-sN}\right) = \sum_{n=0}^{\infty} e^{-sn} \cdot {}^{n+r-1}C_{r-1} p^r q^n$$

$$= p^r \sum_{n=0}^{\infty} {}^{n+r-1}C_{r-1} \left(qe^{-s}\right)^n$$

$$= \left[\frac{p}{1 - qe^{-s}}\right]^r$$

If $L_Z(s)$ is the Laplace transform of Z then,

$$L_Z(s) = L_N[-\ln L_X(s)]$$

where $L_X(s)$ and $L_N(s)$ are Laplace transform of gamma distribution and negative binomial distribution, respectively. substituting the Laplace transforms of N and X in the above equation we get the Laplace transform of compound negative binomial distribution is given by,

$$L_Z(s) = \left\{ \frac{p}{1 - q\left[1 + \frac{s}{\nu}\right]^{-\gamma}} \right\}^r$$

Moments

Differentiating $L_Z(s)$ with respect to s we get,

$$L_Z'(s) = \frac{d}{ds} \left\{ \frac{p}{1 - q\left[1 + \frac{s}{\nu}\right]^{-\gamma}} \right\}^r$$

$$= r \left\{ \frac{p}{1 - q\left[1 + \frac{s}{\nu}\right]^{-\gamma}} \right\}^{r-1} \cdot p \frac{d}{ds} \left[1 - q \left(1 + \frac{s}{\nu}\right)^{-\gamma} \right]^{-1}$$

$$= -r p^r q \gamma \frac{1}{\nu} \left(1 + \frac{s}{\nu}\right)^{-(\gamma+1)} \left[1 - q \left(1 + \frac{s}{\nu}\right)^{-\gamma} \right]^{-(r+1)}$$

Differentiating $L_Z(s)$ with respect to s again,

$$L_Z''(s) = \frac{d}{ds} L_Z'(s)$$

$$= -r p^r q \frac{\gamma}{\nu} \left\{ \left(1 + \frac{s}{\nu}\right)^{-(\gamma+1)} \frac{d}{ds} \left[1 - q \left(1 + \frac{s}{\nu}\right)^{-\gamma} \right]^{-(r+1)} \right.$$

$$\left. + \left[1 - q \left(1 + \frac{s}{\nu}\right)^{-\gamma} \right]^{-(r+1)} \frac{d}{ds} \left(1 + \frac{s}{\nu}\right)^{-(\gamma+1)} \right\}$$

$$= -r p^r q \frac{\gamma}{\nu} \left\{ -(r+1)q \frac{\gamma}{\nu} \left(1 + \frac{s}{\nu}\right)^{-2(\gamma+1)} \left[1 - q \left(1 + \frac{s}{\nu}\right)^{-\gamma} \right]^{-(r+2)} \right.$$

$$\left. - \frac{(\gamma+1)}{\nu} \left(1 + \frac{s}{\nu}\right)^{-(\gamma+2)} \left[1 - q \left(1 + \frac{s}{\nu}\right)^{-\gamma} \right]^{-(r+1)} \right\}$$

$$= r p q \frac{\gamma}{\nu^2} \left(1 + \frac{s}{\nu}\right)^{-(\gamma+2)} \left[1 - q \left(1 + \frac{s}{\nu}\right)^{-\gamma} \right]^{-(r+1)}$$

$$\left\{ (r+1) q \gamma \left(1 + \frac{s}{\nu}\right)^{-\gamma} \left[1 - q \left(1 + \frac{s}{\nu}\right)^{-\gamma} \right]^{-1} + (\gamma+1) \right\}$$

The mean of Z is

$$E(Z) = -L'_Z(s) \mid_{s=0} = \frac{rq\gamma}{p\nu} \tag{5.8}$$

and

$$E(Z^2) = L''_Z(s) \mid_{s=0} = rp^r q \frac{\gamma}{\nu^2} p^{-(r+1)} \left\{ (r+1)q\gamma p^{-1} + (\gamma+1) \right\}$$

$$= \left(\frac{rq\gamma}{p\nu} \right)^2 + \frac{rq\gamma(p+\gamma)}{p^2\nu^2}$$

and the variance of Z is

$$var(Z) = \frac{rq\gamma(p+\gamma)}{p^2\nu^2}$$

For identifiability condition, $E(Z) = 1$, from Eq. (5.8) we have restriction placed on the parameters is,

$$p\nu = rq\gamma$$

therefore under the above restriction the variance of Z is given by, $\sigma^2 = \frac{p+\gamma}{rq\gamma}$ and Laplace transform is

$$L_Z(s) = \left\{ \frac{p}{1 - q\left[1 + \frac{ps}{rq\gamma}\right]^{-\gamma}} \right\}^r$$

Unconditional Bivariate Survival Function

We obtain the unconditional bivariate survival function for jth individual at time $t_{1j} > 0$ and $t_{2j} > 0$ as,

$$S(t_{1j}, t_{2j}) = L_Z(H_1(t_1) + H_2(t_2))$$

$$= \left\{ \frac{p}{1 - q\left[1 + \frac{p(H_{01}(t_{1j}) + H_{02}(t_{2j}))\eta_j}{rq\gamma}\right]^{-\gamma}} \right\}^r$$

where $H_1(t_1)$ and $H_2(t_2)$ are cumulative baseline hazard functions of lifetime random variables T_1 and T_2, respectively.

Cross-ratio Function

The cross-ratio function $\theta^*(t_1, t_2)$ of negative binomial frailty can be written as

$$\theta^*(t_1, t_2) = 1 - \frac{1}{r\gamma} + \frac{\gamma+1}{rq\gamma} \frac{q}{\left[1 - \frac{p}{S(t_1, t_2)^{1/r}}\right]}$$

$$= 1 - \frac{1 - (\gamma + 1)\left[1 - pS(t_1, t_2)^{-\frac{1}{r}}\right]^{-1}}{r\gamma}$$

We know that survival function $S(t_1, t_2)$ is a nonincreasing function from 1 to 0 of $t_1 > 0$ and $t_2 > 0$. Therefore by applying simple mathematical logic we can say $\phi(t_1, t_2)^\gamma$ is increasing function of t_1, t_2. Hence cross-ratio function $\theta^*(t_1, t_2)$ is always positive and decreasing function of t_1, t_2 and decreases between $1 - \frac{1}{r\gamma} + \frac{\gamma+1}{rq\gamma}$ to $1 - \frac{1}{r\gamma}$. This implies that there is always positive association between the survival times t_1 and t_2 and it increases as time t_1, t_2 increases.

5.8 Compound Poisson Frailty with Random Scale

An extension of the compound Poisson frailty model to family data, is to apply a probability distribution to the parameter ρ which was proposed by Moger and Aalen (2005). A probability density of ρ expresses the variation between families. The individuals of a given family are characterized by having a specific value of ρ, so they will have correlated frailties, while individuals from different families are independent. This yields a two-level model, where the frailty has two components: A familial component, for instance, relating to shared genes and environment, and an individual component, which could relate to exposure to individual environment. Thus, the model does not fit into the traditional dichotomy of shared frailty models. We would like to stress the importance of frailty models having clear biological content, corresponding to understand a problem from a substance point of view, as opposed to just making mathematical assumptions. Since compound Poisson distribution is included in the power variance function (PVF) distributions, this corresponds to randomizing a scale parameter in the PVF distributions. Hanagal (2010d) developed compound Poisson frailty with random scale and bivariate exponential of Marshall–Olkin (1967) as baseline distribution.

This section will focus on densities for ρ which are included in the PVF distribution family. Specifically we consider the gamma, inverse Gaussian and positive stable distributions. As given in Hougaard (2000), the distributions can be united in a three-parameter family with parameter set $\alpha \leq 1, \epsilon > 0$, with $\theta \geq 0$ for $\alpha > 0$, and $\theta > 0$ for $\alpha \leq 0$. For $\alpha = 0$ the gamma distributions are obtained. The inverse Gaussian distributions are obtained for $\alpha = 1/2$, and for $\theta = 0$ one gets the positive stable distributions. The positive stable distributions are absolutely continuous and nonnegative, with unimodal densities (Hougaard 1986b). For $\alpha = 1$, a degenerate distribution is obtained, at ϵ, independent of θ. This corresponds to independence within families. This is given by (5.4), with $\eta = -\alpha$, $\rho = -(\epsilon/\alpha)\theta^\alpha$ and $\nu = \theta$. Hence, values of $\alpha < 0$ yield the compound Poisson distributions. The parameterization used in Sect. 5.6 is the most appropriate for $\alpha < 0$, while the parameterization by Hougaard is more easy to use for $\alpha > 0$. The expectation and variance of the distribution of ρ are

$$E(\rho) = \epsilon\theta^{\alpha-1}, \qquad Var(\rho) = \epsilon(1-\alpha)\theta^{\alpha-2}.$$

Thus, the positive stable distribution has no finite expectation or variance. The Laplace transform of ρ is given by

$$L_\rho(s) = \exp\{-\tfrac{\epsilon}{\alpha}[(\theta+s)^\alpha - \theta^\alpha]\}.$$

In the case of the mixed compound Poisson distribution, the unconditional discrete part of Z is given by

$$P(Z=0) = E(\exp(-\rho)) = L_\rho(1).$$

The density of the unconditional continuous part of Z can be calculated in a similar manner by noting that

$$E[\rho^n \exp(-\rho)] = (-1)^n L_\rho^{(n)}(1),$$

where $L^{(n)}(s)$ denotes the nth derivative of the Laplace transform. By inserting the density of ρ into (5.4) and integrating out ρ, the density of Z may be put on the following form:

$$h(z; \eta, \nu, \alpha, \theta, \epsilon) = \exp(-\nu z)\frac{1}{z}\sum_{n=1}^{\infty}\frac{(\nu z)^{n\eta}}{\Gamma(n\eta)n!}(-1)^n L_\rho^{(n)}(1).$$

The derivatives of the Laplace transform for the power variance function distribution for ρ are of the form

$$L_\rho^{(n)}(s) = (-1)^n L_\rho(s)\sum_{j=1}^{n} c_{n,j}(\alpha)\epsilon^j(\theta+s)^{j\alpha-n},$$

as shown in Hougaard (2000). The coefficients $c_{n,j}(\alpha)$ are given by the recursive formula

$$c_{n,1}(\alpha) = \Gamma(n-\alpha)/\Gamma(1-\alpha), \qquad c_{n,n}(\alpha) = 1,$$
$$c_{n,j}(\alpha) = c_{n-1,j-1}(\alpha) + c_{n-1,j}(\alpha)[(n-1)-j\alpha].$$

The Laplace transform of ρ, $L_\rho(s)$, combined with (5.5) yield the expression

$$L_Z(s) = L_\rho\left(1 - \left(\frac{\nu}{\nu+s}\right)^\eta\right)$$

for the Laplace transform of Z. For the PVF distributed ρ, this equals

$$L_Z(s) = \exp\left(-\frac{\epsilon}{\alpha}\left\{\left[\theta + 1 - \left(\frac{\nu}{\nu+s}\right)^{\eta}\right]^{\alpha} - \theta^{\alpha}\right\}\right)$$

if ≤ 1, $\neq 0$,

$$= \left(\frac{\theta}{\theta + 1 - \left(\frac{\nu}{\nu+s}\right)^{\eta}}\right)^{\epsilon} \quad \text{if } = 0.$$

The Laplace transform of the gamma mixture distribution ($\alpha = 0$) is obtained by taking the limit of the general Laplace transform. The positive stable mixture distribution ($\theta = 0$) gives some nice properties when used as a frailty distribution. The Laplace transform of Z in this case is

$$L_Z(s) = \exp\left\{-\frac{\epsilon}{\alpha}\left[1 - \left(\frac{\nu}{\nu+s}\right)^{\eta}\right]^{\alpha}\right\}.$$

Apart from the exponent α, this is of the same form as the Laplace transform of a compound Poisson distribution given in Eq. (5.5), with ϵ/α playing the role of ρ.

Now the survival function of the compound Poisson frailty with random scale is given by

$$S(t) = L_Z(H(t))$$

$$= \exp\left(-\frac{\epsilon}{\alpha}\left\{\left[\theta + 1 - \left(\frac{\nu}{\nu+H(t)}\right)^{\eta}\right]^{\alpha} - \theta^{\alpha}\right\}\right) \quad \text{if } \leq 1, \neq 0,$$

$$= \left(\frac{\theta}{\theta + 1 - \left(\frac{\nu}{\nu+H(t)}\right)^{\eta}}\right)^{\epsilon} \quad \text{if } = 0.$$

The mean and variance of Z can easily be found by means of (5.6) and (5.7), by noting that $E(Z) = E[E(Z|\rho)]$ and that $\text{Var}(Z) = \text{Var}[E(Z|\rho)] + E[\text{Var}(Z|\rho)]$:

$$\beta = E(Z) = \frac{\epsilon\eta}{\nu\theta^{1-\alpha}}, \qquad \text{Var}(Z) = \frac{\epsilon\eta[\theta + \eta(1 - \alpha + \theta)]}{\nu^2\theta^{2-\alpha}}.$$

Note that when a positive stable mixture distribution is used, the frailty distribution Z has no finite expectation or variance. When ρ is not stable distributed ($\theta > 0$), the Laplace transform can be reparameterized by using the expectation β, the squared coefficient of variation is

$$d = \frac{\text{Var}(Z)}{E(Z)^2} = \frac{[\theta + \eta(1 - \alpha + \theta)]}{\nu\theta}$$

as new parameters. The value $d = 0$ corresponds to no heterogeneity.

When individuals in a study belong to families or groups where there may be similarities in risk, then this association can be modeled within the present framework. For simplicity, a paired twins or paired dental implants or paired organs are dependent with hazard function $H_1(t_1) + H_2(t_2)$. Note that gene-specific quantity is shared by each of the twins. The joint survival function given the frailty $Z = z$ is

$$S(t_1, t_2 \mid z) = e^{-z(H_1(t_1) + H_2(t_2))}.$$

From this, we immediately derive the bivariate survival function by integrating Z out

$$
\begin{aligned}
S(t_1, t_2) &= E e^{-Z(H_1(t_1) + H_2(t_2))} \\
&= L(H_1(t_1) + H_2(t_2)) \\
&= \exp\left(-\frac{\epsilon}{\alpha}\left\{\left[\theta + 1 - \left(\frac{\nu}{\nu + H_1(t_1) + H_2(t_2)}\right)^{\eta}\right]^{\alpha} - \theta^{\alpha}\right\}\right) \\
&= \left(\frac{\theta}{\theta + 1 - \left(\frac{\nu}{\nu + H_1(t_1) + H_2(t_2)}\right)^{\eta}}\right)^{\epsilon} \quad \text{if} \ = 0,
\end{aligned}
$$

where $L(.)$ is the Laplace transform of the distribution of Z. Thus, the bivariate survival function is easily expressed by means of the Laplace transform of the frailty distribution, evaluated at the total integrated conditional hazard.

In order to solve the non-identifiability problem, we assume a mean of 1 for the frailty distributions. For the gamma distribution, this can be achieved by setting $\theta = \epsilon$. In the shared PVF model, $E(Z) = 1$ is achieved by setting $\epsilon = \theta^{1-\alpha}$. The shared frailty models are compared to a compound Poisson model where ρ is gamma distributed, yielding a compound Poisson–gamma model. To secure a unit mean for the frailty, we get $\epsilon = \nu\theta/\eta$. In this section, we assume the distribution of frailty as compound Poisson–gamma distribution for the bivariate survival data. The bivariate survival function based on this frailty is given by

$$S(t_1, t_2) = \left(\frac{\theta}{\theta + 1 - \left(\frac{\nu}{\nu + H_1(t_1) + H_2(t_2)}\right)^{\eta}}\right)^{\nu\theta/\eta}.$$

5.9 Frailty Models in Hierarchical Likelihood

The generalized linear model (GLIM) can be extended by incorporating frailty in the linear predictor. This generalized linear mixed model (GLMM) is very useful for accommodating the over-dispersion occurring in the data. Such research has been carried out by Schall (1991), who emphasized the linear logistic regression model with frailty. Schall (1991) proposed an algorithm to estimate the fixed effects, frailty and dispersion components in a GLMM, where this algorithm yields approximate ML and restricted maximum likelihood (REML) estimators for the variance of the frailty terms. Another method adjusting for over-dispersion was developed by Breslow and Clayton (1993), using Laplace's method to obtain the marginal quasi-likelihood (MQL). The integrated quasi-likelihood proposed by Breslow and Clayton (1993), however, cannot be evaluated in closed-form. Therefore, Laplace's method was used to approximate the integral. This approach eventually led to estimating equations based on penalized quasi-likelihood (PQL) for the mean parameter and pseudolikelihood for the variance. The pseudo ML method is used to obtain an estimator by maximizing a likelihood function associated with family of distributions which does not necessarily contain the true distribution. In most cases, the frailty term is assumed to have a Gaussian distribution with mean of zero and a variance of σ^2. Penalized likelihood was specifically exploited by Green and Silverman (1994) to be used for semiparametric regression analysis, whereas Hastie and Tibshirani (1986) applied the penalized likelihood procedure to generalized additive models (GAM).

McGilchrist and Aisbett (1991) and McGilchrist (1993) considered the proportional hazard model

$$h(t; y_i) = h_0(t) \exp(y_i'\beta + u_i), \qquad i = 1, ..., n$$

where y_i is the p-component covariate vector associated with the ith individual or system, β is the p-component regression coefficient vector, and u_i the corresponding individual or system effect in n individuals or systems. Since the frailties $z_i = \exp(u_i)$ are assumed to have a log-normal distribution, then u_i has a normal distribution; relocating u_i (by absorption into the hazard or intercept) leads to a zero mean. McGilchrist (1994) adapted Henderson's (Henderson 1975) and Harville's (Harville 1977) best linear unbiased predictor (BLUP) procedures for mixed normal linear models for use in GLMM.

If the density function of a failure time T_i, conditional on u_i is $g(t_i; \beta \mid u_i)$, then $l_1 = \sum \ln g(t_i; \beta \mid u_i)$ will be the corresponding (conditional) log likelihood function. Then $l(\beta, \mathbf{u}) = l_1 + l_2$ becomes the joint loglikelihood of β and $\mathbf{u} = (u_1, u_2, ..., u_n)'$, where l_2 is the loglikelihood function of the frailty effects. The BLUP procedure avoids having to integrate out the frailty distribution; an important advantage since in most cases, the required numerical integration is not practical (Schall 1991). A similar approach to Henderson's method has been developed by Lee and Nelder (1996), who introduced a class of hierarchical generalized linear models (HGLM) which incorporated random components in the model. In their approach the distribution of frailty could come from any distribution and they paid special attention to the conjugate distribution, where the distribution of frailty is conjugate to that of the response variable. For example, if frailty is assumed to have beta distribution then the conditional distribution of the response given frailty is the binomial distribution or if frailty is assumed to have a inverse gamma distribution then the conditional distribution of the response given frailty is the gamma distribution.

The likelihood function $L(t_1, t_2, \mathbf{u}; \beta, \sigma)$, where σ is the standard deviation of u, is constructed from the product of $L_1(t_1, t_2, \beta \mid \mathbf{u})$, the partial likelihood of paired failure times (T_1, T_2) conditional on frailty, and $L_2(\mathbf{u}, \sigma)$, the likelihood of the frailty. However, the frailty is not directly observable, and the joint likelihood is not a standard likelihood in the conventional sense because it is based on the non-observable random variables **u**. Lee and Nelder (1996) argued that by using hierarchical likelihood (h-likelihood) one avoids integrating out the frailty and also the h-likelihood retains the properties of the likelihood. Also for more complicated problems, such as when the number of parameters goes to infinity, the marginal likelihood cannot be reduced beyond a high-dimensional integral, and numerical integration is no longer feasible or reliable because it is difficult to integrate out the frailty.

Henderson's mixed model equations provide efficient ways of computing the BLUP estimates of β and σ. The ML estimates of β is in fact the same as that arising from the BLUP procedure. Maximizing the density of the residuals with respect to σ produces restricted maximum likelihood (REML) estimates. This estimation procedure using the BLUP technique has been reviewed extensively by Robinson (1991) for normal linear models. His paper mentions that BLUP is an effective method to estimate the frailty, since the random variables **u** are predictable.

Schall (1991) adopted Henderson's procedure to GLMM's. Then McGilchrist (1994) relaxed the exponential family assumption for the conditional distribution of T given u_i, but required the log frailty of u_i to be normally distributed. Lee and Nelder's (1996) HGLM allows for any positive distribution of frailty.

5.10   Frailty Models in Mixture Distributions

Hanagal (2007a, b, 2008a) developed the frailty models in mixture distribution in general. He also obtained the estimation procedures in gamma and positive stable frailty models. The mixture distribution in terms of survival function is

$$
\begin{aligned}
S(t) &= p S_1(t) + (1 - p) S_2(t) \\
     &= p e^{-H_1(t)} + (1 - p) e^{-H_2(t)}.
\end{aligned}
$$

There are two ways of obtaining frailty models. The first one is

$$
\begin{aligned}
S_M(t|z) &= p S_1(t|z) + (1 - p) S_2(t|z) \\
         &= p e^{-z H_1(t)} + (1 - p) e^{-z H_2(t)}.
\end{aligned}
$$

This is called mixture of frailty models or mixture frailty. The second one is

$$
S_F(t|z) = e^{z \ln[p S_1(t) + (1-p) S_2(t)]}.
$$

This is called frailty of the mixture distributions in order to make the distinction between the two types. The same technique can be generalized to mixture of more than two distributions. When we integrate with respect to frailty (Z), we get survival function of mixture distribution in terms of frailty parameter.

Example: Weibull Mixtures

The survival function of two Weibull distributions is

$$
\begin{aligned}
S(t) &= pS_1(t) + (1-p)S_2(t) \\
&= pe^{-\lambda_1 t^{c_1}} + (1-p)e^{-\lambda_2 t^{c_2}}.
\end{aligned}
$$

The mixture frailty is given by

$$
S_M(t|z) = pe^{-z\lambda_1 t^{c_1}} + (1-p)e^{-z\lambda_2 t^{c_2}}. \tag{5.9}
$$

The frailty of the mixture is given by

$$
S_F(t|z) = e^{z \ln[pe^{-\lambda_1 t^{c_1}} + (1-p)e^{-\lambda_2 t^{c_2}}]}. \tag{5.10}
$$

5.10.1 Gamma Frailty in Weibull Mixture

Assuming the distribution of Z as gamma distribution and integrating over Z, in Eq. (5.9), we get Weibull mixture model with gamma mixture frailty, given by

$$
S_M(t) = p\left[1 + \frac{\lambda_1 t^{c_1}}{\alpha}\right]^{-\alpha} + (1-p)\left[1 + \frac{\lambda_2 t^{c_2}}{\alpha}\right]^{-\alpha}.
$$

The pdf corresponding to the above survival function is

$$
f_M(t) = S_{M1}^{\frac{\alpha+1}{\alpha}} p\lambda_1 c_1 t^{c_1-1} + S_{M2}^{\frac{\alpha+1}{\alpha}} (1-p)\lambda_2 c_2 t^{c_2-1},
$$

where $S_{M1} = \left[1 + \frac{\lambda_1 t^{c_1}}{\alpha}\right]^{-\alpha}$ and $S_{M2} = \left[1 + \frac{\lambda_2 t^{c_2}}{\alpha}\right]^{-\alpha}$.

Assuming the distribution of Z as gamma distribution and integrating over Z, in Eq. (5.10), we get Weibull mixture model with gamma frailty, given by

$$
S_F(t) = \left[1 - \frac{\ln[pe^{-\lambda_1 t^{c_1}} + (1-p)e^{-\lambda_2 t^{c_2}}]}{\alpha}\right]^{-\alpha}.
$$

The pdf corresponding to the above survival function is

$$
f_M(t) = S_F^{\frac{\alpha+1}{\alpha}} \frac{p\lambda_1 c_1 t^{c_1-1} e^{-\lambda_1 c_1 t^{c_1-1}} + (1-p)\lambda_2 c_2 t^{c_2-1} e^{-\lambda_2 c_2 t^{c_2-1}}}{[pe^{-\lambda_1 t^{c_1}} + (1-p)e^{-\lambda_2 t^{c_2}}]}.
$$

5.10.2 Positive Stable Frailty in Weibull Mixture

Assuming the distribution of Z as positive stable distribution and integrating over Z, in (5.9), we get Weibull mixture model with positive stable mixture frailty, given by

$$S_M(t) = pe^{-(\lambda_1 t^{c_1})^\alpha} + (1 - p)e^{-(\lambda_2 t^{c_2})^\alpha}.$$

The pdf corresponding to the above survival function is

$$f_M(t) = pe^{-(\lambda_1 t^{c_1})^\alpha} c_1 \alpha \lambda_1^\alpha t^{c_1 \alpha - 1} + (1 - p)e^{-(\lambda_2 t^{c_2})^\alpha} c_2 \alpha \lambda_2^\alpha t^{c_2 \alpha - 1}$$

which is again a mixture of two Weibull distributions. In this case, positive stable frailty model is stable with Weibull mixtures.

Assuming the distribution of Z as positive stable distribution and integrating over Z, in (5.10), we get Weibull mixture model with positive stable frailty, given by

$$S_F(t) = e^{-(-\ln[pe^{-\lambda_1 t^{c_1}} + (1-p)e^{-\lambda_2 t^{c_2}}])^\alpha}.$$

The pdf corresponding to the above survival function is

$$f_F(t) = S_F(t)\alpha(-\ln[pe^{-\lambda_1 t^{c_1}} + (1 - p)e^{-\lambda_2 t^{c_2}}])^{\alpha-1}$$
$$\times \left(\frac{p\lambda_1 c_1 t^{c_1-1}e^{-\lambda_1 t^{c_1}} + (1 - p)\lambda_2 c_2 t^{c_2-1}e^{-\lambda_2 t^{c_2}}}{[pe^{-\lambda_1 t^{c_1}} + (1 - p)e^{-\lambda_2 t^{c_2}}]} \right).$$

5.10.3 PVF Frailty in Weibull Mixture

Assuming the distribution of Z as PVF distribution and integrating over Z, in (5.9), we get Weibull mixture model with PVF mixture frailty, given by

$$S_M(t) = \mu \left[pe^{-\theta(1+\frac{\lambda_1 t^{c_1}}{\theta})^\alpha/\alpha} + (1 - p)e^{-\theta(1+\frac{\lambda_2 t^{c_2}}{\theta})^\alpha/\alpha} \right]$$

where $\mu = e^{\theta/\alpha}$.

The pdf corresponding to the above survival function is

$$f_M(t) = \mu pe^{-\theta(1+\frac{\lambda_1 t^{c_1}}{\theta})^\alpha/\alpha}(1 + \frac{\lambda_1 t^{c_1}}{\theta})^{\alpha-1}\lambda_1 c_1 t^{c_1-1}$$
$$+ \mu(1 - p)e^{-\theta(1+\frac{\lambda_2 t^{c_2}}{\theta})^\alpha/\alpha}(1 + \frac{\lambda_2 t^{c_2}}{\theta})^{\alpha-1}\lambda_2 c_2 t^{c_2-1}.$$

Assuming the distribution of Z as PVF distribution and integrating over Z, in (5.10), we get Weibull mixture model with PVF frailty, given by

$$S_F(t) = \mu \exp\left\{-\theta\left(1 - \frac{\log[pe^{-\lambda_1 t^{c_1}} + (1-p)e^{-\lambda_2 t^{c_2}}]}{\theta}\right)^\alpha / \alpha\right\}.$$

The pdf corresponding to the above survival function is

$$f_F(t) = S_F(t)\left(1 - \frac{\log[pe^{-\lambda_1 t^{c_1}} + (1-p)e^{-\lambda_2 t^{c_2}}]}{\theta}\right)^{\alpha-1}$$
$$\cdot\left(\frac{p\lambda_1 c_1 t^{c_1-1}e^{-\lambda_1 t^{c_1}} + (1-p)\lambda_2 c_2 t^{c_2-1}e^{-\lambda_2 t^{c_2}}}{[pe^{-\lambda_1 t^{c_1}} + (1-p)e^{-\lambda_2 t^{c_2}}]}\right).$$

5.11 Piecewise Gamma Frailty Model

Paik et al. (1994) worked on a generalization of a multivariate frailty model by introducing additional frailty terms for different time intervals. The joint survivor function of the piecewise gamma frailty model is

$$S(t_{i1}, t_{i2}, \ldots, t_{in})$$
$$= \int \cdots \int \prod_{j,k}\{Pr(T_{ij} > t_{ij}|Z_{ij1}, Z_{ij2}, \ldots, Z_{ijk})g(\alpha_i; \mu_1, \nu)d\alpha_i$$
$$\times\; g(\epsilon_{ijk}; \mu_2, \gamma_k)d\epsilon_{ijk}\}$$
$$= \left(\frac{1}{1+\nu A_i}\right)^{\mu_1/\nu} \prod_{j,k}\left(\frac{1}{1+\gamma_k H_{ijk}}\right)^{\mu_2/\gamma_k},$$

where
$H_{ijk} = -\ln S^*(e_{ijk})$ and $A_i = \sum_{j=1}^n \sum_{k=1}^K H_{ijk}$,
$Pr(T_{ij} > t_{ij}|Z_{ij1}, Z_{ij2}, \ldots, Z_{ijk}) = \prod_{k=1}^K \exp\{-Z_{ijk}e_{ijk}\exp(y_{ij}\beta + \phi_k)\}$,
$$e_{ijk} = \begin{cases} a_{k+1} - a_k & \text{if } t_{ij} \geq a_{k+1} \\ t_{ij} - a_k & \text{if } a_k \leq t_{ij} < a_{k+1} \\ 0 & \text{if } t_{ij} < a_k \end{cases}.$$
$0 = a_0 < a_1 < \cdots < a_K = \infty$, α_i and ϵ_{ijk} are independently distributed as gamma $g(\alpha_i; \mu_1, \nu)$ and $g(\epsilon_{ijk}; \mu_2, \gamma_k)$, and $\mu_1 + \mu_2 = 1$,
Z_{ijk} be the unobservable random effect of the jth member of the ith family for the kth time interval where $k = 1, \ldots, K$,
$h_{ijk}^* = \exp(y_{ij}\beta + \phi_k)$ and $S^*(e_{ijk}) = \exp(-e_{ijk}h_{ijk}^*)$ are the baseline hazard and survivor functions, respectively,
y_{ij} is a $1 \times p$ vector of independent variables,
β is a $p \times 1$ vector of unknown parameters of interest, and
$\exp(\phi_k)$ is the underlying hazard for the kth time interval.

The piecewise gamma frailty model includes other models as special cases. First notice that when $\mu_1 = 1$, parameters in the unknown vector γ are not defined. When

$\nu = 0$ and $\mu_1 = 1$, representing a degenerate distribution of α_i at $Z_{ijk} = 1$, the model reduces to the independent piecewise exponential model by Breslow (1974). When $\nu = 0$ and $0 < \mu_1 < 1$, the model is not piecewise exponential but still assumes independence. When $\mu_1 = 1$ and $\nu > 0$, representing a degenerate distribution of ϵ_{ijk}, the model reduces to the gamma frailty model (see Paik et al. 1994).

5.12 Frailty Models Based on Additive Hazard

The additive hazard model describes a different aspect of the association between covariates and the failure time than the proportional hazard model and is more plausible than the latter for many applications (Lin and Ying 1994, Bin 2010). One may use additive hazard model as an alternative to proportional hazards or other nonlinear hazards regression model analysis to describe the effects of covariates on survival time (Hosmer and Royston 2002). O'Neill (1986) shown that use of proportional hazards model can result in serious bias when the additive model is correct (Yin and Cai 2004). However, when the absolute change in risk, instead of the risk ratio, is of primary interest or when the proportional hazard assumption for Cox proportional hazards model is violated, an additive hazard regression model may be more appropriate (Xie et al. 2013).

Frailty models are extensively used in the survival analysis to account for the unobserved heterogeneity in individual risks to disease and death. To analyze the bivariate data on related survival times (e.g. matched pairs experiments, twin or family data), the shared frailty models were suggested. The frailty model is a random effect model for time-to-event data which is an extension of the Cox's proportional hazards model. Bivariate survival data arises whenever each study subjects experience two events. Particular examples include failure times of paired human organs, (e.g. kidneys, eyes, lungs, breasts, etc.) and the first and the second occurrences of a given disease. In the medical literature, several authors considered paired organs of an individual as a two-component system, which work under interdependency circumstances. In industrial applications, these data may come from systems whose survival depend on the survival of two similar components.

Research on the bivariate survival models has grown rapidly several years in the past. Clayton's (1978) random effect model of the bivariate survival was a key innovation. He introduced the notion of the shared relative risk. This model was further developed by Oakes (1982) to analyze the association between two nonnegative random variables. Clayton and Cuzick (1985) added observed covariates to the bivariate survival model with the shared relative risk. Crowder (1985) and Hougaard (1986b) proposed the random effect models of the bivariate Weibull distributions. A shared frailty model with a positive stable distribution of frailty was suggested by Hougaard (1987). He also discussed several other bivariate distributions with biomedical and reliability applications. Oakes (1989) developed a shared frailty model related to the "archimedean distributions" studied by Genest and Mackay (1986). He also proposed a local time-dependent association measure between bivariate life spans and discussed its use for a large class of bivariate survival functions. Vaupel (1991a, b), Vaupel et al. (1991, 1992a, b), Nielsen et al. (1992) studied genetic and environmental influences on longevity using bivariate survival models. Several models are based on the assumption that a common random effect model acts multiplicatively on the hazard rate function. Sometimes the more realistic assumption is that random effect model acts additively on hazard rate function.

Frailty models (Vaupel et al. 1979) are used in the survival analysis to account for the unobserved heterogeneity in the individual risks to disease and death. The frailty model is usually modeled as an unobserved random variable acting multiplicatively on the baseline hazard function. Let a continuous random variable T be a lifetime of an individual. Aalen (1980, 1989) proposed additive hazard model in which covariates acts additively on the baseline hazard and is given below:

$$h(t|\mathbf{X}) = h_0(t) + \mathbf{X}'\boldsymbol{\beta}$$

Another way of writing additive hazard model is given by

$$h(t|\mathbf{X}) = h_0(t) + e^{\mathbf{X}'\boldsymbol{\beta}}$$

where $h_0(t)$ is a baseline hazard function at time $t > 0$, $\mathbf{X}$ is a row vector of covariates, and $\boldsymbol{\beta}$ is a column vector of regression coefficients. Assuming that the frailties are acting additively on the baseline hazard for a given frailty variable $U = u$ at time $t > 0$ is

$$h(t|\mathbf{X}) = h_0(t) + e^{\mathbf{X}'\boldsymbol{\beta} + \mathbf{U}'\boldsymbol{\beta}_U}$$

which is written as

$$h(t \mid z) = h_0(t) + z e^{\mathbf{X}'\boldsymbol{\beta}}, \quad z > 0, \quad -\infty < U < \infty$$

where $z = e^{\mathbf{U}'\boldsymbol{\beta}_U}$. The cumulative hazard rate function is given by

$$H(t \mid z) = H_0(t) + z t e^{\mathbf{X}'\boldsymbol{\beta}}$$

where $H_0(t)$ is the cumulative baseline hazard function at time $t > 0$. The conditional survival function for given frailty at time $t > 0$ is,

$$S(t \mid z) = e^{-\left[H_0(t) + z t e^{\mathbf{X}'\boldsymbol{\beta}}\right]},$$

Integrating over the range of frailty variable Z having density $f(z)$, we get the marginal survival function as

$$S(t) = \int_0^\infty S(t \mid z) f(z) dz$$
$$= \int_0^\infty e^{-\left[H_0(t) + zt e^{X'\beta}\right]} f(z) dz$$
$$= e^{-H_0(t)} L_Z(t e^{X'\beta})$$
$$= S_0(t) L_z(t e^{X'\beta})$$

where $L_Z(.)$ is the Laplace transformation of the distribution of Z and $S_0(t)$ is the baseline survival function of T. Once we get the survival function at time $t > 0$, of lifetime random variable for an individual, we can obtain probability structure and make their inferences based on it.

Hanagal and Pandey (2016) developed the shared frailty model with the gamma distribution as a frailty distribution which is additive to baseline hazard of the generalized log logistic or the generalized Weibull distribution. Hanagal and Pandey (2017) proposed the shared gamma frailty in additive reversed hazard setup.

5.13 Generalized Exponential Frailty Model

Souza and Mayrink (2018) proposed generalized exponential frailty model to analyze kidney infection data. Let Z be a random variable having the generalized exponential (GE) distribution with the density function given by

$$f(z) = \gamma \alpha e^{-\gamma z}(1 - e^{-\gamma z})^{\alpha - 1}, \quad z > 0$$

The Laplace transform of Z if

$$L(s) = \frac{\Gamma(\alpha + 1)\Gamma(s/\gamma + 1)}{\Gamma(\alpha + s/\gamma + 1)}, \quad s > 0$$

The mean and variance of Z are given by

$$E(Z) = [\psi(\alpha + 1) - \psi(1)]/\gamma$$
$$V(Z) = [\psi'(1) - \psi'(\alpha + 1)]/\gamma^2$$

In order to solve non-identifiability problem, we restrict the mean of Z equal to 1 which results $\gamma = 1$. The unconditional survival function of the lifetime variable T is given by

$$S(t) = L_Z(H_0(t)) = \frac{\Gamma(\alpha + 1)\Gamma(H_0(t) + 1)}{\Gamma(\alpha + H_0(t) + 1)}$$

where $H_0(t)$ is the cumulation hazard function of the lifetime T.

5.14 Generalized Gamma Frailty Model

Stacy (1962) introduced generalized gamma distribution (GGD). Later Balakrishnan and Peng (2006) considered this generalized gamma distribution as frailty distribution to analyze coronary heart disease data. The density function of generalized gamma distribution is given by

$$f(z) = \begin{cases} |q|(q^{-2})^{q^{-2}}(\lambda z)^{q^{-2}q/\sigma} \exp[-q^{-2}(\lambda z)^{q/\sigma}]/[\Gamma(q^{-2})\sigma z] \; ; \; q \neq 0 \\ (\sqrt{2\pi}\sigma z)^{-1} \exp[-\{\log(\lambda z)\}^{-2}/(2\sigma^2)] \qquad\qquad ; \; q \neq 0. \end{cases}$$

where $-\infty < q < \infty$ and $\sigma > 0$ are shape parameters and $\lambda > 0$ is a scale parameter. There are many distributions which are special cases of this GGD. For example,

- for $q = 1$, it reduces to Weibull distribution
- for $q = 0$, it reduces to log-normal distribution
- for $q/\sigma = 1$, it reduces to gamma distribution
- for $q^{-2} = 1/2$ and $\sigma/q = -1$, it reduces to positive stable distribution with index 1/2.

The mean of the frailty distribution is

$$E(Z) = \frac{\Gamma(q^{-2}+\sigma/q)}{\Gamma(q^{-2})(q^{-2})^{\sigma/q}\lambda}, \quad q > -1/\sigma.$$

In order to solve the non-identifiability problem, we must have the restriction, $E(Z) = 1$. Under this restriction, we have

$$\lambda = \frac{\Gamma(q^{-2} + \sigma/q)}{\Gamma(q^{-2})(q^{-2})^{\sigma/q}}.$$

Now the density of the frailty distribution can be obtained after substituting the value of λ given above. The variance of the frailty distribution is given by

$$V(Z) = \frac{\Gamma(q^{-2} + 2\sigma/q)\Gamma(q^{-2})}{\Gamma^2(q^{-2} + \sigma/q)}.$$

5.15 Birnbaum–Saunders Frailty Model

The Birnbaum–Saundars (BS) distribution was originally derived as a fatigue model by Birbaum and Saunders (1969). The distribution function of Birnbaum–Saundars (BS) distribution is given by

$$F(z; \alpha, \beta) = \Phi\left[\frac{1}{\alpha}\left\{(\frac{z}{\beta})^{1/2} - (\frac{\beta}{z})^{1/2}\right\}\right], \quad z > 0, \alpha, \beta > 0,$$

where Φ is the standard normal cumulative distribution function, and α and β are the shape and scale parameters, respectively. Balakrishnan and Liu (2018) assume that the frailty random variable Z follows the BS distribution. The density function BS distribution is given by

$$f(z; \alpha, \beta) = \frac{1}{2\sqrt{2\pi}\alpha\beta} \left[(\frac{\beta}{z})^{1/2} + (\frac{\beta}{z})^{3/2} \right]$$

$$\times \exp\left[-\frac{1}{2\alpha^2} \left(\frac{z}{\beta} + \frac{\beta}{z} - 2 \right) \right], \quad z > 0.$$

The mean and variance of Z are

$$E(Z) = \beta(1 + \alpha^2/2)$$
$$V(Z) = (\alpha\beta)^2(1 + 5\alpha^2/4).$$

In order to solve non-identifiability problem in the frailty model, we set the mean of Z equal to one which results

$$\beta = 2/(2 + \alpha^2).$$

Under this restriction one can obtain the distribution function and density function of one parameter BS distribution with parameter α. The variance of Z now reduces to

$$V(Z) = \frac{4\alpha^2 + 5\alpha^4}{\alpha^4 + 4\alpha^2 + 4}.$$

5.16 Frailty Models Based on Lévy Processes

In this section, we consider Lévy process as a frailty distribution. The Lévy process is taken to mean a process with nonnegative, independent, time-homogeneous increments, i.e., a subordinator. The Laplace transform of Lévy process $Z=\{Z(t) : t \geq 0\}$ at time t is given by Lévy–Khinchin formula as below

$$L(s, t) = E \exp\{-sZ(t)\} = \exp\{-t\Phi(s)\} \qquad (5.11)$$

where $s \geq 0$ is the argument of the Laplace transform. The function $\Phi(s)$ is called the Laplace exponent of the Lévy process. The compound Poisson processes, gamma processes, stable processes, etc. are special cases of family of Lévy processes. All nonnegative Lévy processes are limits of compound Poisson processes. For for details on Lévy processes, see Bertoin (1996).

Let $Z(t)$ be the subordinator, and consider processes with a varying 'rate', define the nonnegative deterministic rate function $r(t)$ with integral $R(t) = \int_0^t r(u)du$. Let $Z(R(t))$ be the time-transformed subordinator. Conditional on Z, we define basic failure rate processes $\lambda(t)$ as

$$\lambda(t) = h(t) \int_0^t a(u, t - u) dZ(R(u)).$$

This process will be starting point for all models considered in this section. The function $a(u, s)$ is a weight function determining the extent to which the effect of previous jumps in $Z(t)$ influence the failure rate at time t. The two arguments in $a(u, s)$ depend on two time scales, (i) the timescale of the stochastic process (first argument), and (ii) the time as in distance from the current time (second argument). The deterministic function h determines the 'base' level of the failure rate, and it is absorbed in a. Since most frailty distributions of the classical frailty models are distributions of Lévy processes, the general formulation here incorporates most of these classical models. Notice that, as in the standard frailty model, each individual in the population will have its own realization of the underlying process Z and thus of the hazard process λ. Some models of frailty using Lévy processes are discussed in Singpurwalla (1995), Aalen and Hjort (2002) and Hjort (2003). Gjessing et al. (2003) extend the results of Kebir (1991).

Lévy Processes and Subordinators

The distribution of a Lévy process, i.e. a subordinator Z, is determined by its Laplace exponent Φ, defined in (5.11). Hence, many general results on subordinates are derived in terms of Φ. The function $\Phi(\cdot)$ is increasing and concave, its derivative Φ' decreasing. We have the general representation

$$\Phi(s) = ds + \int_0^\infty (1 - e^{-sx}) \pi(dx),$$

where d is called the drift coefficient. At time t, the distribution of $Z(t)$ is shifted to the right by an amount td. The measure $\pi(dx)$ has support on $(0, \infty)$ and satisfies the condition $\int_0^\infty (1 \wedge x)\pi(dx) < \infty$. It is called the Lévy measure of the process Z. When $\int_0^\infty \pi(dx) = \rho < \infty$, i.e. when $(\frac{1}{\rho})\pi$ is a probability measure on $(0, \infty)$, we can write

$$\Phi(s) = ds + \rho(1 - L_0(s)),$$

where $L_0(s)$ is the Laplace transform of $(1/\rho)\pi$. For the derivatives we have

$$\Phi'(s) = d + \int_0^\infty x e^{-sx} \pi(dx),$$

$$\Phi''(s) = -\int_0^\infty x^2 e^{-sx} \pi(dx),$$

which both exist for $s > 0$. Clearly, $\lim_{s \to \infty} \Phi'(s) = d$. When $s = 0$, we obtain the relationships

$$EZ(t) = \Phi'(0)t = (d + \int_0^\infty x\pi(dx))t,$$

$$VarZ(t) = -\Phi''(0)t = \int_0^\infty x^2\pi(dx)t,$$

which in some cases will be infinite.

References

Aaberge, R., Kravdel, O., Wennemo, T.: Unobserved heterogeneity in models of marriage dissolution. Disscussion Paper 42, Cental Bureau of Statistics, Norway (1989)

Aalen, O.O.: A model for non-parametric regression analysis of counting processes. Lect. Notes Stat. **2**, 1–25 (1980)

Aalen, O.O.: Heterogeneity in survival analysis. Stat. Med. **7**, 1121–1137 (1988)

Aalen, O.O.: A linear regression model for the analysis of lifetimes. Stat. Med. **8**(8), 907–925 (1989)

Aalen, O.O.: Modelling heterogeneity in survival analysis by the compound Poisson distribution. Ann. Appl. Prob. **2**, 951–972 (1992)

Aalen, O.O., Hjort, N.L.: Frailty models that yield proportional hazards. Stat. Prob. Lett. **58**, 335–342 (2002)

Aalen, O.O., Hjort, N.L.: Frailty models that yield proportional hazards. Stat. Probab. Lett. **58**, 335–342 (2002)

Aalen, O.O., Tretli, S.: Analyzing incidence of tests cancer by means of a frailty model. Cancer Causes Control **10**, 285–292 (1999)

Balakrishnan, N., Liu, K.: Semi-parametric likelihood inference for Birnbaum-Saunders frailty model. REVSTAT **16**(2), 231–255 (2018)

Balakrishnan, N., Peng, Y.: Generalized gamma frailty model. Stat. Med. **25**, 2797–2816 (2006)

Barndorff-Nielsen, O.E.: A note on electrical networks. Adv. Appl. Probab. **26**, 63–67 (1994)

Bertoin, J.: Levy Processes. Cambridge University Press, Cambridge (1996)

Bin, H.: Additive hazards model with time-varying regression coefficients. Acta Math. Sci. **30B**(4), 1318–1326 (2010)

Birbaum, Z.W., Saunders, S.C.: A new family of life distributions. J. Appl. Probab. **55**(2), 319–327 (1969)

Breslow, N.E.: Covariate analysis of censored survival data. Biometrics **30**, 89–100 (1974)

Breslow, N.E., Clayton, D.G.: Approximate inference in generalized linear models. J. Am. Stat. Assoc. **88**, 9–23 (1993)

Callegaro, A., Lacobelli, S.: The cox shared frailty model with log-skew-normal frailties. Stat. Model. **12**(5), 399–418 (2012)

Chen, P., Zhang, J., Zhang, R.: Estimation of the accelerated failure time frailty model under generalized gamma frailty. Comput. Stat. Data Anal. **62**, 171–180 (2013)

Chhikara, R.S., Folks, J.L.: The inverse gaussian distribution. Marcel Dekker, New York (1996)

Clayton, D.G., Cuzick, J.: Multivariate generalizations of the proportional hazard model (with discussion). J. R. Stat. Soc., A **148**, 82–117 (1985)

Clayton, D.G.: A model for association in bivariate life tables and its application in epidemiological studies of familial tendency in chronic disease incidence. Biometrika **65**, 141–151 (1978)

Cosco, T.D., Armstrong, J.J., Stephan, B.C.M., Brayne, C.B.: Sucussful aging and frailty: mutually exclusive paradgms or two ends of a shared continuum? Can. Gariatrics J. **18**(1), 35–36 (2015)

Crowder, M.: A distributional model for repeated failure time measurements. R. Stat. Soc., B **47**, 447–452 (1985)

Duchateau, L., Janssen, P.: The Frailty Model. Springer, New York (2008)

Enky, D.G., Noufaily, A., Farrington, P.: A time-varying shared frailty model with application to infectious diseases. Ann. Appl. Stat. **8**(1), 3430–3447 (2014)

Fan, J.J., Hsu, L., Prentice, R.L.: Dependence estimation over a finite bivariate failure region. Lifetime Data Anal. **6**, 343–355 (2000)

Farrington, C.P., Unkel, S., Izquierdo, K.A.: The relative frailty variance and shared frailty models. J. R. Stat. Soc. (Ser. B) **74**(4), 673–696 (2012)

Fine, J.P., Glidden, D.V., Lee, K.E.: A simple estimator for a shared frailty regression model. J. R. Stat. Soc. B **65**, 317–329 (2003)

Gacula, M.C., Kubala, J.J.: Statistical models for shelf life failures. Jr. Food Sci **40**, 404–409 (1975)

Genest, C., Mackay, R.J.: The joy of copulas: bivariate distributions with given marginals. Am. Stat. **40**, 280–283 (1986)

Gjessing, H.K., Aalen, O.O., Hjort, N.L.: Frailty models based on Levy processes. Adv. Appl. Probab. **35**, 532–550 (2003)

Glidden, D.V.: Checking the adequacy of the gamma frailty model for multivariate failure times. Biometrika **86**, 381–394 (1999)

Govindarajulu, U.S., Lin, H., Lunetta, K.L., D'Agostino, R.B.: Frailty models: applications to biomedical and gentic studies. Stat. Med. **30**(22), 2754–2764 (2011)

Green, P.J., Silverman, B.W.: Nonparametric Regression and Generalized Linear Models. A Roughness Penalty Approach. Chapman & Hall, London (1994)

Hanagal, D.D., Bhambure, S.M.: Modeling Australian twin data using shared positive stable frailty models based on reversed hazard rate. Commun. Stat., Theory Methods **46**(8), 3754–3771 (2017)

Hanagal, D.D., Kamble, A.T.: Bayesian estimation in shared compound negative binomial frailty models. Res. Rev.: J. Stat. Math. Sci. **2**(1), 53–67 (2016)

Hanagal, D.D., Pandey, A.: Shared inverse gaussian frailty models based on additive hazards. Commun. Stat., Theory Methods **46**(22), 11143–11162 (2017)

Hanagal, D.D.: Positive stable frailty regression models in mixture distributions. In: Proceedings of 3rd International Conference on Reliability and Safety Engineering, December 17–19: held at Indian Institute of Technology, pp. 350–356. Udaipur, India (2007a)

Hanagal, D.D.: Gamma frailty regression models in mixture distributions. Econ. Qual. Control. **22**(2), 295–302 (2007b)

Hanagal, D.D.: A power variance function frailty regression model in bivariate survival data. IAPQR Trans. **32**(2), 117–129 (2007c)

Hanagal, D.D.: Frailty regression models in mixture distributions. J. Stat. Plan. Inference **138**(8), 2462–2468 (2008)

Hanagal, D.D.: Modeling heterogeneity for bivariate survival data by power variance function distribution. J. Reliab. Stat. Stud. **2**, 14–27 (2009)

Hanagal, D.D.: Correlated compound Poisoon frailty model for the bivariate survival data. Int. J. Stat. Manag. Syst. **5**, 127–140 (2010a)

Hanagal, D.D.: Modeling heterogeneity for bivariate survival data by compound Poisson distribution. Model. Assist. Stat. Appl. **5**(1), 01–09 (2010b)

Hanagal, D.D.: Modeling heterogeneity for bivariate survival data by Weibull distribution. Stat. Pap. **51**(4), 947–958 (2010c)

Hanagal, D.D.: Modeling heterogeneity for bivariate survival data by the compound Poisson distribution with random scale. Stat. Probab. Lett. **80**, 1781–1790 (2010d)

Hanagal, D.D., Bhambure, S.M.: Analysis of kidney infection data using positive stable frailty models. Adv. Reliab. **1**, 21–39 (2014)

Hanagal, D.D., Dabade, A.D.: Modeling Hetrogeneity in bivariate survival data by compound Poisson distribution using Bayesian approach. Int. J. Stat. Manag. Syst. **7**(1–2), 36–84 (2012)

Hanagal, D.D., Dabade, A.D.: Compound negative binomial shared frailty models for bivariate survival data. Stat. Probab. Lett. **83**, 2507–2515 (2013)

Hanagal, D.D., Kamble, A.T.: Bayesian estimation in shared positive stable frailty models. J. Data Sci. **13**, 615–640 (2014)

Hanagal, D.D., Kamble, A.T.: Bayesian estimation in shared compound Poisson frailty models. J. Reliab. Stat. Stud. **8**(1), 159–180 (2015)

Hanagal, D.D., Pandey, A.: Shared gamma frailty models based on additive hazards. J. Indian Soc. Probab. Stat. **17**(2), 161–184 (2016)

Harville, D.A.: Maximum likelihood approaches to variance component estimation and related problems. J. Am. Stat. Assoc. **72**, 320–340 (1977)

Hastie, T., Tibshirani, R.: Generalized additive models. Stat. Sci. **1**, 297–318 (1986)

Henderson, C.R.: Best linear unbiased estimation and prediction under a selection model. Biometrics **31**, 423–447 (1975)

Hijort, N.L.: Topic in non-parametric bayesian studies (with discussion): Highly structured stochastic systems. In: Green, E.J., Hijort, N.L., Richardson, S. (eds.), Oxford University Press, London (2006)

Hosmer, D.W., Royston, P.: Using Aalen's linear hazards model to investigate time-varying effects in the proportional hazards regression model. Strat. J. **2**(4), 331–350 (2002)

Hougaard, P.: Life table methods for heterogeneous populations: distributions describing heterogeneity. Biometrika **71**, 75–83 (1984)

Hougaard, P.: A class of multivariate failure time distributions. Biometrika **73**, 671–678 (1986a)

Hougaard, P.: Survival models for hetrogeneous populations derived from stable distributions. Biometrika **73**, 387–396 (1986b)

Hougaard, P.: Modeling multivariate survival. Scand. J. Stat. **14**, 291–304 (1987)

Hougaard, P.: Analysis of Multivariate Survival Data. Springer, New York (2000)

Kau, J.B., Keenan, D.C., Li, X.: An analysis of mortgage termination risks: a shared frailty approach with MSA level random effects. J. R. Estate Financ. Econ. **42**(1), 51–67 (2011)

Kebir, Y.: On hazard rate processes. Nav. Res. Logist. **38**, 865–876 (1991)

Lee, Y., Nelder, J.A.: Hierarchical generalized linear models. J. R. Stat. Soc., B **58**, 619–678 (1996)

Liang, K.Y.: Estimating effects of probands characteristic in familial risk: 1. Adjustments for censoring and correlated ages at onset. Genet. Epidemiol. **8**, 329–338 (1991)

Lin, D.Y., Ying, Z.: Semiparametric analysis of the additive risk model. Biometrika **81**(1), 61–71 (1994)

Marshall, A.W., Olkin, I.: A Multivariate Exponential Distribution. J. Am. Stat. Assoc. **62**, 30–44 (1967)

Mauguen, A., Rachet, B., Pelissier, S.M., MacGrogan, G., Laurent, A., Laurent, A., Rondeau, V.: Dyanamic prediction of risk of death using history of cancer recurrences in joint frailty models. Stat. Med **32**(30), 5366–5380 (2013)

Mazroui, Y., Pelissier, S.M., MacGrogan, G., Brouste, V., Rondeau, V.: Multivariate frailty models for two types of recurrent events with a dependent terminal event: application to breast cancer data. Biom. J. **55**(6), 866–884 (2013)

McGilchrist, C.A.: Estimation in genralized mixed models. J. R. Stat. Soc., B **56**, 61–69 (1994)

McGilchrist, C.A.: REML estimation for survival models with frailty. Biometrics **49**, 221–225 (1993)

McGilchrist, C.A., Aisbett, C.W.: Regression with frailty in survival analysis. Biometrics **47**, 461–466 (1991)

Moger, T.A., Aalen, O.O.: A distribution for multivariate frailty based on the compound Poisson distribution with random scale. Lifetime Data Anal. **11**, 41–59 (2005)

Molenberghs, G., Verbeke, G.: On Weibull-Gamma frailty model, its infinite moments, and its connection to generalized log-logistic, logistic, Cauchy, and extreme value distributions. Jr. Stat Plann inference **141**(2), 861–868 (2011)

Nelsen, R.B.: An introduction to copulas, 2nd edn. Springer, New York (2006)

Oakes, D.: A model for association in bivariate survival data. J. R. Stat. Soc., B **44**, 414–493 (1982)

Oakes, D.: Bivariate survival models induced by frailties. J. Am. Stat. Assoc. **84**, 487–493 (1989)

O'Neill, T.J.: Inconsistency of misspecified proportional hazardsmodel. Stat. Prob. Lett. **4**, 219–222 (1986)

Paik, M., Tsai, W., Ottman, R.: Multivariate survival analysis using piecewise gamma frailty. Biometrics **50**, 975–988 (1994)

Preter, H.D., Looy, D.V., Mortelmans, D.: Retirement timing of dual earner couples in 11 European countries? a comparison of Cox and shared frailty models. J. Fam. Econ. Issues **36**(3), 396–407 (2015)

Robinson, G.K.: That BLUP is a good thing: the estimation of random effects. Stat. Sci. **6**, 15–51 (1991)

Schall, R.: Estimation in generalized linear models with random effects. Biometrika **78**, 719–727 (1991)

Seshadri, V.: The inverse gaussian distribution: Statistical theory and applications. Springer Science, New York (1999)

Shih, J.H.: A goodness-of-fit test for association in a bivariate survival model. Biometrika **85**, 189–200 (1998)

Singpurwalla, N.D.: Survival in dynamic environments. Stat. Sci. **10**, 86–103 (1995)

Souza, W.B., Mayrink, V.D.: Semiparametric generalized exponential frailty model for clustered survival data. Ann. Inst. Stat. Math. **71**(3), 679–701 (2018)

Unkel, S., Farrington, C.P., Whitaker, H.J., Pebody, R.: Time varying frailty models and the estimation of heterogeneities in transmission of infectious diseases. J. R. Stat. Soc. (Ser. C) **63**(1), 141–158 (2013)

Unkel, S., Farrington, C.P.: A new measure of time-varying association for shared frailty models with bivariate current status data. Biostatistics **13**(4), 665–679 (2012)

Vaupel, J.W., Yashin, A.I., Hauge, M., Harvald, B., Holm, N.Y., Liang, X.: Strategies of Modelling Genetics in Survival Analysis: What Can We Learn from Twin Data? Paper Presented at PAA Meeting, April 30- May 2, Denver (1992b)

Vaupel, J.W., Yashin, A.I., Hauge, M., Harvald, B., Holm, N.Y., Liang, X.: Survival Analysis in Genetics: Danish Twins Data Applied to Gerontological Question. Klein, J.P., Goel, P.K. (eds.), Survival Analysis: State of Art, 3rd edn., pp. 121–138. Kluwer Academic Publisher, Dordrecht (1991)

Vaupel, J.W., Yashin, A.I., Hauge, M., Harvald, B., Holm, N.Y., Xue, L.: Survival Analysis in Genetics: Danish Twins Data Applied to Gerontological Question. Klein, J.P., Goel, P.K. (eds.), Survival Analysis: State of Art. Kluwer, Dordrecht (1992a)

Vaupel, J.W.: Relatives risks: frailty models of life history data. Theor. Popul. Biol. **37**(1), 220–234 (1991a)

Vaupel, J.W.: Kindred lifetimes: Frailty models in population gentics. In: Adem, J., Lam, D.A., Hermalin, A.I., Smouse, P.E. (eds.) Convergent Questions in Genetics and Demography, 3rd edn. Oxford University Press, Oxford (1991b)

Vaupel, J.W., Manton, K.G., Stallard, E.: The impact of heterogeneity on individual frailty on the dynamic of mortality. Demography **16**(3), 439–454 (1979)

Vilmann, H., Kirkeby, S., Kronborg, D.: Histomorphometrical analysis of the influence of soft diet on masticatory muscle development in the muscular dystrophic mouse. Arch. Oral Biol. **35**(1), 37–42 (1990)

Xie, X., Strickler, H.D., Xue, X.: Additive hazard regression models: an application to the natural history of human papillomavirus. Comput. Math. Methods Med. **2013**, 1–7 (2013)

Xu, L., Zhang, J.: An EM-like algorithm for the semiparametric accelerated failure time gamma frailty model. Comput. Stat. Data Anal. **54**(6), 1467–1474 (2010)

Yin, G., Cai, J.: Additive hazards model with multivariate failure time data. Biometrika **91**(4), 801–818 (2004)

Chapter 6
Estimation Methods for Shared Frailty Models

6.1 Introduction

In this chapter, we discuss the different methods of estimation for shared frailty models which are used more often and they have a lot of applications. Hanagal (2005b, 2006a, b, c, d) has obtained an estimation of the parameters and test for regression coefficients under different bivariate Weibull baseline with gamma frailty model. Hanagal (2005a, 2006c) has proposed an estimation of the parameters, test for frailty and test for regression coefficients under different bivariate Weibull with positive stable frailty model. Hanagal (2007c, 2009b) has developed the estimation of the parameters, test for frailty and test for regression coefficients under the bivariate Weibull baseline with the PVF frailty model. Hanagal (2007a, b, 2008a) discussed shared frailty models with mixture distributions. Hanagal (2008b, 2010b) has obtained the estimation of the parameters, test for frailty and test for regression coefficients under the bivariate Weibull baseline with lognormal and Weibull frailty models. Hanagal (2010a) has obtained the estimation of the parameters and test for regression coefficients under the bivariate Weibull baseline with compound Poisson frailty model. Hanagal (2010c) has obtained the estimation of the parameters and test for regression coefficients under bivariate Weibull baseline using compound Poisson frailty with a random scale model. Hanagal (2009a) has presented different frailty models under different bivariate Weibull baseline models.

Androulakis et al. (2012) applied penalized likelihood approach to a general likelihood function for data organized in clusters, which corresponds to a class of frailty models, which includes the Cox model and the gamma frailty model as special cases. In the penalized likelihood, they employ Breslow's estimate for the cumulative hazard function and analyzed the non-Hodgkins lymphoma (NHL) data organized in clusters. Ha et al. (2014) proposed a unified procedure via a penalized h-likelihood (HL) for variable selection of fixed effects in a general class of sub-distribution hazard frailty models, in which random effects may be shared or correlated. Mauguen et al. (2013a, b) proposed two different discrimination measures to take into account

© Springer Nature Singapore Pte Ltd. 2019   123
D. D. Hanagal, *Modeling Survival Data Using Frailty Models*,
Industrial and Applied Mathematics, https://doi.org/10.1007/978-981-15-1181-3_6

cluster membership. They calculated measures at three levels: between groups, within groups, and overall. Rondeau et al. (2011) compared several forms of cure rate frailty models to model correlated failure time models. They illustrated cure rate frailty models with breast cancer data and colorectal cancer data using maximum likelihood estimates. Ha et al. (2013) considered three penalty functions (least absolute shrinkage and selection operator (LASSO), smoothly clipped absolute deviation (SCAD), and h-likelihood) in their variable selection procedure. They implemented the proposed method with a slight modification to existing h-likelihood estimation approaches. Berg and Drepper (2016) developed inference for shared frailty survival models with left-truncated data. Halstead et al. (2011) proposed Bayesian analysis of shared frailty models to examine the survival of adult females of the giant gerter snake in the Sacramento Valley, California, USA, and also examine the effects of individual and habitat characteristics on daily risk of mortality. Souza and Mayrink (2018) proposed frailty model for clustered survival data by assuming a generalized exponential (GE) distribution for the latent frailty effect. They proposed EM-based algorithm for the GE frailty model.

6.2 Inference for the Shared Frailty Model

The conditional joint survival distribution of failure times $T_1, T_2, \ldots, T_n$ given the frailty z is given by

$$P(T_1 > t_1, \ldots, T_n > t_n | z) = P(T_1 > t_1 | z) p(T_2 > t_2 | z) \cdots P(T_n > t_n | z)$$

$$= \exp\left\{-z \sum_{j=1}^{n} H_0(t_j) \exp(\beta Y_j)\right\}. \tag{6.1}$$

Integrating out the frailty variable, we get unconditional joint survival function as given below.

$$S(t_1, \ldots, t_n) = P(T_1 > t_1, \ldots, T_n > t_n)$$

$$= \int_0^\infty P(T_1 > t_1, \ldots, T_n > t_n | z) f(z) dz$$

$$= \int_0^\infty \exp\left\{-z \sum_{j=1}^{n} H_0(t_j) \exp(\beta Y_j)\right\} f(z) dz$$

$$= L\left[\sum_{j=1}^{n} H_0(t_j) \exp(\beta Y_j)\right], \tag{6.2}$$

where L is the Laplace transform of the Z and $H_0(t) = \int_0^t h_0(z) dz$.

Assume that the frailty distribution follows any one of the three distributions, namely gamma, the lognormal, and the positive stable distributions. For other distributions, see Hougaard (2000) and Ohman and Eberly (2001).

From (6.2), one can derive the likelihood function for one group as follows: if the failure time is observed for the jth individual at time t_j, its probability is given by $P(T_j = t_j, T_1 > t_1, \ T_2 > t_2, \ldots)$

$$= -\frac{\partial S(t_1, \ldots, t_n)}{\partial t_j}$$

$$= -h_0(t_j) \exp(\beta Y_j) L^{(1)} \left(\sum_{j=1}^{n} H_0(t_j) \exp(\beta Y_j) \right), \tag{6.3}$$

where $L^{(1)}(s)$ is the first derivative of $L(s)$ with respect to s. Let $D. = \sum \delta_j$ be the total number of failures in the group and θ be the parameter of the frailty distribution. Then, using Eq. (6.3), the likelihood for one group is given by

$$(-1)^{D.} \left\{ \prod_{j=1}^{n} h_0(t_j)^{\delta_j} \exp(\delta_j \beta Y_j) \right\} L^{(D.)} \left(\sum_{j=1}^{n} H_0(t_j) \exp(\beta Y_j) \right). \tag{6.4}$$

The likelihood function for all individuals is obtained by multiplying the group likelihoods together. Specifically, if D_i denotes the number of failures in the ith group, and $D = \sum_{i=1}^{G} D_i$, then the likelihood function is given by

$$(-1)^{D} \prod_{i=1}^{G} \left\{ \prod_{j=1}^{n_i} h_0(t_{ij})^{\delta_{ij}} \exp(\delta_{ij} \beta Y_{ij}) \right\} L^{(D_i)} \left(\sum_{j=1}^{n_i} H_0(t_{ij}) \exp(\beta Y_{ij}) \right). \tag{6.5}$$

Assuming a parametric form for h_0, one can estimate the parameters by differentiating the loglikelihood function. If a parametric from is not assumed for h_0, there are many estimation methods available in the semiparametric model. These methods are described below.

In the likelihood function (6.5), insert the nonparametric expressions for $H_0(t)$, $H_0(t) = \sum_{t_k \leq t} h_{0k}$, assuming a discrete contribution h_{0k} at each time of failure. Here, t_k is the kth smallest failure time, regardless of the subgroup, M is the number of distinct failures, and d_k is the number of failures at t_k, $k = 1, \ldots, M$. Thus, one can get the function with parameters $\beta, \theta, h_{01}, \ldots, h_{0M}$. Then follow the usual method for estimation: differentiate the loglikelihood with respect to all parameters and use the Newton–Raphson method to obtain estimates. This method takes much more iterations for convergence than other methods, so it is not preferable when we deal with a frailty distribution. However, for the data set with complicated dependence structures, one may end up with the likelihood function which cannot be handled by simpler methods. In this case, the full conditional approach may be the only resolution.

6.3   The EM Algorithm

The EM algorithm, which is a simpler method, can also be used for estimation since we can treat the frailty as covariates. Klein (1992) developed the estimation based on the EM algorithm for the gamma frailty. A similar method was developed by Wang et al. (1995) for the positive stable frailty. Shu and Klein (1999) also offered SAS macros for the gamma and the positive stable frailty models on the Internet. In the E-step of the algorithm, the expected value of L_{full} is computed given the current estimates of the parameters and the observable data. In the M-step, plug estimates of frailties into the modified partial likelihood, update the estimates of β and h_0; plug into L_{full}, update the estimate θ. In the M-step, estimates of parameters which maximize the expected value of L_{full} from the E-step are obtained. Now define the full likelihood as the product of the conditional and the density of frailties.

$$L_{full} = \prod_{i=1}^{G} \prod_{j=1}^{n_i} (z_i)^{\delta_{ij}} h_0(t_{ij})^{\delta_{ij}} \exp(\delta_{ij}\beta Y_{ij}) \exp\{-z_i H_0(t_{ij}) \exp(\beta Y_{ij})\} f(z_i).$$

(6.6)

More specifically, the steps of the EM algorithm are as follows:

(1) Provide initial values of β, h_0, and θ.
(2) In the E-step, plug values of β, h_0, and θ into the full likelihood (6.6) and calculate the conditional expectation of z_i and $\ln(z_i)$ given the observable data. Parner (1997) suggested a general formula for the expectation of frailties,

$$E(z_i) = -\frac{L^{(D_i+1)}[\sum_j \hat{H}_0(t_{ij}) \exp(\hat{\beta}Y_{ij})]}{L^{(D_i)}[\sum_j \hat{H}_0(t_{ij}) \exp(\hat{\beta}Y_{ij})]}, \quad i = 1, \ldots, G.$$

(6.7)

In this step, the unobserved terms in the loglikelihood are removed by substitution with the mean value given the observations.
(3) In the M-step, plug the expectation of frailties into the modified partial likelihood, update the estimates of β and h_0; plug into Eq. (6.6), update the estimate of θ. In this case, the partial likelihood turns out to be

$$L(\beta) = \prod_{k=1}^{M} \frac{\exp(\hat{z}_k(\beta s_k))}{[\sum_{l \in R(t_k)} \hat{z}_l \exp(\beta Y_l)]^{d_k}},$$

(6.8)

where t_k is the kth smallest failure time, regardless of subgroup, d_k is the number of failures at t_k, D_k is the set of all individuals who fail at time t_k, and $s_k = \sum\limits_{j \in D_k} Y_j$.

Furthermore, the maximum likelihood estimate of h_{0_k} is

$$\hat{h}_{0_k} = \frac{d_k}{\sum\limits_{l \in R(t_k)} \hat{z}_l \exp(\hat{\beta} Y_l)}, \quad k = 1, \ldots, M. \tag{6.9}$$

Here, the frailty values are considered fixed and known.
(4) Repeat the E-step and M-step until the estimates converge.

The standard errors of the estimates of h_0, β, and θ can be obtained from the inverse of the observed information matrix.

6.4 The Gamma Frailty Model

The density function of the frailty is

$$f(z) = \frac{z^{1/\theta-1} \exp(-z/\theta)}{\Gamma(1/\theta)\theta^{1/\theta}} \tag{6.10}$$

with the Laplace transform $L(s) = (1 + \theta s)^{-1/\theta}$. Thus the mean of the frailty is 1, which is the desired property of the frailty distribution; the variance is θ, which reflects the degree of dependence in the data. Large θ indicates strong dependence. From Eq. (6.2), it is easily seen that the marginal hazard is

$$\frac{h_0(t_j) \exp(\beta Y)}{1 + \theta H_0(t_j) \exp(\beta Y)}. \tag{6.11}$$

For two randomly selected individuals with covariate values Y and Y^*, the marginal hazards are not proportional over time and the relative risk is given by

$$\exp(\beta(Y - Y^*)) \frac{1 + \theta H_0(t) \exp(\beta Y^*)}{1 + \theta H_0(t) \exp(\beta Y)}, \tag{6.12}$$

which depends on time through $H_0(t)$. From Eq. (6.12), it is clear that the relative risk starts at $\exp(\beta(Y - Y^*))$ because no failure occurs, and converges to 1 as $t \to \infty$ since $H_0(t) \to \infty$ in this case. If we are interested in the relative risk at a given time t, we can calculate it by replacing θ, β, and $H_0(t)$ with their estimates in Eq. (6.12).

The pth derivative of the Laplace transform is

$$L^{(p)}(s) = (-1)^p \theta^p (1 + \theta s)^{-1/\theta - p} \Gamma\left(\frac{1}{\theta} + p\right) / \Gamma\left(\frac{1}{\theta}\right).$$

Following Eq. (6.5), the likelihood for all individuals is given by

$$(-1)^D \prod_{i=1}^{G} \frac{\theta^{D_i} \Gamma(1/\theta + D_i)}{\Gamma(1/\theta)} \left\{ \prod_{j=1}^{n_i} h_0(t_{ij})^{\delta_{ij}} \exp(\delta_{ij} \beta Y_{ij}) \right\}$$

$$\times \left\{ 1 + \theta \sum_{j=1}^{n_i} H_0(t_{ij}) \exp(\beta Y_{ij}) \right\}^{-1/\theta - D_i}.$$

From the EM algorithm, the full likelihood is

$$\prod_{i=1}^{G} \prod_{j=1}^{n_i} h_o(t_{ij})^{\delta_{ij}} \exp(\delta_{ij} \beta Y_{ij}) \exp\{-z_i H_0(t_{ij}) \exp(\beta Y_{ij})\}$$

$$\times \prod_{i=1}^{G} \frac{z_i^{1/\theta + D_i - 1} \exp(-z_i/\theta)}{\Gamma(1/\theta)\theta^{1/\theta}}.$$

The estimates of β and $H_0(t)$ in the model are obtained without frailty. This corresponds to setting $\theta = 0$. Use them as initial estimates of β and $H_0(t)$ with $\theta = 0$ as an initial estimate for θ. For the E-step, obtain the expectation of frailty z_i. We can get it using Eq. (6.7) directly.

$$E(Z_i) = \frac{1 + D_i \hat{\theta}}{1 + \hat{\theta} \sum_j^{n_i} \hat{H}_0(t_{ij}) \exp(\hat{\beta} Y_{ij})}.$$

Based on L_{full}, the distribution of z_i given the observable data is still a gamma with shape parameter $\tilde{\alpha}_i = 1/\theta + D_i$ and scale parameter $\tilde{\theta}_i = 1/\theta + \sum_j H_0(t_{ij})$ $\exp(\beta Y_{ij})$. Hence, it can be proved that for the gamma (α, θ),

$$E(z) = \alpha/\theta, \qquad E(\ln(z)) = \psi(\alpha) - \ln \theta,$$

where $\psi(\alpha)$ is the digamma function $\Gamma'(\alpha)/\Gamma(\alpha)$. Then, for the E-step, the expectation of z_i and the expectation of $\ln(z_i)$ are $\tilde{\alpha}_i/\tilde{\theta}_i$ and $\psi(\tilde{\alpha}_i) - \ln(\tilde{\theta}_i)$, respectively. The formula in Eq. (6.7) gives us exactly the same result for $E(z_i)$. For the M-step, obtain the estimate of β based on Eq. (6.8). The estimate of h_{0k} is given by Eq. (6.9) for $k = 1, \ldots, M$, and the estimate of θ is derived by maximizing the likelihood of θ.

$$L(\theta) = \Gamma(1/\theta)^{-G} \theta^{-G/\theta} \prod_{i=1}^{G} \hat{z}_i^{1/\theta + D_i - 1} \exp(-\hat{z}_i/\theta).$$

Information matrix can be derived; then plug in the estimates of $\beta, h_{01}, \ldots, h_{0M}, \theta$. The variance–covariance matrix is obtained by the observed information matrix.

6.5 The Positive Stable Frailty Model

Assume that frailty has a positive stable distribution with a parameter θ. We restrict $0 < \theta \leq 1$ to get a distribution with positive numbers. The Laplace transform is $L(s) = \exp(-s^{\theta})$. The marginal distribution of T_j is given by

$$P(T_j > t) = \exp\{-H_0(t_j)^{\theta} \exp(\theta \beta Y)\}.$$

Thus, the integrated hazard and the hazard function are $H_0(t_j)^{\theta} \exp(\theta \beta Y)$, and $\theta h_0(t_j) H_0(t_j)^{\theta-1} \exp(\theta \beta Y)$, respectively. For the marginal distributions of two individuals with covariate values Y and Y^*, the relative risk is the constant $\exp(\theta \beta (Y - Y^*))$.

The pth derivative of Laplace transform is

$$L^{(p)}(s) = (-1)^p \exp(-s^{\theta}) \sum_{m=1}^{p} c_{p,m} \theta^m s^{m\theta-p},$$

where $c_{p,m}$ is a polynomial in θ of degree m and is defined recursively by

$$c_{p,p} = 1, \quad c_{p,1} = \Gamma(p - \theta)/\Gamma(1 - \theta),$$

and

$$c_{p,m} = c_{p-1,m-1} + c_{p-1,m}\{(p - 1) - m\theta\}.$$

From Eq. (6.5), the likelihood function for all individuals is given by

$$\prod_{i=1}^{G} \left\{ \prod_{j=1}^{n_i} h_0(t_{ij})^{\delta_{ij}} \exp(\delta_{ij} \beta Y_{ij}) \right\} \exp\left\{ -\left[\sum_{j=1}^{n_i} H_0(t_{ij}) \exp(\beta Y_{ij}) \right]^{\theta} \right\}$$

$$\times \sum_{m=1}^{D_i} c_{D_i,m} \theta^m \left[\sum_{j=1}^{n_i} H_0(t_{ij}) \exp(\beta Y_{ij}) \right]^{m\theta - D_i}. \tag{6.13}$$

One can use the EM algorithm for estimation. For the E-step, using the general formula Eq. (6.7), the expectation of frailty z_i is given by

$$E(z_i) = \frac{\sum_{m=1}^{D_i+1} c_{D_i+1,m} \theta^m [\sum_j H_0(t_{ij}) \exp(\beta Y_{ij})]^{m\theta - D_i - 1}}{\sum_{m=1}^{D_i} c_{D_i,m} \theta^m [\sum_j H_0(t_{ij}) \exp(\beta Y_{ij})]^{m\theta - D_i}}.$$

For the M-step, one has trouble in estimating θ because its likelihood function, involving the positive stable density, is really complicated. Wang et al. (1995) suggested a practical algorithm for providing values for θ and searching for the value which maximizes Eq. (6.13).

6.6 Modified EM (MEM) Algorithm for Gamma Frailty Models

The KM–EM algorithm (Klein and Moeschberger 2003) developed an estimate to estimate gamma frailty models. Therneau et al. (2000) and Ripatti and Palmgren (2000) obtained a penalized partial likelihood (PPL) method. If the frailties $\mathbf{Z} = \{z_i, i = 1, \ldots, G\}$ were observed, then the survival times $\mathbf{T} = (t_{i1}, \ldots, t_{in_i})$ are independently conditioned on z_i. The loglikelihood function for the complete data $\mathbf{Y} = (\mathbf{T}, \delta, \mathbf{Y}, \mathbf{Z})$ is

$$
L_F(\theta, \beta, \lambda_0) = \sum_{i=1}^{G} \left[\ln g(z_i) + \sum_{j=1}^{n_i} \{\delta_{ij} \ln(\lambda(t_{ij}|Y_{ij})z_i) - z_i \Lambda(t_{ij}|Y_{ij})\} \right],
$$

where $L_F(.)$ is decomposed into two parts $L_F(\theta, \beta, \lambda_0) = L_1(\theta) + L_2(\beta, \lambda_0)$, where

$$
L_1(\theta) = -G\left\{ \frac{\ln \theta}{\theta} + \ln \Gamma\left(\frac{1}{\theta}\right) \right\} + \sum_{i=1}^{G} \left\{ \left(\frac{1}{\theta} + D_i - 1\right) \ln z_i - \frac{z_i}{\theta} \right\},
$$

$$
L_2(\beta, \lambda_0) = \sum_{i=1}^{G} \sum_{i=1}^{n_i} \{\delta_{ij} \ln \lambda(t_{ij}|Y_{ij}) - z_i \Lambda(t_{ij}|Y_{ij})\}.
$$

The expected value of complete data loglikelihood $L_F(\theta, \beta, \lambda_0)$ is computed, given the current parameter estimates and the observed data in the E-step. The maximum likelihood estimates are obtained by maximizing the expected value of $L_F(\theta, \beta, \lambda_0)$ in the M-step.

In the E-step, the expectation of z_i and $\log z_i$ are calculated given the data and current estimates (β, θ). The frailties z_i are i.i.d. gamma random variables with shape parameter $A_i = 1/\theta + D_i$ and scale parameter $C_i = 1/\theta + \sum_{j=1}^{n_i} \Lambda_0(t_{ij}) \exp(\beta Y_{ij})$. Thus,

$$
E[z_i] = \frac{A_i}{C_i} \quad \text{and} \quad E[\ln z_i] = \psi(A_i) - \ln(C_i),
$$

where

$$
\psi(\alpha) = \frac{d \ln \Gamma(\alpha)}{d\alpha}.
$$

is the digamma function. The expectation of $L_2(\beta, \lambda_0)$ is

$$E(L_2(\beta, \lambda_0)|\delta_{ij}, t_{ij}, Y_{ij}; z_i) = \sum_{i=1}^{G} \sum_{j=1}^{n_i} \left\{ \delta_{ij} [\ln \lambda(t_{ij}|Y_{ij})] - \frac{A_i}{C_i} \Lambda(t_{ij}|Y_{ij}) \right\}.$$

(6.14)

Let $\alpha = 1/\theta$. The expected loglikelihood

$$E(L_1(\alpha)|\delta_{ij}, t_{ij}, Y_{ij}; z_i)$$

$$= G \times [\alpha \ln \alpha - \ln \Gamma(\alpha)] + \alpha \sum_{i=1}^{G} \left[\frac{(\psi(A_i) - \ln C_i)(A_i - 1)}{\alpha} - \frac{A_i}{C_i} \right].$$

Let $Y = [\frac{(\psi(A_i) - \ln C_i)(A_i - 1)}{\alpha} - A_i/C_i]/G$. Then equivalently, we can just maximize

$$m(\alpha) = \alpha \ln \alpha - \ln \Gamma(\alpha) + \alpha Y.$$

The derivatives are $m'(\alpha) = \ln \alpha + 1 + Y - \psi(\alpha)$ and $m''(\alpha) = 1/\alpha - \psi(1, \alpha)$, where

$$\psi(\alpha) = \frac{d \ln \Gamma(\alpha)}{d\alpha} \quad \text{and} \quad \psi(1, \alpha) = \frac{d^2 \ln \Gamma(\alpha)}{d\alpha^2}.$$

The Newton–Raphson step to obtain the MLE of α can be achieved by

$$\alpha_{k+1} = \alpha_k - \frac{m'(\alpha_k)}{m''(\alpha_k)}.$$

The MEM algorithm avoids complicated matrix computation and can handle large data set with thousands of groups and distinct event times. A profile likelihood EM algorithm suggested by Klein and Moeschberger (2003) and Nielson et al. (1992) can be also implemented. The profile likelihood of parameter θ is defined as

$$PL(\theta) = \sup_{\beta_\theta} L(\theta, \beta_\theta).$$

For each fixed value of θ in a specific range, the EM algorithm described above is used to obtain an estimate of β_θ. The value of the profile likelihood is then given by $L(\theta, \beta_\theta)$. The value of θ which maximizes this quantity is, then, the MLE.

Applications and Discussions

McGilchrist and Aisbett (1991) analyze the data on the recurrence times from the time of insertion of the catheter to infection for kidney patients with portable dialysis equipment. The observation is censored when catheters may be removed for reasons other than an infection. There are 38 patients and each has exactly two observations. The risk variables are age, sex (0 = male, 1 = female), and disease type coded as 0 = Glomerulo Nephritis (GN), 1 = Acute Nephritis (AN), 2 = Polycystic Kidney

Table 6.1 Parameter estimates of (β, θ) with standard errors

Variable	EM algorithm		PPL	
	Estimate	S.E.	Estimate	S.E.
Age	0.0035	0.0111	0.0034	0.0111
Sex	−1.4746	0.3578	−1.4715	0.3579
GN	0.0908	0.4066	0.0894	0.4068
AN	0.3520	0.4001	0.3518	0.4002
PKD	−1.4237	0.6307	−1.4277	0.6309
θ	0.0043	0.6607	5×10^{-7}	N/A

Disease (PKD), and 3 = Other. The five regression variables fitted are age, sex, and presence/absence of disease types GN, AN, and PKD.

Gamma frailty model is fitted to compare both the MEM algorithm and the PPL methods. Because the lognormal distribution was used for the frailty by McGilchrist and Aisbett (1991), the parameter estimates are different. From Table 6.1, we see that the parameter estimates from the MEM algorithm, especially the standard errors, are very close to the values from the PPL method.

The modified EM algorithm incorporates the standard statistical procedures to find out the MLE, then multiple imputation is used to find the standard errors. This approach avoids the calculation of inverse of matrix. In the simulation study, the three estimation methods produced similar parameter estimates when the number of groups is small, say less than 100. The EM algorithms give the standard error for the frailty parameter estimate $\hat{\theta}$, but the PPL method does not. For a medium number of groups, from one thousand and ten thousand, the KM–EM algorithm cannot run because the calculation of inverse of the matrix exhausts computer resources. Yu (2006) pointed out that the MEM algorithm is the only method that can handle such data set when the number of groups gets even larger (greater than 100,000). In summary, the three methods produce similar results and are competitive when the number of groups is small or medium. The MEM algorithm is preferred for a huge data set. In the case of the gamma frailty model, the EM algorithm and PPL approach give the same results. This was proved theoretically by Duchateau and Janssen (2008).

References

Androulakis, E., Koukouvinos, C., Vonta, F.: Estimation and variable selection via frailty models with penalized likelihood. Stat. Med. **31**(20), 2223–2239 (2012)

Berg, G.J., Drepper, B.: Inference for shared-frailty survival models with left-truncated data. Econ. Rev. **35**(6), 1075–1098 (2016)

Duchateau, L., Janssen, P.: The Frailty Model. Springer, New York (2008)

Ha, I.D., pan, J., Oh, S., Lee, Y.: Variable selection in general frailty models using penalized h-likelihood. J. Comput. Graph. Stat. **23**(4), 1044–1060 (2013)

Ha, I.D., Lee, M., Oh, S., Jeong, J.H., Sylvester, R., Lee, Y.: Variable selection in subdistribution hazard frailty models with competing risks. Stat. Med. **33**(26), 4590–4604 (2014)

Halstead, B.J., Wylie, G.D., Coates, P.S., Valcarcel, P., Casazza, M.L.: Bayesian shared frailty models for regional inference about wildlife survival. Anim. Conserv. **15**(2), 127–128 (2011)

Hanagal, D.D.: A positive stable frailty regression model in bivariate survival data. J. Indian Soc. Probab. Stat. **9**, 35–44 (2005a)

Hanagal, D.D.: Bivariate Weibull regression with gamma frailty for censored data. In: Proceedings of 1st International Conference on Reliability and Safety Engineering, December 21–23: held at Indian Institute of Technology, pp. 13–20. Bhuvaneshwar, India (2005b)

Hanagal, D.D.: A gamma frailty regression model in bivariate survival data. IAPQR Trans. **31**, 73–83 (2006a)

Hanagal, D.D.: Bivariate Weibull regression model with gamma frailty for the survival data. Stat. Methods, (Special issue on National Seminar on Modelling and Analysis of Life Time Data), pp. 37–51 (2006b)

Hanagal, D.D.: Bivariate Weibull regression with positive stable frailty for censored data. In: Proceedings of 2nd International Conference on Reliability and Safety Engineering, December 18–20: held at Indian Institute of Technology, pp. 184–192. Chennai, India (2006c)

Hanagal, D.D.: Weibull extension of bivariate exponential regression model with gamma frailty for survival data. Econ. Qual. Control. **21**, 165–174 (2006d)

Hanagal, D.D.: Positive stable frailty regression models in mixture distributions. In: Proceedings of 3rd International Conference on Reliability and Safety Engineering, December 17–19: held at Indian Institute of Technology, pp. 350–356. Udaipur, India (2007a)

Hanagal, D.D.: Gamma frailty regression models in mixture distributions. Econ. Qual. Control **22**(2), 295–302 (2007b)

Hanagal, D.D.: A power variance function frailty regression model in bivariate survival data. IAPQR Trans. **32**(2), 117–129 (2007c)

Hanagal, D.D.: Frailty regression models in mixture distributions. J. Stat. Plan. Inference **138**(8), 2462–2468 (2008a)

Hanagal, D.D.: Modelling heterogeneity for bivariate survival data by the lognormal distribution. Stat. Probab. Lett. **78**(9), 1101–1109 (2008b)

Hanagal, D.D.: Weibull extension of bivariate exponential regression model with different frailty distributions. Stat. Pap. **50**, 29–49 (2009a)

Hanagal, D.D.: Modeling heterogeneity for bivariate survival data by power variance function distribution. J. Reliab. Stat. Stud. **2**, 14–27 (2009b)

Hanagal, D.D.: Modeling heterogeneity for bivariate survival data by compound Poisson distribution. Model. Assist. Stat. Appl. **5**(1), 01–09 (2010a)

Hanagal, D.D.: Modeling heterogeneity for bivariate survival data by Weibull distribution. Stat. Pap. **51**(4), 947–958 (2010b)

Hanagal, D.D.: Modeling heterogeneity for bivariate survival data by the compound Poisson distribution with random scale. Stat. Probab. Lett. **80**, 1781–1790 (2010c)

Hougaard, P.: Analysis of Multivariate Survival Data. Springer, New York (2000)

Klein, J.P.: Semiparametric estimation of random effects using the Cox model based on EM algorithm. Biometrics **48**, 795–806 (1992)

Klein, J.P., Moeschberger, M.L.: Survival Analysis, 2nd edn. Springer, New York (2003)

Mauguen, A., Collette, S., Pignon, J.P., Rondeau, V.: Concordance measures in shared frailty models: application to clustered data in cancer prognosis. Stat. Med. **32**(27), 4803–4820 (2013a)

Mauguen, A., Rachet, B., Pelissier, S.M., MacGrogan, G., Laurent, A., Rondeau, v.: Dynamic prediction of risk of death using histry of cancer recurrencies in joint frailty models. Stat. Med. **32**(30), 5366–5380 (2013b)

McGilchrist, C.A., Aisbett, C.W.: Regression with frailty in survival analysis. Biometrics **47**, 461–466 (1991)

Nielson, G.G., Gill, R.D., Anderson, P.K., Sorensen, T.I.A.: A counting process approach to maximum likelihood estimation in frailty models. Scand. J. Stat. **19**(1), 25–43 (1992)

Ohman, P., Eberly, L.: A shifted frailty distribution for correlated time to event data. Research report. Department of Statistics, University of Florida, Gainesville (2001)

Parner, E.: Inference in semi-parametric frailty models. Ph.D. Thesis. University of Aarhus, Denmark (1997)

Ripatti, S., Palmgren, J.: Estimation of multivariate frailty models using penalized likelihood. Biometrics **56**, 1016–1022 (2000)

Rondeau, V., Schaffner, E., Corbiere, F., Gonzalez, J.R., Pelessier, S.M.: Cure frailty models for survival data: application to recurrences for breast cancer and to hospital readmissions for colorectal cancer. Stat. Methods Med. Res. **22**(3), 243–260 (2011)

Shu, Y., Klein, J.P.: A SAS micro for the positive stable frailty model. In: American Statistical Association Proceedings of Statistical Computing Section, pp. 47–52, (1999)

Souza, W.B., Mayrink, V.D.: Semiparametric generalized exponential frailty model for clustered survival data. Ann. Inst. Stat. Math. **71**(3), 679–701 (2018)

Therneau, T.M., Grambsch, P.M., Pankratz, V.S.: Penalized survival models and frailty. Technical Report, 66, Mayo Foundation (2000)

Wang, S.T., Klein, J.P., Moeschberger, M.L.: Semi-parametric estimation of covariate effects using the positive stable frailty model. Appl. Stoch. Model. Data Anal. **11**, 121–133 (1995)

Yu, B.: Estimation of shared frailty models by a modified EM algorithm. Comput. Stat. and Data Anal. **50**(2), 463–474 (2006)

Chapter 7
Analysis of Survival Data in Shared Frailty Models

7.1 Introduction

Therneau and Grambsch (2000) have given some data analysis on frailty models using SPLUS and SAS software packages. In this chapter, we analyze some more data which was discussed in Chap. 1 using R package which has free open access to everyone.

7.2 Analysis for Bone Marrow Transplantation (BMT) Data

Consider the data set on bone marrow transplantation (BMT) given in Sect. 1.2. We analyze the data using gamma frailty and Gaussian frailty models for the parametric baseline models using R statistical package. Let us consider lognormal distribution as the baseline model which has the highest loglikelihood among parametric family. The following is the R program.

```
bmt=read.table(file="C:/David/Book2/Data/BMT2.txt",header=T)
library(survival)
fit1=survreg(Surv(T,I)~PAge+PSex+hospital+g,data=bmt,
dist='lognormal')
summary(fit1)
```

Here, the variable of interest (response variable, T) is time to death or relapse, I is an indicator (1-dead or relapsed, 0-alive or disease-free). PAge, PSex, hospital, and g are the covariates indicating patient age, patient sex (1-male, 0-female), and disease group (1-ALL, 2-AML-low risk, 3-AML-high risk). The output of the R program is given below.

© Springer Nature Singapore Pte Ltd. 2019
D. D. Hanagal, *Modeling Survival Data Using Frailty Models*,
Industrial and Applied Mathematics, https://doi.org/10.1007/978-981-15-1181-3_7

```
Call:
survreg(formula = Surv(T, I) ~ PAge + PSex + hospital + g,
    data = bmt, dist = "lognormal")

            Value Std. Error      z        p
(Intercept)  7.6086     0.6347  11.99  4.11e-33
PAge        -0.0190     0.0162  -1.17  2.42e-01
PSex         0.4147     0.3034   1.37  1.72e-01
hospital     0.3008     0.1361   2.21  2.71e-02
g           -0.3512     0.1936  -1.81  6.96e-02
Log(scale)   0.7553     0.0703  10.75  5.89e-27

Scale= 2.13

Log Normal distribution
Loglik(model)= -1008.1    Loglik(intercept only)= -1014
        Chisq= 11.84 on 4 degrees of freedom, p= 0.019
Number of Newton-Raphson Iterations: 3
n= 274
```

From the output of the R program, it is observed that the test for the regression parameters equal to zero is rejected with a chi-square value of 11.84 for 4 df and p-value is 0.019. Hospital is the most effective variable which is related to the survival of patients with p-value 0.027. The loglikelihood (intercept only) is −1014 for the lognormal distribution as a baseline. For other baseline distributions, the loglikelihood (intercept only) for Weibull baseline is −1024.1 and for loglogistic baseline is −1017.1. Among these three distributions, lognormal has the highest loglikelihood with value −1014. R package does not have gamma distribution as a baseline model for the survival function. Now we introduce the frailty component in the above regression model. First, we introduce gamma frailty and then Gaussian frailty models. R package does not have a positive stable, power variance function, Weibull as a frailty distribution. The following is the R program for the gamma frailty model.

```
fit2=survreg(Surv(T,I)~PAge+PSex+hospital+g+frailty(pat),
data=bmt,dist='lognormal')
summary(fit2)
```

In the above R command, the patient is the frailty variable which has gamma distribution by default when not specified. The output of the R program is given below.

```
Call:
survreg(formula = Surv(T, I) ~ PAge + PSex + hospital + g
    + frailty(pat), data = bmt, dist = "lognormal")
```

```
                Value Std. Error       z        p
(Intercept)    7.1304     0.6964  10.240 1.32e-24
PAge          -0.0116     0.0200  -0.579 5.63e-01
PSex           0.3341     0.3301   1.012 3.12e-01
hospital       0.1870     0.1463   1.278 2.01e-01
g             -0.0864     0.2360  -0.366 7.14e-01
Log(scale)    -1.1182     0.0606 -18.453 4.96e-76

Scale= 0.327

Log Normal distribution
Loglik(model)= -719.6   Loglik(intercept only)= -1014
        Chisq= 588.81 on 115.5 degrees of freedom, p= 0
Number of Newton-Raphson Iterations:  8 38
n= 274
```

From the output of the R program, it is observed that the test for the regression parameters equal to zero is rejected with chi-square value 588.81 for 115.5 df and the p-value is 0. The effect of frailty component is significant as compared to without the frailty term. Now the loglikelihood has been increased to -719.6 from -1008.1. The chi-square value is 577 for 1 df and p-value is 0. The following is the R program for the Gaussian frailty model.

```
fit3=survreg(Surv(T,I)~PAge+PSex+hospital+g+frailty(pat,
dist='gauss'),data=bmt,dist='lognormal')
summary(fit3)
```

In the above R command, the patient is the frailty variable which has Gaussian distribution. The output of the R program is given below.

```
Call:
survreg(formula = Surv(T, I) ~ PAge + PSex + hospital + g
    + frailty(pat, dist = "gauss"), data = bmt,
    dist = "lognormal")

                Value Std. Error       z        p
(Intercept)    6.7119     0.6054   11.09 1.46e-28
PAge          -0.0169     0.0156   -1.09 2.77e-01
PSex           0.2363     0.2916    0.81 4.18e-01
hospital       0.1976     0.1279    1.55 1.22e-01
g             -0.2008     0.1880   -1.07 2.85e-01
Log(scale)    -1.1215     0.0606  -18.52 1.50e-76

Scale= 0.326

Log Normal distribution
Loglik(model)= -721.3   Loglik(intercept only)= -1014
```

```
        Chisq= 585.28 on 122.4 degrees of freedom, p= 0
Number of Newton-Raphson Iterations:   5 27
n= 274
```

In the frailty model for the nonparametric Cox's proportional hazards model, there is a problem of convergence while estimating the parameters for this data. The following are the R commands without output for this data.

```
fit4=coxph(Surv(T,I)~PAge+PSex+hospital+g+frailty(pat),data=bmt)
fit5=coxph(Surv(T,I)~PAge+PSex+hospital+g+frailty(pat,
dist='gauss'),data=bmt)
```

7.3   Analysis for Acute Leukemia Data

Consider the data set on remission duration from a clinical trial for acute leukemia given in Sect. 1.3. Here, the variable of interest is time to relapse for placebo and 6-MP patients. The cens is a relapse indicator (0-censored, 1-relapse), status is the covariate indicating the remission status at randomization (1-partial, 2-complete). We analyze the data using ordinary Cox's proportional hazards (PH) model, gamma frailty, and Gaussian frailty models for the nonparametric Cox's PH model using the R statistical package. The following are the R commands with output.

```
> fit1=coxph(Surv(time,cens)~status,data=remission)
> summary(fit1)
Call:
coxph(formula = Surv(time, cens) ~ status, data = remission)

  n= 42

          coef exp(coef) se(coef)    z Pr(>|z|)
status -0.2070    0.8130   0.4143 -0.5    0.617

        exp(coef) exp(-coef) lower .95 upper .95
status      0.813       1.23     0.361     1.831

Rsquare= 0.006    (max possible= 0.988 )
Likelihood ratio test= 0.24  on 1 df,    p=0.6231
Wald test            = 0.25  on 1 df,    p=0.6174
Score (logrank) test = 0.25  on 1 df,    p=0.6168

> fit1$loglik
[1] -93.18427 -93.06351

> fit2=coxph(Surv(time,cens)~status+frailty(pat),
```

```
  data=remission)
> summary(fit2)

Call:
coxph(formula = Surv(time, cens) ~ status + frailty(pat),
    data = remission)

  n= 42
              coef   se(coef) se2    Chisq DF p
status       -0.207 0.414     0.414  0.25  1  0.62
frailty(pat)                         0.00  0  0.95

         exp(coef) exp(-coef) lower .95 upper .95
status      0.813      1.23      0.361     1.83


Iterations: 6 outer, 23 Newton-Raphson
     Variance of random effect= 5e-07   I-likelihood = -93.1
Degrees of freedom for terms= 1 0
Rsquare= 0.006   (max possible= 0.988 )
Likelihood ratio test= 0.24  on 1 df,    p=0.623
Wald test            = 0.25  on 1 df,    p=0.617
> fit2$loglik
[1] -93.18427 -93.06350


> fit3=coxph(Surv(time,cens)~status+frailty(pat,dist='gauss'),
  data=remission)
> summary(fit3)

Call:
coxph(formula = Surv(time, cens) ~ status + frailty(pat,
    dist = "gauss"), data = remission)

  n= 42
                          coef   se(coef) se2    Chisq DF   p
status                   -0.208 0.415     0.414  0.25  1.00 0.62
frailty(pat, dist = "gaus                       0.02  0.03 0.64

         exp(coef) exp(-coef) lower .95 upper .95
status      0.812      1.23      0.36      1.83


Iterations: 10 outer, 34 Newton-Raphson
     Variance of random effect= 0.00130
Degrees of freedom for terms= 1 0
Rsquare= 0.007   (max possible= 0.988 )
Likelihood ratio test= 0.29  on 1.03 df,    p=0.603
Wald test            = 0.25  on 1.03 df,    p=0.628


> fit3$loglik
[1] -93.18427 -93.03973
```

The log partial-likelihood when the vector $\beta = 0$ is –93.18427. In the ordinary Cox's PH model, the final fit is –93.06351 and in the gamma frailty model, the

variance of the random effect is estimated to be almost close to zero, corresponding
0 df. A likelihood ratio test for the frailty is twice the difference between the log
partial-likelihood with the frailty term integrated out, shown as "I-likelihood" in the
printout, and the loglikelihood of a no-frailty model, or $2(93.1 - 93.063) = 0.074$.
It has one degree of freedom with p-value $= 0.785$. The third fit is Gaussian frailty
fit which chooses the estimate of the random effect using an REML criterion. The
REML method has a slightly larger estimated frailty variance 0.0013 as compared to
gamma frailty variance which is close to zero. The integrated likelihood is not printed
for Gaussian frailty. Now we analyze the data with parametric baseline models. The
following are the R commands with output.

```
> fit4=survreg(Surv(time,cens)~status,data=remission,
  dist='lognormal')
> fit4
Call:
survreg(formula = Surv(time, cens) ~ status, data = remission,
    dist = "lognormal")

Coefficients:
(Intercept)        status
   2.045857      0.238918

Scale= 1.109509

Loglik(model)= -115.2   Loglik(intercept only)= -115.4
        Chisq= 0.33 on 1 degrees of freedom, p= 0.56
n= 42

> fit5=survreg(Surv(time,cens)~status+frailty(pat),
  data=remission, dist='lognormal')
> fit5
Call:
survreg(formula = Surv(time, cens) ~ status + frailty(pat),
    data = remission, dist = "lognormal")

                coef  se(coef) se2    Chisq DF   p
(Intercept)    2.046 0.747     0.745  7.51  1.00 0.0061
status         0.239 0.415     0.414  0.33  1.00 0.5700
frailty(pat)                          0.05  0.07 0.5600

Scale= 1.11

Iterations: 10 outer, 31 Newton-Raphson
      Variance of random effect= 0.00263   I-likelihood = -55.7
Degrees of freedom for terms= 1.0 1.0 0.1 1.0
Likelihood ratio test=0.43  on 1.1 df, p=0.535  n= 42
> fit5$loglik
[1] -115.3930 -115.1776

> fit6=survreg(Surv(time,cens)~status+frailty(pat,
```

```
      dist='gauss'),data=remission,dist='lognormal')
> fit6
Call:
survreg(formula = Surv(time, cens) ~ status + frailty(pat,
    dist = "gauss"), data = remission, dist = "lognormal")

                      coef  se(coef) se2   Chisq DF    p
(Intercept)          2.046 0.747    0.746 7.51  1.00 0.0061
status               0.239 0.414    0.414 0.33  1.00 0.5600
frailty(pat, dist = "gaus                 0.02  0.03 0.6300


Scale= 1.11

Iterations: 10 outer, 28 Newton-Raphson
      Variance of random effect= 0.00130
Degrees of freedom for terms= 1 1 0 1
Likelihood ratio test=0.38  on 1 df, p=0.549  n= 42
> fit6$loglik
[1] -115.3930 -115.2024
```

It is observed from the above R output that the loglikelihood (intercept only) for the lognormal distribution is −115.4. For the other parametric distribution, the loglikelihood for Weibull is −116.4 and for loglogistic, it is −115.4 and we take here lognormal distribution as the baseline model to analyze frailty models. The estimate of the variance for gamma frailty is 0.00263 and for Gaussian frailty is 0.0013. The loglikelihood of a no-frailty model (in gamma), or $2(115.4 − 115.17) = 0.46$. It has one degree of freedom with p-value $= 0.497$. Similarly, the loglikelihood of a no frailty (in Gaussian), or $2(115.4 − 115.20) = 0.4$ which is chi-square for one df with p-value $= 0.527$. So far, there is a clear cut way to say which frailty distribution is best.

7.4   Analysis for HLA Data

Consider the data set on kidney dialysis (HAL) given in Sect. 1.7. Here, the variable of interest is time to graft rejection. The cens is a relapse indicator (1-censored, 0-graft rejected). HAL is the covariate indicating the HAL matching (1-good, 0-poor). We analyze the data using ordinary Cox's proportional hazards (PH) model, gamma frailty, and Gaussian frailty models for the nonparametric Cox's PH model using the R statistical package. The following are the R commands with output.

```
> fit1=coxph(Surv(time,cens==1)~HAL,data=hal)
> summary(fit1)
Call:
coxph(formula = Surv(time, cens == 1) ~ HAL,
    data = hal)

  n= 34
```

```
          coef exp(coef)  se(coef)      z Pr(>|z|)
HAL -1.0812    0.3392    0.4257 -2.54   0.0111 *
---
Signif. codes:  0 ***  0.001  **  0.01  *  0.05  .  0.1      1

     exp(coef) exp(-coef) lower .95 upper .95
HAL    0.3392      2.948    0.1473     0.7812

Rsquare= 0.183    (max possible= 0.99 )
Likelihood ratio test= 6.89  on 1 df,    p=0.008688
Wald test            = 6.45  on 1 df,    p=0.01108
Score (logrank) test = 7  on 1 df,    p=0.008167

> fit1$loglik
[1] -78.58933 -75.14636

> fit2=coxph(Surv(time,cens==1)~HAL+frailty(pat),data=hal)
> summary(fit2)
Call:
coxph(formula = Surv(time, cens == 1) ~ HAL + frailty(pat),
   data = hal)

  n= 34
              coef  se(coef)  se2   Chisq DF   p
HAL          -1.36  0.49    0.463   7.68 1.00 0.0056
frailty(pat)                      27.54 9.45 0.0015

     exp(coef) exp(-coef) lower .95 upper .95
HAL    0.257       3.89     0.0984     0.672

Iterations: 6 outer, 55 Newton-Raphson
     Variance of random effect= 0.925    I-likelihood = -73.4
Degrees of freedom for terms= 0.9 9.4
Rsquare= 0.671    (max possible= 0.99 )
Likelihood ratio test= 37.8  on 10.3 df,    p=5.34e-05
Wald test            = 7.68  on 10.3 df,    p=0.69

> fit3=coxph(Surv(time,cens==1)~HAL+frailty(pat,dist='gauss'),
   data=hal)
> summary(fit3)
Call:
coxph(formula = Surv(time, cens == 1) ~ HAL + frailty(pat,
   dist = "gauss"), data = hal)

  n= 34
                      coef  se(coef)  se2   Chisq DF p
HAL                  -1.52  0.515   0.475   8.76  1 0.00310
frailty(pat, dist = "gaus                   34.17 11 0.00034

     exp(coef) exp(-coef) lower .95 upper .95
HAL    0.218       4.59     0.0795     0.598

Iterations: 8 outer, 47 Newton-Raphson
```

```
      Variance of random effect= 1.79
Degrees of freedom for terms=  0.9 11.0
Rsquare= 0.723    (max possible= 0.99 )
Likelihood ratio test= 43.6   on 11.8 df,    p=1.57e-05
Wald test             = 8.76   on 11.8 df,    p=0.712


> fit4=coxph(Surv(time,cens==1)~HAL+frailty(pat,dist='gauss',
  method='aic'),data=hal)
> summary(fit4)
Call:
coxph(formula = Surv(time, cens == 1) ~ HAL + frailty(pat,
    dist = "gauss", method = "aic"), data = hal)

  n= 34
                        coef  se(coef)  se2   Chisq DF   p
HAL                    -2.37  0.727    0.699  10.6  1.0 1.1e-03
frailty(pat, dist = "gaus                       75.1 15.1 5.9e-10


      exp(coef) exp(-coef) lower .95 upper .95
HAL      0.0936       10.7    0.0225      0.39


Iterations: 10 outer, 118 Newton-Raphson
      Variance of random effect= 19.3
Degrees of freedom for terms=  0.9 15.1
Rsquare= 0.803    (max possible= 0.99 )
Likelihood ratio test= 55.3   on 16.1 df,    p=3.34e-06
Wald test             = 10.6   on 16.1 df,    p=0.836
```

The log partial-likelihood when the vector $\beta = 0$ is –78.59. In the ordinary Cox's PH model, the final fit is –75.14 and in the gamma frailty model, the variance of the random effect is estimated to be 0.925, corresponding 9.45 df. HAL matching is a significant covariate in all the models. A likelihood ratio test for the frailty is twice the difference between the log partial-likelihood with the frailty term integrated out, shown as "I-likelihood" in the printout, and the loglikelihood of a no-frailty model, or $2(75.14 - 73.4) = 3.48$. It has one degree of freedom with p-value = 0.062. The frailty variable (patient) is not significantly related to time to graft rejection. The third fit is Gaussian frailty fit which chooses the estimate of the random effect using a REML criterion. The fourth fit is Gaussian frailty fit which uses Akaike's information criterion (AIC) to choose the variance of random effect, that is, it maximizes the value of (LR test - df)—two quantities that are printed on the last line. The estimate of the variance of random effect is 19.3 as compared to the REML method which is 1.79. The AIC method has a larger estimated frailty variance. The REML method has a slightly larger estimated frailty variance 1.79 as compared to gamma frailty variance which is 0.925. The integrated likelihood is not printed for Gaussian frailty. Now we analyze the data with parametric baseline models. The following are the R commands with output.

```
> fit5=survreg(Surv(time,cens==1)~HAL,data=hal,dist='lognormal')
```

```
> summary(fit5)

Call:
survreg(formula = Surv(time, cens == 1) ~ HAL, data = hal,
    dist = "lognormal")
             Value Std. Error     z        p
(Intercept)  3.060      0.121 25.23 2.04e-140
HAL          0.556      0.183  3.03  2.43e-03
Log(scale)  -0.653      0.135 -4.83  1.36e-06

Scale= 0.521

Log Normal distribution
Loglik(model)= -119.1   Loglik(intercept only)= -123.1
        Chisq= 8.07 on 1 degrees of freedom, p= 0.0045
Number of Newton-Raphson Iterations: 4
n= 34

> fit6=survreg(Surv(time,cens==1)~HAL+frailty(pat),data=hal,
  dist='lognormal')
> summary(fit6)

Call:
survreg(formula = Surv(time, cens == 1) ~ HAL + frailty(pat),
    data = hal, dist = "lognormal")
             Value Std. Error     z        p
(Intercept)  3.120      0.176 17.76 1.35e-70
HAL          0.492      0.105  4.67 2.98e-06
Log(scale)  -1.351      0.133 -10.16 2.98e-24

Scale= 0.259

Log Normal distribution
Loglik(model)= -97   Loglik(intercept only)= -123.1
        Chisq= 52.2 on 13.8 degrees of freedom, p= 2.2e-06
Number of Newton-Raphson Iterations: 10 39
n= 34

> fit7=survreg(Surv(time,cens==1)~HAL+frailty(pat,dist='gauss'),
  data=hal,dist='lognormal')
> summary(fit7)

Call:
survreg(formula = Surv(time, cens == 1) ~ HAL + frailty(pat,
    dist = "gauss"), data = hal, dist = "lognormal")
             Value Std. Error     z        p
(Intercept)  3.039      0.121 25.02 4.02e-138
HAL          0.489      0.106  4.62  3.78e-06
Log(scale)  -1.327      0.139 -9.52  1.70e-21

Scale= 0.265

Log Normal distribution
```

```
Loglik(model)= -98.2    Loglik(intercept only)= -123.1
        Chisq= 49.81 on 12.3 degrees of freedom, p= 1.9e-06
Number of Newton-Raphson Iterations:   6 23
n= 34
```

It is observed from the above R output that the loglikelihood (intercept only) for the lognormal distribution is −123.1. For the other parametric distribution, the loglikelihood for Weibull is −128.1 and for loglogistic, it is −123.5 and we take here, the lognormal distribution (which has the highest loglikelihood) as the baseline model to analyze frailty models. The covariate HAL matching is significant in all the parametric regression models. The estimates of the variance for gamma frailty and for Gaussian frailty are not printed in the R output. The loglikelihood of a no-frailty model (in gamma), or $2(119.1 - 97.0) = 44.2$. It has one degree of freedom with p-value $= 0.0$. Similarly, the loglikelihood of a no frailty (in Gaussian), or $2(119.1 - 98.2) = 41.8$ which is chi-square for one df with p-value $= 0.0$. From both frailty models, it is observed from the R output that the frailty variable (patient) is very highly significantly related to the time to graft rejection.

7.5   Analysis for Kidney Infection Data

Consider the data set on kidney infection given in Sect. 1.5. Here, the variable of interest is the first or second recurrence time. The cens is a recurrence indicator (0-censored, 1-recurrence occurred). The covariates are age, sex (0-male, 1-female), and three disease indicator variables GN, AN, and PKD. Therneau and Grambsch (2000) analyzed this data using gamma and Gaussian frailty models. When all the three covariates are included in the gamma frailty, the variance of the random effect is essentially zero. When the disease variable is dropped out of the random effects model, the estimate of the variance of the random effect is 0.408. The LR test for no frailty gives chi-square value 5.4 for one df with p-value of 0.02. Now we analyze the data with parametric baseline models and compare the results with nonparametric models. The following are the R commands with output.

```
> fit1=survreg(Surv(time,cens)~age+gender+disease,data=kidney1,
  dist='lognormal')
> summary(fit1)

Call:
survreg(formula = Surv(time, cens) ~ age + gender + disease,
    data = kidney1, dist = "lognormal")
                Value Std. Error       z        p
(Intercept)  3.346170     0.4728  7.0771 1.47e-12
age         -0.000918     0.0114 -0.0805 9.36e-01
gender       1.476469     0.3172  4.6543 3.25e-06
```

```
diseaseAN     -0.620735      0.4097 -1.5153 1.30e-01
diseaseGN     -0.322634      0.4124 -0.7824 4.34e-01
diseasePKD     0.695716      0.5735  1.2132 2.25e-01
Log(scale)     0.104581      0.0914  1.1446 2.52e-01

Scale= 1.11

Log Normal distribution
Loglik(model)= -326   Loglik(intercept only)= -337.1
        Chisq= 22.24 on 5 degrees of freedom, p= 0.00047
Number of Newton-Raphson Iterations: 4
n= 76

> fit2=survreg(Surv(time,cens)~age+gender+disease+frailty(id),
  data=kidney1,dist='lognormal')
> summary(fit2)

Call:
survreg(formula = Surv(time, cens) ~ age + gender + disease +
    frailty(id), data = kidney1, dist = "lognormal")
                 Value Std. Error      z       p
(Intercept)    3.55693      0.5700  6.240 4.38e-10
age           -0.00331      0.0129 -0.257 7.97e-01
gender         1.48908      0.3763  3.957 7.59e-05
diseaseAN     -0.63131      0.4624 -1.365 1.72e-01
diseaseGN     -0.31810      0.4615 -0.689 4.91e-01
diseasePKD     0.80826      0.6549  1.234 2.17e-01
Log(scale)    -0.26487      0.1049 -2.526 1.15e-02

Scale= 0.767

Log Normal distribution
Loglik(model)= -302.5   Loglik(intercept only)= -337.1
        Chisq= 69.2 on 20.2 degrees of freedom, p= 2.8e-07
Number of Newton-Raphson Iterations: 10 33
n= 76
```

It is observed from the above R output that the loglikelihood (intercept only) for the lognormal distribution is −337.1. For the other parametric distribution, the loglikelihood for Weibull is −338.6 and for loglogistic, it is −339.1 and we take here the lognormal distribution (which has the highest loglikelihood) as the baseline model to analyze frailty models. The covariate gender and disease AN are significant factors in all the lognormal regression models. We analyze the data using the gamma frailty model only. The loglikelihood of a no-frailty model, or $2(326.0 - 302.5) = 47$. It has one degree of freedom with p-value $= 0.0$. From the gamma frailty model, it is observed from the R output that the frailty variable (patient) is very highly significantly related to the recurrence time.

7.6   Analysis of Litters of Rats

Consider the data set on litters of rats given in Sect. 1.6. Here, the variable of interest is the follow-up time. The status is an indicator (0-tumor, 1-censored). The covariate is the treatment indicator. Therneau and Grambsch (2000) analyzed this data using gamma and Gaussian frailty models. They observed that the estimate of the variance of the random effect is highest when Gaussian frailty with the AIC method is used. Now, we analyze the data with gamma frailty and test for no frailty in the gamma frailty model under Cox's PH model.

```
> fit1=coxph(Surv(time,status==1)~ind,data=rats)
> summary(fit1)
Call:
coxph(formula = Surv(time, status == 1) ~ ind, data = rats)

  n= 150

      coef exp(coef) se(coef)     z Pr(>|z|)
ind 0.9047    2.4713   0.3175 2.849  0.00438 **
---
Signif. codes:  0  ***  0.001  **  0.01  *  0.05  .  0.1     1

    exp(coef) exp(-coef) lower .95 upper .95
ind     2.471     0.4046     1.326     4.605

Rsquare= 0.052   (max possible= 0.916 )
Likelihood ratio test= 7.98  on 1 df,    p=0.004741
Wald test           = 8.12  on 1 df,    p=0.004379
Score (logrank) test = 8.68  on 1 df,    p=0.003217

> fit1$loglik
[1] -185.6556 -181.6677

> fit2=coxph(Surv(time,status==1)~ind+frailty(litter),data=rats)
> summary(fit2)
Call:
coxph(formula = Surv(time, status == 1) ~ ind + frailty(litter),
    data = rats)

  n= 150
                coef se(coef) se2   Chisq DF    p
ind             0.914 0.323    0.319  8.01  1.0 0.0046
frailty(litter)                      17.69 14.4 0.2400

    exp(coef) exp(-coef) lower .95 upper .95
ind      2.50      0.401      1.32       4.7

Iterations: 6 outer, 24 Newton-Raphson
    Variance of random effect= 0.499   I-likelihood = -180.8
Degrees of freedom for terms=  1.0 14.4
```

```
Rsquare= 0.222    (max possible= 0.916 )
Likelihood ratio test= 37.6  on 15.4 df,    p=0.00124
Wald test            = 8.01  on 15.4 df,    p=0.934
```

The log partial-likelihood without frailty in the first fit with covariate is −181.6 and log partial-likelihood with gamma frailty in the second fit with covariate is −180.8. The LR test for no frailty with chi-square value 1.6 for one 1 df and p-value is 0.2. Next, we analyze the data using parametric models.

```
> fit3=survreg(Surv(time,status==1)~ind,data=rats,dist='weibull')
> summary(fit3)

Call:
survreg(formula = Surv(time, status == 1) ~ ind, data = rats,
    dist = "weibull")
            Value Std. Error     z        p
(Intercept)  4.983    0.0833 59.81 0.00e+00
ind         -0.239    0.0891 -2.68 7.42e-03
Log(scale)  -1.333    0.1439 -9.26 2.01e-20

Scale= 0.264

Weibull distribution
Loglik(model)= -242.3   Loglik(intercept only)= -246.3
        Chisq= 8 on 1 degrees of freedom, p= 0.0047
Number of Newton-Raphson Iterations: 7
n= 150

> fit6=survreg(Surv(time,status==1)~ind+frailty(litter),
  data=rats,dist='weibull')
> summary(fit6)

Call:
survreg(formula = Surv(time, status == 1) ~ ind
    + frailty(litter), data = rats, dist = "weibull")
            Value Std. Error     z        p
(Intercept)  5.021    0.1339 37.49 1.53e-307
ind         -0.200    0.0679 -2.95 3.16e-03
Log(scale)  -1.712    0.1262 -13.57 6.20e-42

Scale= 0.181

Weibull distribution
Loglik(model)= -204.3   Loglik(intercept only)= -246.3
        Chisq= 83.88 on 37.9 degrees of freedom, p= 2.5e-05
Number of Newton-Raphson Iterations: 10 30
n= 150

> fit7=survreg(Surv(time,status==1)~ind+frailty(litter,
  dist='gauss'),data=rats,dist='weibull')
```

```
> summary(fit7)

Call:
survreg(formula = Surv(time, status == 1) ~ ind +
    frailty(litter,dist = "gauss"), data = rats,
    dist = "weibull")
              Value Std. Error      z        p
(Intercept)   4.871      0.0636  76.54 0.00e+00
ind          -0.182      0.0665  -2.74 6.13e-03
Log(scale)   -1.649      0.1459 -11.30 1.25e-29

Scale= 0.192

Weibull distribution
Loglik(model)= -225.7   Loglik(intercept only)= -246.3
        Chisq= 41.06 on 16.4 degrees of freedom, p= 0.00068
Number of Newton-Raphson Iterations:  8 37
n= 150
```

It is observed from the above R output that the loglikelihood (intercept only) for the Weibull distribution is −246.3. For the other parametric distribution, the loglikelihood for lognormal is −247.1 and for loglogistic, it is −246.5 and we take here the Weibull distribution (which has the highest loglikelihood) as the baseline model to analyze frailty models. The covariate treatment indicator is a significant factor in all the Weibull regression models. We analyze the data using gamma frailty and Gaussian frailty models. The LR of a no-frailty model (in gamma) is $2(242.3 − 204.3) = 78$. It has chi-square one degree of freedom with p-value $= 0.0$. The LR of a no frailty (in Gaussian) is $2(242.3 − 225.7) = 33.2$. It has chi-square one degree of freedom with p-value $= 0.0$. From the Gaussian and gamma frailty models, it is observed from the R output that the frailty variable (litter) is very highly significantly related to the recurrence time.

7.7 Analysis for Diabetic Retinopathy Data

Consider the data set on diabetic retinopathy given in Sect. 1.8. Here, the variable of interest is the follow-up time. The status is an indicator (0-tumor, 1-censored). We consider two covariates in the analysis, one is laser type (treatment) and the second is the type of diabetes (1-juvenile, 2-adult). Therneau and Grambsch (2000) analyzed this data using gamma and Gaussian frailty models. They observed that the estimate of the variance of the random effect is the highest when Gaussian frailty with the AIC method is used. Now, we analyze the data with Gaussian and gamma frailties and test for no frailty in the parametric regression model.

```
> fit1=survreg(Surv(time,status)~treat+adult, data=diabetics,
    dist='lognormal')
> summary(fit1)
```

```
Call:
survreg(formula = Surv(time, status) ~ treat + adult,
    data = diabetics, dist = "lognormal")
                Value Std. Error       z        p
(Intercept)   4.74357    0.5122  9.2608 2.03e-20
treat        -0.28471    0.2291 -1.2425 2.14e-01
adult         0.00771    0.2314  0.0333 9.73e-01
Log(scale)    0.66247    0.0637 10.4034 2.39e-25

Scale= 1.94

Log Normal distribution
Loglik(model)= -842.1   Loglik(intercept only)= -842.9
        Chisq= 1.55 on 2 degrees of freedom, p= 0.46
Number of Newton-Raphson Iterations: 3
n= 394

> fit2=survreg(Surv(time,status)~treat+adult+frailty(id),
  data=diabetics,dist='lognormal')
> summary(fit2)

Call:
survreg(formula = Surv(time, status) ~ treat + adult +
  frailty(id), data = diabetics, dist = "lognormal")
                Value Std. Error       z        p
(Intercept)   4.8461     0.5601  8.652 5.08e-18
treat        -0.2352     0.2511 -0.936 3.49e-01
adult        -0.1146     0.2524 -0.454 6.50e-01
Log(scale)   -0.0183     0.0578 -0.317 7.51e-01

Scale= 0.982

Log Normal distribution
Loglik(model)= -701.3   Loglik(intercept only)= -842.9
        Chisq= 283.18 on 126.1 degrees of freedom, p= 4.3e-14
Number of Newton-Raphson Iterations:  8 31
n= 394

> fit3=survreg(Surv(time,status)~treat+adult+frailty(id,
  dist='gauss'), data=diabetics,dist='lognormal')
> summary(fit3)

Call:
survreg(formula = Surv(time, status) ~ treat + adult +
  frailty(id, dist = "gauss"), data = diabetics,
  dist = "lognormal")
                Value Std. Error       z        p
(Intercept)   4.3241     0.4454  9.709 2.76e-22
treat        -0.2531     0.2015 -1.256 2.09e-01
adult        -0.0102     0.2032 -0.050 9.60e-01
Log(scale)    0.0585     0.0663  0.882 3.78e-01

Scale= 1.06
```

```
Log Normal distribution
Loglik(model)= -726.9    Loglik(intercept only)= -842.9
        Chisq= 231.98 on 106.1 degrees of freedom, p= 2.2e-11
Number of Newton-Raphson Iterations:   6 23
n= 394
```

It is observed from the above R output that the loglikelihood (intercept only) for the lognormal distribution is −842.9. For the other parametric distribution, the loglikelihood for Weibull is −848 and for loglogistic, it is −845.6 and we take here the lognormal distribution (which has the highest loglikelihood) as the baseline model to analyze frailty models. No covariates are significant factors in all the lognormal regression models. We analyze the data using the gamma frailty and Gaussian frailty models. The LR of a no-frailty model (in gamma) is $2(842.1 − 701.3) = 281.6$. It has chi-square one degree of freedom with p-value $= 0.0$. The LR of a no frailty (in Gaussian) is $2(842.1 − 726.9) = 230.4$. It has chi-square one degree of freedom with p-value $= 0.0$. From the Gaussian and gamma frailty models, it is observed from the R output that the frailty variable (patient) is very highly significantly related to the follow-up time.

Reference

Therneau, T.M., Grambsch, P.M.: Modeling Survival Data: Extending the Cox Model. Springer, New York (2000)

Chapter 8
Tests of Hypotheses in Frailty Models

8.1 Introduction

In this chapter, we discuss some well-known tests for frailty which are used more often and they have a lot of applications. In frailty models, there is a clear need for inference on the heterogeneity parameter which measures the association between the survival outcomes in a specific cluster. The model specification of frailty models typically requires the heterogeneity parameter to be positive or, in case of homogeneity, to be zero. Therefore hypothesis testing problems for homogeneity against heterogeneity are described by a one-sided alternative hypothesis and, under the null hypothesis, the parameter is at the boundary of the parameter space which is $(0, \infty)$. Geerdens et al. (2013) constructed goodness-of-fit tests for gamma frailties. Mazroui et al. (2016) proposed joint frailty model for two types of recurrent events and a dependent terminal event to account for potential dependencies between events with potentially time-varying coefficients and applied this model to breast cancer data. They developed likelihood ratio tests to test time dependency and the association of covariates. In this chapter, three different test procedures are discussed. We first discuss tests for gamma frailty based on likelihood ratio and score tests and analyze diabetic retinopathy data. In Sect. 8.3, we discuss the logrank test for testing $\beta = 0$ in parametric and nonparametric setup for uncensored and censored data and we give some numerical examples. In the last section, we discuss a test for homogeneity, i.e., all frailties have common distribution and we analyze kidney infection data.

8.2 Tests for Gamma Frailty Based on Likelihood Ratio and Score Tests

Tests for heterogeneity in frailty models are subject to inequality constraints in an alternative hypothesis. Hence the classical likelihood ratio asymptotic chi-square distribution theory is no longer valid.

© Springer Nature Singapore Pte Ltd. 2019
D. D. Hanagal, *Modeling Survival Data Using Frailty Models*,
Industrial and Applied Mathematics, https://doi.org/10.1007/978-981-15-1181-3_8

Chernoff (1954) studied the asymptotic distributional behavior of the test statistic. Self and Liang (1987) considered likelihood ratio tests for independent and identically distributed observations. Silvapulle and Silvapulle (1995) study one-sided score tests, see also Verbeke and Molenberghs (2003) in the context of mixed linear models. Vu and Zhou (1997) derive general theoretical results. More information is contained in the overview paper by Sen and Silvapulle (2002).

Nguti et al. (2004) considered the following hypotheses testing for the random effect having the variance θ

$$H_0 : \theta = 0 \quad \text{versus} \quad H_a : \text{`} > 0$$

The likelihood ratio test for the above hypotheses testing problem does not follow the classical chi-square limit theory. Vaida and Xu (2000) state that for the likelihood ratio test, there is a correction for the null distribution, which is no longer a chi-square distribution. This has been discussed in similar setups by Stram and Lee (1994) and Self and Liang (1987) in the context of mixed effects models. Duchateau et al. (2002) simulate the limit distribution of the likelihood ratio test and conjecture that the simulated distribution is a 50:50 mixture of a χ_0^2 and a χ_1^2 distribution. Bjarnason and Hougaard (2000) use this model to study the Fisher information.

8.2.1   The Model and the Main Results

Consider a set of n independent and identically distributed random vectors $T_i = (T_{i1}, T_{i2})$, $i = 1, 2, ..., n$. Assume that each vector is a cluster of size two. Assume that the lifetimes T_{i1} and T_{i2} conditional on the frailty variables Z_i (for $Z_i = z$), are independent with a Weibull $(z\lambda, \gamma)$ distribution, i.e., the conditional hazard is

$$h(t|z) = z\lambda\gamma t^{\gamma-1}$$

with $\lambda > 0$ and $\gamma > 0$, where Z_i has the gamma density

$$f(z) = z^{\frac{1}{\theta}-1} \exp\left(-\frac{z}{\theta}\right) / [\Gamma(1/\theta)\theta^{\frac{1}{\theta}}].$$

The dependence between T_{i1} and T_{i2} is caused by the frailty variables $Z_1, ..., Z_n$ representing unobserved common risk factors. The frailty variables are assumed to be independent with mean 1 and variance $\text{Var}(Z_i) = \theta$. Given $Z_i = z$, the conditional survival function of (T_{i1}, T_{i2}) is

$$S(t_1, t_2|z) = P(T_{i1} > t_1, T_{i2} > t_2|Z = z)$$
$$= \exp\{-z\lambda(t_1^{\gamma} + t_2^{\gamma})\}.$$

The unconditional survival function is

$$S(t_1, t_2) = E[\exp\{-z\lambda(t_1^\gamma + t_2^\gamma)\}].$$

The corresponding joint density is

$$f(t_1, t_2) = \frac{(1+\theta)\lambda^2\gamma^2 t_1^{\gamma-1} t_2^{\gamma-1}}{[1 + \theta\lambda(t_1^\gamma + t_2^\gamma)]^{\frac{1}{\theta}+2}}.$$

For $\theta > 0$, which implies heterogeneity between clusters, the components of the vector (T_{i1}, T_{i2}) are correlated which is the correlation within cluster. To quantify the within cluster dependence, one can use Kendall's coefficient of concordance which, in terms of the joint density and survival function, is given by

$$4 \int_0^\infty \int_0^\infty f(t_1, t_2) S(t_1, t_2) dt_1 dt_2 - 1,$$

see Hougaard (2000, p. 132) and Bjarnason and Hougaard (2000). For this model, Kendall's coefficient of concordance is $\theta/(2+\theta)$ which is zero for $\theta = 0$ (homogeneity between clusters). Moreover, one can easily obtain that

$$\lim_{\theta \to 0} f(t_1, t_2) = (\lambda\gamma t_1^{\gamma-1} e^{-\lambda t_1^\gamma})(\lambda\gamma t_2^{\gamma-1} e^{-\lambda t_2^\gamma}),$$

i.e., T_{i1} and T_{i2} are independent Weibull distributed random variables. The likelihood for the data is given by

$$\prod_{i=1}^n \frac{(1+\theta)\lambda^2\gamma^2 T_{i1}^{\gamma-1} T_{i2}^{\gamma-1}}{[1 + \theta\lambda(T_{i1}^\gamma + T_{i2}^\gamma)]^{\frac{1}{\theta}+2}}$$

with corresponding loglikelihood

$$L = \sum_{i=1}^n [2\ln\lambda + 2\ln\gamma + \ln(1+\theta) + (\gamma-1)(\ln T_{i1} + \ln T_{i2})$$

$$- \left(\frac{1}{\theta}+2\right)\ln(1 + \theta\lambda(T_{i1}^\gamma + T_{i2}^\gamma))].$$

To test the within cluster dependence, we consider the testing problem $H_0 : \theta = 0$ against $H_a : \theta > 0$. For further discussion, it is convenient to work with the following transformed Weibull parameters: $\eta = -\ln\lambda$ and $\alpha = -\ln\gamma$; or $\lambda = \exp(-\eta)$ and $\gamma = \exp(-\alpha)$. Further, we use τ as a shorthand notation for the set of model parameters (θ, η, α) and $\nu = (\eta, \alpha)$ for the set of nuisance parameters.

The corresponding likelihood ratio statistic is

$$\Lambda = 2(\max L(\tau) - \max L_0(\tau))$$

where $\max L(\tau)$ and $\max L_0(\tau)$ are maximum loglikelihoods under H_a and H_0, respectively.

8.2.2   Analysis of Diabetic Retinopathy

Claeskens et al. (2005) establish the limiting distribution of the likelihood ratio statistic when covariate information is present. The asymptotic distribution of the related score test was also discussed by Claeskens et al. (2005). The diabetic retinopathy data (Huster et al. 1989) was used to test the heterogeneity by considering time to blindness in each eye of 197 patients with diabetic retinopathy. One eye of each patient is randomly selected for treatment and the other eye is observed without treatment. The data are bivariate right censored data with a treatment indicator as a covariate. They assumed Weibull distribution as a baseline for this data with scale parameter λ and shape parameter γ and the positive stable frailty distribution with parameter θ. They obtained the parameter estimates and their standard errors which are presented in Table 8.1.

The null and full loglikelihood models values are -846.499 and -841.272, respectively. The -2loglikelihood is 10.454 which is the likelihood ratio statistic. The p-value for the one-sided likelihood ratio test equals 0.0006. This implies heterogeneity is present by the construction of a profile likelihood-based confidence interval for θ. For a given value of θ, maximize $L(\theta, \lambda, \gamma, \beta)$ with respect to λ, γ, and β, for a given θ. Claeskens et al. (2006) and Morgan (1992) obtained the profile likelihood-based confidence interval. They obtained 95% confidence limits for θ (0.32, 1.20) which does not include zero, hence heterogeneity is present in the data.

8.3   Logrank Tests for Testing $\beta = 0$

The logrank test proposed from different viewpoints by Savage (1956), Mantel (1966), Peto and Peto (1972) among others is the optimal nonparametric test for testing the null hypothesis $\beta = 0$ in the proportional hazards model

$$h_i(t) = \exp(\beta y_i + \gamma w_i)b_0(t) \tag{8.1}$$

for a (different) unknown baseline hazard function $b_0(t)$. For example, y is the treatment assigned by randomization in a clinical trial and w is an unknown covariate. The test for $\beta = 0$ has been considered explicitly by numerous authors, for example, Lagakos and Schoenfeld (1984), Morgan (1986), and Struthers and Kalbfleisch (1986). Oakes and Jeong (1998) used the notation and some results from the theory of frailty models (see example Vaupel et al. 1979; Hougaard 1984; Oakes 1989) to connect this work with that of Gill (1980), Harrington and Fleming (1982), and others on weighted logrank tests.

Table 8.1 Diabetic retinopathy study: Parameter estimates (standard errors)

Model	θ	λ	γ	β
Full	0.712(0.145)	0.011(0.190)	0.888(0.006)	0.382(0.046)
Null	–	0.015(0.126)	0.799(0.005)	0.280(0.027)

Oakes and Jeong (1998) used the concept of the efficacy $e(U)$ (cf Pitman (1979), Chap. 5) of a test statistic $U(\beta)$ of the null hypothesis $\beta = 0$. The $U(\beta)$ is the derivative of a correctly or incorrectly specified loglikelihood function in β. Let $\mu(\beta) = E_\beta U$ and assume that $\mu(0) = 0$. Note that expectations and variances are always taken under the null hypothesis $\beta = 0$ unless indicated otherwise by subscript. Then

$$e(U) = \lim_{n\to\infty} \frac{1}{n} \frac{\{\mu'(0)\}^2}{\mathrm{var}\{U(0)\}}.$$

When U is an asymptotically efficient test, for example, when it is based on the score statistic $U(\beta)$ from the true loglikelihood, the efficacy equals the unit Fisher information. The asymptotic relative efficiency (ARE) of a test statistic $\overline{U}$ to another test U of the same hypothesis against the same class of alternatives is the ratio of their efficaciousness. It is well-known that when U is an efficient test, this ratio is just $\rho^2(\overline{U}, U)$, the squared correlation between the two test statistics under the null hypothesis.

Parametric Tests for Uncensored Samples

Oakes and Jeong (1998) proposed parametric test in uncensored samples for testing $\beta = 0$. Suppose that the baseline hazard $b_0(t)$ in Eq. (8.1) is known and that the value of the covariate w_i is observed for every individual as well as that of y_i. The loglikelihood in (β, γ) is

$$l(\beta) = \sum \ln h(t) + \sum \ln S(t)$$
$$= \beta \sum y_i + \gamma \sum w_i + n \ln b_0(t_i) - \sum \exp(\beta y_i + \gamma w_i) B_i,$$

where $B_i = B(t_i) = \int_0^{t_i} b_0(u_i) du_i$. The scores in (β, γ) are

$$\frac{\partial l}{\partial \beta} = \sum y_i - \sum y_i \theta_i z_i B_i = U_1^{(p)}(\beta),$$

where $\theta = exp(\beta y_i)$ and $z_i = exp(\gamma w_i)$; the superscript p denoting "parametric",

$$\frac{\partial l}{\partial \gamma} = \sum w_i - \sum w_i \theta_i z_i B_i,$$

and the observed information matrix has elements

$$-\frac{\partial^2 l}{\partial \beta^2} = \sum y_i^2 \theta_i z_i B_i,$$
$$-\frac{\partial^2 l}{\partial \beta \partial \gamma} = \sum y_i w_i \theta_i z_i B_i,$$

$$-\frac{\partial^2 l}{\partial \gamma^2} = \sum w_i^2 \theta_i z_i B_i.$$

Viewed as random variables, each term $\theta_i z_i B_i$ has a unit exponential distribution, so the elements of the unit Fisher information matrix are simply $\mathcal{I}_{\beta\beta}^{(p)} = n^{-1} \sum y_i^2, \mathcal{I}_{\beta\gamma}^{(p)} = n^{-1} \sum y_i w_i \to 0, \mathcal{I}_{\gamma\gamma}^{(p)} = n^{-1} \sum w_i^2$. Hence β and γ are asymptotically orthogonal, and the effective limiting unit Fisher information for β is $\lim n^{-1} var[U_1^{(p)}(0)] = \lim \mathcal{I}_1^p(\beta) = \lim n^{-1} \sum y_i^2$ whether or not γ is known.

Suppose now that the w_i are not observed such that the Z_i are independent and identically distributed random variables with a common distribution that has Laplace transform $p(s) = E \exp(-sZ)$. The survivor function and density for subject i are respectively $S_i(t, \beta) = p(\theta_i B)$ and $f_i(t, \beta) = -\theta_i p'(\theta_i B)b_0(t)$. The total loglikelihood is (recalling that $\sum y_i = 0$)

$$l(\beta) = -\left[\sum \ln\{-p'(\theta_i \beta_i)\} + \sum \ln b_0(t_i)\right].$$

The unit Fisher information at $\beta = 0$ is

$$\mathcal{I}_2^{(p)}(0) = n^{-1} \sum y_i^2 \left[\int \frac{\{Bp''(B)\}^2}{-p'(B)} dB - 1\right].$$

See Oakes and Jeong (1998). Since both $U_2^{(p)}$ and $U_1^{(p)}$ are score statistics from correctly specified loglikelihoods, the former based on less data than the later, their relative efficacy $e(2 : 1)$ is the ratio of the two information, namely

$$e(2 : 1) = \int \frac{\{Bp''(B)\}^2}{-p'(B)} dB - 1.$$

Oakes and Jeong (1998) considered the score test obtained under the incorrect assumption that the $w_i = 1$, the proportional hazards model. The density of T_i under this model would be $f_i(t) = -\theta_i p(B_i)^{\theta_i - 1} p'(B_i)b_0(t)$. The score statistic evaluated at $\beta = 0$ is

$$U_3^{(p)} = \sum y_i \ln p(B_i).$$

It is easily shown that $var(U_3^{(p)}) = \sum y_i^2$. The ARE of this test relative to the test based on $U_2^{(p)}$, which is best for this model, is

$$e(3 : 2) = e(U_3^{(p)})/e(U_2^{(p)}) = \rho^2(U_2^{(p)}, U_3^{(p)})$$
$$= \frac{[\int B\{p'(B)\}^2/p(B)dB]^2}{\int \{Bp''(B)\}^2/\{-p'(B)\}dB - 1}.$$

The ARE of $U_3^{(p)}$ relative to $U_1^{(p)}$ is

$$e(3:1) = e(3:2)e(2:1) = \left[\int \frac{B\{p'(B)\}^2}{p(B)} dB \right]^2.$$

Oakes and Jeong (1998) also considered nonparametric tests of the hypothesis $\beta = 0$ and also based on censored samples.

8.4 Test for Heterogeneity in Kidney Infection Data

McGilchrist and Aisbett (1991) presented data for the recurrence times (in days) of infections of 38 kidney patients from insertion of a catheter until it had to be removed owing to infection. In this data, there are three covariates: age, gender (1 for males and 2 for females), and type of disease ($0 = GN, 1 = AN, 2 = PKD$, and $3 = $ other). The survival time of the jth recurrence ($j = 1, 2$) in the ith patient ($i = 1, \cdots, 38$) is denoted by t_{ij}. Given the above covariates y_{ij} and the unobserved frailties z_i, the hazard function is modeled as

$$\lambda(t_{ij}|y_{ij}, z_i) = z_i \lambda_0(t_{ij}) \exp(\beta' y_{ij}), \tag{8.2}$$

where $\lambda_0(\cdot)$ denotes for the baseline hazard function and β is the regression parameter. This model supports the assumption that the frailties of the 38 different individuals are independent and frailty is common for the two recurrent times of the individuals. This data set has been used by several authors to investigate the effect of frailty in the survival data. For example, see Hougaard (2000), Ibrahim et al. (2001), and Therneau and Grambsch (2000).

In most articles the frailties, z_i are assumed to be i.i.d. which, however, is not always true. Lee and Lee (2003) considered that the heterogeneity of the frailty distribution was based on noticing the differences between the two recurrent times for the individuals. They found that some patients have very large deviations and others have relatively small ones, which suggests that the 38 patients might have come from a heterogeneous population and should be classified into several groups to make a more correct inference. Therefore, Lee and Lee (2003) claim that this phenomenon is a result of the heterogeneity of the frailty distribution.

In order to check the heterogeneity of the frailty distribution, Lee and Lee (2003) assume that the $\ln Z_i$ in Eq. (8.2) follow a normal distribution with mean zero and variance σ^2, provided all the frailties follow a common distribution. The hypotheses is to be tested as

$$H_0 : \sigma_i^2 = \sigma^2, \ i = 1, 2, ..., n \ \text{ versus } \ H_1 : \alpha_i^2 \neq \alpha^2 \ \text{ at least for one } \ i.$$

Lee and Lee (2003) rearrange the estimated frailties, $\hat{z}_i$'s, according to the magnitude of the differences between the two recurrent times, regardless of censoring. More precisely, letting $\Delta_i = |t_{i1} - t_{i2}|$, the interval size, Lee and Lee (2003) assume z_i to be associated with its interval size Δ_i, viz., $z_i := z_i(\Delta_i)$, and rearrange the $\hat{z}_i$'s in order corresponding to the magnitude of Δ_i. The censoring times are treated like event times for simplicity. Then apply the cusum of squares test based on the ordered $\hat{z}_i$'s and construct the cusum of squares test statistic:

$$T_n := \max_{1 \le k \le n} D_k := \frac{1}{\sqrt{n}\hat{k}_n} \max_{1 \le k \le n} \left| \sum_{t=1}^{k} \hat{z}_t^2 - \frac{k}{n} \sum_{t=1}^{n} \hat{z}_t^2 \right|$$

where

$$\hat{k}_n^2 = n^{-1} \sum_{t=1}^{n} \hat{z}_t^4 - \left(n^{-1} \sum_{t=1}^{n} \hat{z}_t^2 \right)^2.$$

Then we reject H_0 if T_n is large.

Employ the cusum of squares test since it is simple to construct and useful not only for testing for a variance change but also for detecting the location where the change point occurs. Also, it is a distribution-free test and can be used for any underlying distributions. As a matter of fact, it is well-known that for any i.i.d. r.v.'s x_i with a fourth moment,

$$S_n := \frac{1}{\sqrt{n}\hat{\tau}_n} \max_{1 \le k \le n} \left| \sum_{t=1}^{k} x_t^2 - \frac{k}{n} \sum_{t=1}^{n} x_t^2 \right|,$$

where

$$\hat{\tau}_n^2 = n^{-1} \sum_{t=1}^{n} x_t^4 - \left(n^{-1} \sum_{t=1}^{n} x_t^2 \right)^2$$

converges in law to the sup of a standard Brownian bridge due to Donsker's invariance principle (cf. Billingsley 1968). Thus given the critical values, any significance level is easily obtained from an existing table. For example, for the significance level $\alpha = 0.05$, the associated critical value is 1.358. For the details regarding the cusum of squares test, see Inclan and Tiao (1994) and the articles cited therein.

Lee and Lee (2003) observe that there is one significant variance change in the frailties at $\Delta_i = 122$, that is, the 33rd patient ($k = 25$). This indicates that the frailty tends to have a different variation depending on the interval size. They considered a new model to fit the data based on this fact. This justifies that the new model explains the kidney infection data better than the original method.

Models and Methods

Consider the following two models:

Model I: This model refers to the frailty model in Eq. (8.2), where the $\ln Z_i$ follow a normal distribution with mean zero and variance σ^2.

Table 8.2 Regression estimates (standard error) from Model I and Model II

		Disease		
Age $\hat{\beta}_1$	Sex $\hat{\beta}_2$	Type = 0 $\hat{\beta}_3$	Type = 1 $\hat{\beta}_4$	Type = 2 $\hat{\beta}_5$
Model I: $\hat{\sigma}^2 = 0.483$				
0.0052 (0.0147)	−1.6790 (0.4582)	0.1807 (0.5354)	0.3936 (0.5368)	−1.1400 (0.8099)
Model II: $\hat{\sigma}_1^2 = 0.0003$, $\hat{\sigma}_2^2 = 1.494$				
0.0046 (0.0116)	−1.8252 (0.3999)	0.4530 (0.4493)	0.2444 (0.4184)	−1.0230 (0.7800)

Model II: The proposed model is based on the variance change test. Assume that the frailties are classified into two groups, say, Group 1 ($\Delta_i < 122$) and Group 2 ($\Delta_i \geq 122$) and assume

$$\ln Z_i \sim \begin{cases} N(0, \sigma_1^2) & \Delta_i < 122 \\ N(0, \sigma_2^2) & \Delta_i \geq 122 \end{cases}.$$

The parameters of the two models are estimated using the best linear unbiased prediction (BLUP) estimation using an iterative Newton–Raphson method (cf. McGilchrist and Aisbett 1991). The variance of the frailties are computed from restricted maximum likelihood (REML) equations which allow ties in survival times.

Now fit Model II to the kidney infection data. From Table 8.2, one can see that Group 1 has no frailty effects; the estimated variance of 0.0003 is almost negligible. Group 2 has a frailty effect among the patients. This shows that covariates are sufficient to explain individual heterogeneity and there is no need to consider the frailties in Group 1. But in Group 2, the presence of random effects accommodate extra individual variation. Note that although both Models I and II yield almost the same $\hat{\beta}$, Model II produces a smaller variance for the regression parameter. This indicates that Model II outperforms Model I, and Model II gives us a clue as to the phenomenon of the various interval sizes.

Therneau and Grambsch (2000) argued that ignoring patient 21, the Cox's proportional hazards model without considering the frailty is well fitted to the kidney infection data. This implies that any nonzero estimated frailties are entirely due to this observation. Lee and Lee (2003) also analyzed the kidney infection data deleting patient 21. The results of this analysis are shown in Table 8.3.

The estimate of β_5 has a positive sign in Model I, whereas it had a negative sign before (but the other estimates keep their signs). Also, its absolute value changes from 1.1400 to 0.1881, which is a somewhat large change. This indicates that patient 21 influences greatly the estimation of β_5 in Model I. Meanwhile, in Model II, the estimates are not much affected by patient 21. This indicates that there is no substantial evidence to justify viewing this observation as an outlier at least in estimating the regression parameter based on Model II.

Table 8.3 Regression estimates (standard error) with patient 21 removed

		Disease		
Age $\hat{\beta}_1$	Sex $\hat{\beta}_2$	Type = 0 $\hat{\beta}_3$	Type = 1 $\hat{\beta}_4$	Type = 2 $\hat{\beta}_5$
Model I: $\hat{\sigma}^2 = 0.363$				
0.0017 (0.0142)	−1.9744 (0.4400)	0.2329 (0.5166)	0.5625 (0.5203)	0.1881 (0.8069)
Model II: $\hat{\sigma}_1^2 = 3.839 \times 10^{-8}$, $\hat{\sigma}_2^2 = 0.491$				
0.0021 (0.0118)	−1.8608 (0.3835)	0.3230 (0.4468)	0.3828 (0.4265)	−1.1579 (0.6971)

One can see that the removal of the observation affected substantially the variance of estimated frailties. As seen in Table 8.3, the variance is decreased in both Models I and II. This phenomenon is guessable since the REML solution is always sensitive to small changes in data. Actually, without patient 21, the variance of estimated frailties in Group 1 changes from 3.0×10^{-4} to 3.8×10^{-8}, which implies that assuming the frailty in Group 1 is even more meaningless than in the case with patient 21 included. This reduction in the variance effect is also seen in Group 2, but the variance is still significant, which supports the existence of frailties and is opposed to the result based on Model I.

References

Billingsley, P.: Covergence of Probability Measures. Wiley, New York (1968)

Bjarnason, H., Hougaard, P.: Fisher information for two gamma frailty bivariate Weibull models. Lifetime Data Anal. **6**, 59–71 (2000)

Chernoff, H.: On the distribution of likelihood ratio. Ann. Math. Stat. **25**, 573–578 (1954)

Claeskens, G., Nguti, R., Janssen, P.: One-sided tests in shared frailty models. (Preprint) (2006)

Claeskens, G., Nguti, R., Janssen, P.: One-sided tests in shared frailty models. Preprint, Unpublished (2005)

Duchateau, L., Janssen, P., Lindsey, P., Legrand, C., Nguti, R., Sylvester, R.: The shared frailty model and the power for heterogeneity tests in multicenter trials. Comput. Stat. Data Anal. **40**, 603–620 (2002)

Geerdens, C., Claeskens, G., Janssen, P.: Goodness-of-fit tests for the frailty distribution in proportional hazards models with shared frailty. Biostatistics **14**(3), 433–446 (2013)

Gill, R.D.: Censoring and stochastic integrals. Mathematical Centre Tracks 124: Mathematische Centre, Amsterdam (1980)

Harrington, D., Fleming, T.R.: A class of rank test procedures for censored survival data. Biometrika **69**, 553–566 (1982)

Hougaard, P.: Analysis of Multivariate Survival Data. Springer, New York (2000)

Hougaard, P.: Life table methods for heterogeneous populations: distributions describing heterogeneity. Biometrika **71**, 75–83 (1984)

Huster, W.J., Brookmeyer, R., Self, S.G.: Modelling paired survival data with covariates. Biometrics **45**, 145–156 (1989)

Ibrahim, J.G., Chen, M.H., Sinha, D.: Bayesian Survival Analysis. Springer Inc, New York (2001)

Inclan, C., Tiao, G.C.: Use of cumulative sums of squares for retrospective detection of changes of variances. J. Am. Stat. Assoc. **89**, 913–923 (1994)

Lagakos, S.W., Schoenfeld, D.: Properties of proportional hazards score tests under misspecified regression models. Biometrics **40**, 1037–1048 (1984)

Lee, S., Lee, S.: Testing heterogeneity for frailty distribution in shared frailty model. C. Stat. Theor. Methods. **32**(11), 2245–2253 (2003)

Mantel, N.: Evaluation of survival data and two new rank order statistics arising in its consideration. Cancer Chemother. Rep. **50**, 163–170 (1966)

Mazroui, Y., Mauguen, A., Pelissier, S.M., MacGrogan, G., Brouste, V., Rondeau, V.: Time varying coefficients in a multivariate frailty model: application to breast cancer recurrences of several types and death. Lifetime Data Anal. **22**(2), 191–215 (2016)

McGilchrist, C.A., Aisbett, C.W.: Regression with frailty in survival analysis. Biometrics **47**, 461–466 (1991)

Morgan, B.J.T.: Analysis of Quantal Response Data. Chapman & Hall, London (1992)

Morgan, T.M.: Omitting covariates from the proportional hazards model. Biometrics **42**, 993–995 (1986)

Nguti, R., Claeskens, G., Janssen, P.: Likelihood ratio tests for a shared frailty model: a non-standard problem. Technical Report, 309. Limburgs Central University, Belgium (2004)

Oakes, D.: Bivariate survival models induced by frailties. J. Am. Stat. Assoc. **84**, 487–493 (1989)

Oakes, D., Jeong, J.H.: Frailty models and rank tests. Lifetime Data Anal. **4**, 209–228 (1998)

Peto, R., Peto, J.: Asymptotically efficient rank invariant test procedures (with discussion). J. R. Stat. Soc., A **135**, 185–206 (1972)

Pitman, E.J.G.: Some basic theory of statistical inference. Chapman and Hall, London (1979)

Savage, I.R.: Contributions to the theory of rank order statistics-the two sample case. Ann. Math. Stat. **27**, 590–615 (1956)

Self, S.G., Liang, K.Y.: Asymptotic properties of maximum likelihood estimators and likelihood ratio tests under nonstandard conditions. J. Am. Stat. Assoc. **82**, 605–610 (1987)

Sen, P.K., Silvapulle, M.J.: An appraisal of some aspects of statistical inference under inequality constraints. J. Stat. Plan. Inference **107**, 3–43 (2002)

Silvapulle, M.J., Silvapulle, P.: A score test against one-sided alternatives. J. Am. Stat. Assoc. **90**, 342–349 (1995)

Stram, D.O., Lee, J.W.: Variance components testing in the longitudinal mixed effects models. Biometrics **50**, 1171–1177 (1994)

Struthers, C. Kalbfleisch, J.D.: Misspecified proportional hazard models. Biometrika, **73**, 363–369 (1986)

Therneau, T.M., Grambsch, P.M.: Modeling Survival Data: Extending the Cox Model. Springer, New York (2000)

Vaida, F., Xu, R.: Proportional hazards model with random effects. Stat. Med. **19**, 3309–3324 (2000)

Vaupel, J.W., Manton, K.G., Stallard, E.: The impact of heterogeneity on individual frailty on the dynamic of mortality. Demography **16**(3), 439–454 (1979)

Verbeke, G., Molenberghs, G.: The use of score tests for inference on variance components. Biometrics **59**, 254–262 (2003)

Vu, H.T.V., Zhou, S.: Generalization of likelihood ratio tests under nonstandard conditions. Ann. Stat. **25**, 897–916 (1997)

Chapter 9
Shared Gamma Frailty Models

9.1 Introduction

The shared gamma frailty model is a more widely used frailty distribution in the literature. In this chapter, we consider frailty distribution as gamma distribution because as the gamma variates are positive, it fits the nonnegative criterion of frailties with no transformation. The gamma frailty distribution is discussed in detail in Chap. 5, Sect. 5.1. The cross ratio function is constant for the gamma frailty model (see Clayton 1978). When there is no variability in the distribution of frailty variable Z that implies Z has a degenerate distribution and when the distribution of Z is not degenerate the dependence is positive.

Hanagal (2005, 2006) discussed the positive stable frailty and gamma frailty regression models in the bivariate survival data and Hanagal (2007a) also presented the gamma frailty regression models in the mixture distributions. Hanagal (2007b) proposed a power variance function frailty model with bivariate Weibull as the baseline distribution. Hanagal (2008) proposed a bivariate Weibull regression model with heterogeneity (frailty or random effect) which is generated by the log-normal distribution. Hanagal (2010) deals with modeling heterogeneity for bivariate survival data by the compound Poisson distribution with random scale. Hanagal (2011, 2017) gave extensive literature review on different frailty models. Shared frailty models are the most commonly used frailty models in literature, where individuals in the same cluster share a common frailty. Hanagal and Dabade (2012, 2013a, b, c, d, 2014, 2015), Hanagal and Kamble (2014a, b), Hanagal and Bhambure (2014, 2015, 2016) and Hanagal and Pandey (2014, 2015a, 2015b, 2016, 2017) and Hanagal et al. (2017a, b) analyzed kidney infection data using shared gamma and inverse Gaussian frailty models with different baseline distributions for the multiplicative model. Hanagal and Bhambure (2014) and Hanagal and Kamble (2014c) developed shared positive stable frailty model with different baseline distributions for the multiplicative model to analyze kidney infection data. Hanagal and Kamble (2015, 2016) analyzed kidney infection data using shared compound Poisson and compound negative binomial frailty models.

© Springer Nature Singapore Pte Ltd. 2019
D. D. Hanagal, *Modeling Survival Data Using Frailty Models*,
Industrial and Applied Mathematics, https://doi.org/10.1007/978-981-15-1181-3_9

Suppose n individuals are observed for the study and let a bivariate random variable (T_{1j}, T_{2j}) represent the first and the second the survival times of the jth individual $(j = 1, 2, \ldots, n)$. Also suppose that there are k observed covariates collected in a row vector $\mathbf{X}_j = (X_{1j}, \ldots, X_{kj})$ for the jth individual where X_{aj} $(a = 1, 2, \ldots, k)$ represents the value of the ath observed covariate for the jth individual. Here we assume that the first and the second survival times for each individual share the same value of the covariates. Let Z_j be shared frailty for the jth individual. Assuming that the frailties are acting multiplicatively on the baseline hazard function and both the survival times of individuals are conditionally independent for given frailty, the conditional hazard function for the jth individual at the ith $(i = 1, 2)$ survival time $t_{ij} > 0$ for given frailty $Z_j = z_j$ has the form,

$$h(t_{ij} \mid z_j, \mathbf{X}_j) = z_j h_0(t_{ij}) e^{\mathbf{X}_j \beta}$$

where $h_0(t_{ij})$ is the baseline hazard at time $t_{ij} > 0$ and $\beta = (\beta_1, \ldots, \beta_k)'$ is a column vector of order k, of the regression coefficients. The conditional cumulative hazard function for the jth individual at the ith survival time $t_{ij} > 0$ for a given frailty $Z_j = z_j$ is,

$$H(t_{ij} \mid z_j, \mathbf{X}_j) = z_j H_0(t_{ij}) \eta_j$$

where $\eta_j = e^{\mathbf{X}_j \beta}$ and $H_0(t_{ij})$ is the cumulative baseline hazard rate at time $t_{ij} > 0$. The conditional survival function for the jth individual at the ith survival time $t_{ij} > 0$ for a given frailty, $Z_j = z_j$ is,

$$
\begin{aligned}
S(t_{ij} \mid z_j, \mathbf{X}_j) &= e^{-H(t_{ij} \mid z_j, \mathbf{X}_j)} \\
&= e^{-z_j H_0(t_{ij}) \eta_j}
\end{aligned}
$$

Under the assumption of independence, the bivariate conditional survival function for a given frailty $Z_j = z_j$ at time $t_{1j} > 0$ and $t_{2j} > 0$ is,

$$
\begin{aligned}
S(t_{1j}, t_{2j} \mid z_j, \mathbf{X}_j) &= S(t_{1j} \mid z_j, \mathbf{X}_j) S(t_{2j} \mid z_j, \mathbf{X}_j) \\
&= e^{-z_j (H_{01}(t_{1j}) + H_{02}(t_{2j})) \eta_j}
\end{aligned}
$$

where $H_{01}(t_{1j})$ and $H_{02}(t_{2j})$ are the cumulative baseline hazard rates at times $t_{1j} > 0$ and $t_{2j} > 0$ respectively.

The unconditional bivariate survival function at time $t_{1j} > 0$ and $t_{2j} > 0$ can be obtained by integrating over the frailty variable Z_j having the probability function $f_Z(z_j)$, for the jth individual.

$$
\begin{aligned}
S(t_{1j}, t_{2j} \mid \mathbf{X}_j) &= \int_{Z_j} S(t_{1j}, t_{2j} \mid z_j) f_Z(z_j) dz_j \\
&= \int_{Z_j} e^{-z_j (H_{01}(t_{1j}) + H_{02}(t_{2j})) \eta_j} f_Z(z_j) dz_j
\end{aligned}
$$

$$= L_{Z_j}[(H_{01}(t_{1j}) + H_{02}(t_{2j}))\eta_j]$$

where $L_{Z_j}(.)$ is the Laplace transform of the frailty variable of Z_j for the jth individual. Here onwards we represent $S(t_{1j}, t_{2j} \mid \mathbf{X}_j)$ as $S(t_{1j}, t_{2j})$. When Z follows gamma distribution with single parameter θ as discussed in Chap. 5, the above bivariate survival function can be written incorporating gamma frailty for the random variable Z as follows:

$$S(t_{1j}, t_{2j}) = [1 + \theta \eta_j \{ (H_{01}(t_{1j}) + H_{02}(t_{2j})) \}]^{-\frac{1}{\theta}} \quad (9.1)$$

where $H_{01}(t_{1j})$ and $H_{02}(t_{2j})$ are the cumulative baseline hazard functions of the lifetime random variables T_{1j} and T_{2j}, respectively.

The bivariate distribution in the presence of covariates, when the frailty variable is degenerate is given by,

$$S(t_{1j}, t_{2j}) = e^{-\left(\eta_j \{ (H_{01}(t_{1j}) + H_{02}(t_{2j})) \} \right)} \quad (9.2)$$

According to different assumptions on the baseline distributions we get different shared gamma frailty models.

9.2 Baseline Distributions

9.2.1 Generalized Log-Logistic Distribution

The log-logistic distribution is very useful in a wide variety of applications, especially in the analysis of survival data (O'Quigley and Struthers 1982; Bennett 1983; Cox and Snell 1989). The log-logistic distribution is very similar in shape to the log-normal distribution, however, it has the advantage of having simple algebraic expressions for its survivor and hazard functions and a closed-form for its distribution function. It is therefore, more convenient than the log-normal distribution in handling censored data. However, due to the symmetry of the log-logistic distribution, it may be inappropriate for modeling censored survival data, especially for the cases where the hazard rate is skewed or heavily tailed. In this chapter we use a generalization of the log-logistic distribution and refer to this as the generalized log-logistic distribution given in Mohammed et al. (1990). The generalized log-logistic distribution reflects the skewness and the structure of the heavy tail and generally shows some improvement over the log-logistic distribution.

Mohammed et al. (1990) show that the distribution function of generalized logistic is given by,

$$F(x) = \frac{1}{\beta(m, n)} \int_0^{F_0(x)} u^{m-1}(1 - u)^{n-1} du$$

where $\beta(m, n)$ is the complete beta function and

$$F_0(x) = (1 + e^{-x})^{-1}, -\infty < x < \infty$$

is the logistic distribution function. We call $F(x)$ the generalized logistic distribution with parameters (m, n), and use the notation $X \sim GLD(m, n)$.

The logarithmic transformation $X = \gamma ln(\lambda T)$ applied to $GLD(m, 1)$ to obtain the generalized log-logistic distribution $GLLD(m, 1)$. The distribution function of T is,

$$F(t) = (1 + (\lambda t)^{-\gamma})^{-m}, t, m, \lambda > 0, \gamma \geq 1. \tag{9.3}$$

Similarly logarithmic transformation $X = \gamma ln(\lambda T)$ applied to $GLD(1, n)$ to obtain the generalized log-logistic distribution $GLLD(1, n)$. The distribution function of T is,

$$F(t) = 1 - (1 + (\lambda t)^{\gamma})^{-n}, t, n, \lambda > 0, \gamma \geq 1. \tag{9.4}$$

A random variable T with c.d.f. as given by Eqs. (9.3) and (9.4) are generalized log-logistic distribution with parameters $(m, 1)$ and $(1, n)$, respectively. We call Eq. (9.3) as generalized log-logistic type I and Eq. (9.4) as generalized log-logistic type II. Let us now consider for the sake illustration only one generalized log-logistic type II distribution.

Now rearranging the parameters, the survival function of the generalized log-logistic distribution type II is,

$$S(t) = (1 + (\lambda t)^{\gamma})^{-\alpha}.$$

The corresponding hazard rate and cumulative hazard rate are respectively as follows,

$$h(t) = \alpha \left(\frac{\lambda \gamma (\lambda t)^{\gamma - 1}}{1 + (\lambda t)^{\gamma}} \right)$$

$$H(t) = \alpha ln(1 + (\lambda t)^{\gamma})$$

When $\alpha = 1$, this distribution reduces to log-logistic distribution.

9.2.2 Generalized Weibull Distribution

In survival analysis, Weibull distribution is the most popular distribution to model lifetime data. We use the generalized Weibull distribution as a baseline distribution. If a continuous random variable T follows the generalized Weibull distribution then the survival function, the cumulative hazard rate function, and the hazard rate are respectively,

$$S(t) = 1 - (1 - e^{-\lambda t^\gamma})^\alpha \quad t > 0, \alpha > 0, \lambda > 0, \gamma > 0$$

$$H(t) = -ln(1 - (1 - e^{-\lambda t^\gamma})^\alpha)$$

$$h(t) = \frac{\alpha \lambda \gamma t^{\gamma-1} e^{-\lambda t^\gamma} (1 - e^{-\lambda t^\gamma})^{\alpha-1}}{1 - (1 - e^{-\lambda t^\gamma})^\alpha}$$

If $\gamma = 1, \alpha = 1$, the failure rate is constant (exponential), $\gamma \neq 1, \alpha = 1$, the failure rate is monotonic (Weibull), $\gamma < 1, \alpha < 1$, the failure rate is decreasing, $\gamma > 1, \alpha > 1$, the failure rate is increasing, $\gamma > 1, \alpha < 1$, the failure rate is bathtub or increasing and $\gamma < 1, \alpha > 1$, the failure rate is unimodal or decreasing. The generalized Weibull family can be used effectively in the analysis of the survival data. The family is versatile, accommodating monotone, unimodal, and bathtub-shaped hazard functions. The scaled total time on test (TTT) transform can be used to identify the shape of the hazard function. The family has closed-form expressions for the distribution functions and the hazard functions, and is closed under proportional hazards modeling. Because of its analytic tractability, the likelihood-based inference in the regular case and an alternative method based on a "modified likelihood" can be easily implemented see Mudholkar et al. (1993, 1995, 1996). Furthermore, it permits testing the goodness of fit of the Weibull distributions as sub models, which is not possible in most of the models with non-monotone hazard functions proposed in the literature.

9.2.3 Generalized Rayleigh Distribution

Burr (1942) introduced twelve different forms of cumulative distribution functions for modeling lifetime data. Recently, Surles and Padgett (2001) (see also Surles and Padgett (2004)) introduced the two-parameter Burr type X distribution and named it as the generalized Rayleigh distribution. Note that the two-parameter generalized Rayleigh distribution is a particular case of the generalized Weibull distribution, originally proposed by Mudholkar and Srivastava (1993) (see also Mudholkar, Srivastava and Freimer (1995)). The generalized Rayleigh (GR) distribution has a shape and a scale parameter. It is observed by Raquab and Kundu (2006) that for a shape parameter ≤ 0.5 the probability density function (PDF) of the GR distribution is a decreasing function and it is the right-skewed unimodal function for a shape parameter >0.5. The hazard function of GR distribution can be either bathtub shape or an increasing function depending on the shape parameter. Surles and Padgett (2001) showed that the two-parameter GR distribution can be used quite effectively in modeling strength data and also modeling general lifetime data. In survival analysis, the two-parameter generalized Rayleigh distribution can be used quite effectively in modeling strength data and also in modeling general lifetime data.

If a continuous random variable T follows the two-parameter generalized Rayleigh distribution, then the survival function, the hazard function, and the cumulative hazard function are, respectively,

$$S(t) = \begin{cases} 1 - \left(1 - e^{-(\lambda t)^2}\right)^{\alpha} & ; \ t > 0, \alpha > 0, \lambda > 0 \\ 1 & ; \ otherwise, \end{cases}$$

$$h(t) = \begin{cases} \dfrac{2\alpha\lambda^2 t e^{-(\lambda t)^2}\left(1 - e^{-(\lambda t)^2}\right)^{\alpha-1}}{1 - \left(1 - e^{-(\lambda t)^2}\right)^{\alpha}} & ; \ t > 0, \alpha > 0, \lambda > 0 \\ 0 & ; \ otherwise, \end{cases}$$

$$H(t) = \begin{cases} -\log\left[1 - \left(1 - e^{-(\lambda t)^2}\right)^{\alpha}\right] & ; \ t > 0, \alpha > 0, \lambda > 0 \\ 0 & ; \ otherwise, \end{cases}$$

where α and λ are, respectively, the shape and the scale parameters. In the case of $\alpha > 1/2$ the hazard function is an increasing function of time and when $\alpha \leq 1/2$, then hazard function is of a bathtub type.

9.2.4   Weighted Exponential Distribution

Gupta and Kundu (2009) introduced a shape parameter to an exponential family and named it as the weighted exponential distribution. The class of weighted exponential distributions has a shape and a scale parameter. The weighted exponential model can be observed as a hidden truncation model, as was observed in the case of skew-normal distribution by Arnold and Beaver (2000). The hazard function of weighted exponential distribution is an increasing function. This is suitable for modeling lifetime data when wear-out and aging are present. Therefore, it can be used quite effectively to analyze positively skewed data and it can be quite conveniently applied for censored data often arising in practice.

A continuous random variable T is said to follow the weighted exponential distribution if its survival function is,

$$S(t) = \begin{cases} \dfrac{\alpha+1}{\alpha}\left[e^{-(\lambda t)} - \dfrac{e^{-(\alpha+1)\lambda t}}{\alpha+1}\right] & ; \ t > 0, \alpha > 0, \lambda > 0 \\ 1 & ; \ otherwise, \end{cases}$$

where α and λ are, respectively, the shape and the scale parameters of the distribution. The hazard function and cumulative hazard function are, respectively,

$$h(t) = \begin{cases} \dfrac{(\alpha+1)\lambda\left(1-e^{-\alpha\lambda t}\right)}{\left[(\alpha+1)-e^{-\alpha\lambda t}\right]} & ;\ t > 0,\ \alpha > 0,\ \lambda > 0 \\ 0 & ;\ otherwise, \end{cases}$$

$$H(t) = \begin{cases} (\alpha+1)\lambda t + \log\alpha - \log\left[(\alpha+1)e^{\alpha\lambda t} - 1\right] & ;\ t > 0,\ \alpha > 0,\ \lambda > 0 \\ 0 & ;\ otherwise. \end{cases}$$

In this case the hazard function will be an increasing function for all $\alpha > 0$ (see Jones (2004)). Exponential distribution can be obtained only as a limiting distribution ($\alpha \to \infty$ and $\lambda = 1$).

9.2.5 Extended Weibull Distribution

The third baseline distribution we have considered is the extended Weibull distribution introduced by Xie et al. (2002). The extended Weibull distribution has shape and scale parameters. The model can be seen as a generalization of the Weibull distribution. The shape of the hazard function depends on a shape parameter γ. When $\gamma > 1$, for any $t > 0$, the hazard function $h(t)$ is an increasing function. When $\gamma < 1$, the hazard function has a bathtub shape property.

A continuous random variable T is said to follow the extended Weibull distribution if its survival function is,

$$S(t) = \begin{cases} e^{\alpha\lambda\left[1-e^{\left(\frac{t}{\alpha}\right)^{\gamma}}\right]} & ;\ t > 0,\ \gamma > 0,\ \alpha > 0,\ \lambda > 0 \\ 1 & ;\ otherwise, \end{cases}$$

where γ is shape parameter and λ and α are scale parameters of the distribution. The hazard function and cumulative hazard function are, respectively,

$$h(t) = \begin{cases} \lambda\gamma\left(\frac{t}{\alpha}\right)^{\gamma-1} e^{\left(\frac{t}{\alpha}\right)^{\gamma}} & ;\ t > 0,\ \gamma > 0,\ \alpha > 0,\ \lambda > 0 \\ 0 & ;\ otherwise, \end{cases}$$

$$H(t) = \begin{cases} \lambda\alpha\left[e^{\left(\frac{t}{\alpha}\right)^{\gamma}} - 1\right] & ;\ t > 0,\ \gamma > 0,\ \alpha > 0,\ \lambda > 0 \\ 0 & ;\ otherwise. \end{cases}$$

For the extended Weibull distribution, hazard function is an increasing function if $\gamma \geq 1$ and it is bathtub-shaped when $\gamma < 1$.

When scale parameter α becomes very large or approaches infinity, we have the standard two-parameter Weibull distribution with a shape parameter γ and a scale parameter $\frac{\alpha^{\gamma-1}}{\lambda}$.

9.3 Gamma Frailty with Baseline Distributions

Substituting cumulative hazard function for the generalized log-logistic type II, the generalized Weibull, generalized Rayleigh, weighted exponential, and extended Weibull baseline distributions in Eqs. (9.1) and (9.2), we get the unconditional bivariate survival functions at time $t_{1j} > 0$ and $t_{2j} > 0$ as,

$$S(t_{1j}, t_{2j}) = [1 + \theta \eta_j \{\alpha_1 ln(1 + (\lambda_1 t_{1j})^{\gamma_1}) + \alpha_2 ln(1 + (\lambda_2 t_{2j})^{\gamma_2})\}]^{-\frac{1}{\theta}} \quad (9.5)$$

for the case of generalized log-logistic type II baseline distribution with frailty.

$$S(t_{1j}, t_{2j}) = [1 - \theta \eta_j (ln[1 - (1 - e^{-\lambda_1 t_{1j}^{\gamma_1}})^{\alpha_1}] + ln[1 - (1 - e^{-\lambda_2 t_{2j}^{\gamma_2}})^{\alpha_2}])]^{-\frac{1}{\theta}} \quad (9.6)$$

for the case of generalized Weibull baseline distribution with frailty.

$$S(t_{1j}, t_{2j}) = \left[1 - \theta \left(\log\left[1 - \left(1 - e^{(\lambda_1 t_{1j})^2}\right)^{\alpha_1}\right] + \log\left[1 - \left(1 - e^{(\lambda_2 t_{2j})^2}\right)^{\alpha_2}\right]\right) \eta_j\right]^{-\frac{1}{\theta}} \quad (9.7)$$

for the case of the generalized Rayleigh baseline distribution with frailty,

$$S(t_{1j}, t_{2j}) = \left[1 + \theta \left(H_{01}(t_{1j}) + H_{02}(t_{2j})\right) \eta_j\right]^{-\frac{1}{\theta}}, \quad (9.8)$$

where,

$$H_{01}(t_{1j}) = (\alpha_1 + 1)\lambda_1 t_{1j} + \log \alpha_1 - \log[(\alpha_1 + 1)e^{\alpha_1 \lambda_1 t_{1j}} - 1]$$

and

$$H_{02}(t_{2j}) = (\alpha_2 + 1)\lambda_2 t_{2j} + \log \alpha_2 - \log[(\alpha_2 + 1)e^{\alpha_2 \lambda_2 t_{2j}} - 1]$$

for the case of the weighted exponential baseline distribution with frailty, and

$$S(t_{1j}, t_{2j}) = \left[1 + \theta(\lambda_1 \alpha_1 (e^{\left(\frac{t_{1j}}{\alpha_1}\right)^{\gamma_1}} - 1) + \lambda_2 \alpha_2 (e^{\left(\frac{t_{2j}}{\alpha_2}\right)^{\gamma_2}} - 1))\eta_j\right]^{-\frac{1}{\theta}} \quad (9.9)$$

for the case of the extended Weibull baseline distribution with frailty.

$$S(t_{1j}, t_{2j}) = exp(-\eta_j \{\alpha_1 ln(1 + (\lambda_1 t_{1j})^{\gamma_1}) + \alpha_2 ln(1 + (\lambda_2 t_{2j})^{\gamma_2})\}) \quad (9.10)$$

for the case of generalized log-logistic type II baseline distribution without frailty

$$S(t_{1j}, t_{2j}) = exp(\eta_j (ln[1 - (1 - e^{-\lambda_1 t_{1j}^{\gamma_1}})^{\alpha_1}] + ln[1 - (1 - e^{-\lambda_2 t_{2j}^{\gamma_2}})^{\alpha_2}]))$$

$$(9.11)$$

for the case of generalized Weibull baseline distribution without frailty

$$S(t_{1j}, t_{2j}) = e^{\eta_j \left(\log\left[1-\left(1-e^{(\lambda_1 t_{1j})^2}\right)^{\alpha_1}\right] + \log\left[1-\left(1-e^{(\lambda_2 t_{2j})^2}\right)^{\alpha_2}\right] \right)} \tag{9.12}$$

for the case of the generalized Rayleigh baseline distribution without frailty,

$$S(t_{1j}, t_{2j}) = e^{-\eta_j \left(H_{01}(t_{1j}) + H_{02}(t_{2j}) \right)}, \tag{9.13}$$

where $H_{01}(t_{1j})$ and $H_{02}(t_{2j})$ are given in equation (2.11) for the case of the weighted exponential baseline distribution without frailty, and

$$S(t_{1j}, t_{2j}) = e^{-\eta_j \left(\lambda_1 \alpha_1 \left[e^{\left(\frac{t_{1j}}{\alpha_1}\right)^{\gamma_1}} - 1 \right] + \lambda_2 \alpha_2 \left[e^{\left(\frac{t_{2j}}{\alpha_2}\right)^{\gamma_2}} - 1 \right] \right)} \tag{9.14}$$

for the case of the extended Weibull baseline distribution without frailty.

Here onwards we call Eqs. (9.5), (9.6), (9.7), (9.8), (9.9), (9.10), (9.11), (9.12), (9.13), and (9.14) as Model I, Model II, Model III, Model IV, Model V, Model VI, Model VII, Model VIII, Model IX, and Model X, respectively. Model I to Model V the models with frailty and Model VI to Model X are the models without frailty.

To every bivariate distribution function $F(t_1, t_2)$ with absolute marginal distribution functions $F(t_1)$ and $F(t_2)$, corresponds a unique function,

$$C : [0, 1] \times [0, 1] \rightarrow [0, 1],$$

is called a copula such that

$$F(t_1, t_2) = C(F(t_1), F(t_2)) \quad for \quad (t_1, t_2) \in (0, \infty) \times (0, \infty)$$

For a given copula C, there exists a unique survival copula $\overline{C}$, such that

$$\overline{C}(u, v) = u + v - 1 + C(1 - u, 1 - v)$$

and

$$S_{T_1, T_2}(t_1, t_2) = \overline{C}(S_{T_1}(t_1), S_{T_2}(t_2))$$

Here S_{T_1, T_2}, S_{T_1} and S_{T_2} are the survival functions. Conversely it is possible to construct a bivariate survival function using copula having the desired marginal survivals and a chosen dependence structure, see Nelsen (2006) for details. The joint bivariate survival function (9.5) to (9.9) can be expressed in terms of survival copula as,

$$\overline{C}(u, v) = \left[u^{-\theta} + v^{-\theta} - 1 \right]^{-1/\theta} \tag{9.15}$$

where $u = S_{T_1}(\cdot)$ and $v = S_{T_2}(\cdot)$

For Model I

$$S_{T_i}(t_i) = [1 + \theta\eta\{\alpha_i ln(1 + \lambda_i t_i^{\gamma_i})]^{-\frac{1}{\theta}}, i = 1, 2.$$

For Model II

$$S_{T_i}(t_i) = [1 - \theta\eta ln[1 - (1 - e^{-\lambda_i t_i^{\gamma_i}})^{\alpha_i}]]^{-\frac{1}{\theta}}, i = 1, 2.$$

for Model III

$$S_{T_i}(t_{ij}) = \left[1 - \theta\left(\log\left[1 - \left(1 - e^{(\lambda_i t_{ij})^2}\right)^{\alpha_i}\right]\right)\eta_j\right]^{-\left(\frac{1}{\theta}\right)}, i = 1, 2,$$

for Model IV

$$S_{T_i}(t_{ij}) = \left[1 + \theta\left((\alpha_i + 1)\lambda_i t_{ij} + ln\alpha_i - ln[(\alpha_i + 1)e^{\alpha_i \lambda_i t_{ij}} - 1]\right)\eta_j\right]^{-\frac{1}{\theta}}, i = 1, 2,$$

and
for Model V

$$S_{T_i}(t_{ij}) = \left[1 + \theta(\lambda_i\alpha_i(e^{\left(\frac{t_{ij}}{\alpha_i}\right)^{\gamma_i}} - 1)))\eta_j\right]^{-\frac{1}{\theta}}, i = 1, 2.$$

The above Eq. (9.15) is often called as Clayton Archimedean copula.

9.4 Likelihood Specification and Bayesian Estimation of Parameters

Suppose there are n individuals under study, whose first and second observed failure times are represented by (t_{1j}, t_{2j}). Let c_{1j} and c_{2j} be the observed censoring times for the jth individual $(j = 1, 2, 3, \ldots, n)$ for first and second recurrence times, respectively. We also assume that independence between censoring schemes and lifetimes of individuals.

The contribution of bivariate lifetime random variable of the jth individual in likelihood function is given by,

$$L_j(t_{1j}, t_{2j}) = \begin{cases} f_1(t_{1j}, t_{2j}), & t_{1j} < c_{1j}, t_{2j} < c_{2j}, \\ f_2(t_{1j}, c_{2j}), & t_{1j} < c_{1j}, t_{2j} > c_{2j}, \\ f_3(c_{1j}, t_{2j}), & t_{1j} > c_{1j}, t_{2j} < c_{2j}, \\ f_4(c_{1j}, c_{2j}), & t_{1j} > c_{1j}, t_{2j} > c_{2j}. \end{cases}$$

and the likelihood function is,

$$L(\psi, \beta, \theta) = \prod_{j=1}^{n_1} f_1(t_{1j}, t_{2j}) \prod_{j=1}^{n_2} f_2(t_{1j}, c_{2j}) \prod_{j=1}^{n_3} f_3(c_{1j}, t_{2j}) \prod_{j=1}^{n_4} f_4(c_{1j}, c_{2j}) \quad (9.16)$$

where θ, ψ and β are respectively the frailty parameter, the vector of baseline parameters and the vector of regression coefficients. For without frailty model likelihood function is,

$$L(\psi, \beta) = \prod_{j=1}^{n_1} f_1(t_{1j}, t_{2j}) \prod_{j=1}^{n_2} f_2(t_{1j}, c_{2j}) \prod_{j=1}^{n_3} f_3(c_{1j}, t_{2j}) \prod_{j=1}^{n_4} f_4(c_{1j}, c_{2j})$$

(9.17)

The counts n_1, n_2, n_3 and n_4 are the number of individuals for which first and the second failure times (t_{1j}, t_{2j}) lie in the ranges $t_{1j} < c_{1j}, t_{2j} < c_{2j}$; $t_{1j} < c_{1j}, t_{2j} > c_{2j}$; $t_{1j} > c_{1j}, t_{2j} < c_{2j}$ and $t_{1j} > c_{1j}, t_{2j} > c_{2j}$ respectively and

$$f_1(t_{1j}, t_{2j}) = \frac{\partial^2 S(t_{1j}, t_{2j})}{\partial t_{1j} \partial t_{2j}} = (1+\theta) h_{01}(t_{1j}) h_{02}(t_{2j}) S(t_{1j}, t_{2j})^{\frac{\theta+2}{\theta}} \eta_j^2$$

$$f_2(t_{1j}, c_{2j}) = -\frac{\partial S(t_{1j}, c_{2j})}{\partial t_{1j}} = h_{01}(t_{1j}) S(t_{1j}, c_{2j})^{\frac{\theta+1}{\theta}} \eta_j$$

$$f_3(c_{1j}, t_{2j}) = -\frac{\partial S(c_{1j}, t_{2j})}{\partial t_{2j}} = h_{02}(t_{2j}) S(c_{1j}, t_{2j})^{\frac{\theta+1}{\theta}} \eta_j$$

$$f_4(c_{1j}, c_{2j}) = S(c_{1j}, c_{2j})$$

Substituting hazard functions $h_{01}(t_{1j})$, $h_{02}(t_{2j})$ and survival function $S(t_{1j}, t_{2j})$ for the above ten models into the last relations we get the likelihood function given by Eq. (9.16) for Model I to Model V and (9.17) for Model VI and Model X.

Unfortunately, computing the maximum likelihood estimators (MLEs) involves solving the high dimensional optimization problems. As the method of maximum likelihood fails to estimate the parameters due to the convergence problem in the iterative procedure, we use the Bayesian approach. The traditional maximum likelihood approach to estimation is commonly used in survival analysis, but it can encounter difficulties with frailty models. Moreover, standard maximum likelihood-based inference methods may not be suitable for small sample sizes or situations in which there is heavy censoring (see Kheiri et al. (2007)). Thus, in our problem a Bayesian approach, which does not suffer from these difficulties, is a natural one, even though it is relatively computationally intensive.

The Bayesian approach to statistics treats unknown parameters of the models as random variables with some distributions known as prior distributions. In the Bayesian estimation, we obtain posterior mean using the Markov Chain Monte Carlo (MCMC) method which uses computer simulation techniques to obtain a Markov sequence with ergodic properties in such a way that it has a limiting distribution. The distribution of a parameter can be updated by combining its prior distribution and the likelihood function called the posterior density of a parameter. So if $L(y \mid \theta)$ is the likelihood function and $p(\theta)$ is the prior density of a parameter, then the posterior density function $\pi(\theta \mid y)$ is given by $\pi(\theta \mid y) \propto L(y \mid \theta) p(\theta)$.

In our case the joint posterior density function of parameters for given failure times is given by,

$$\pi(\lambda_1, \gamma_1, \lambda_2, \gamma_2, \theta, \underline{\beta}|t_1, t_2) \propto L(t_1, t_2|\lambda_1, \gamma_1, \lambda_2, \gamma_2, \theta, \underline{\beta})g_1(\lambda_1)g_2(\gamma_1)g_3(\lambda_2)g_4(\gamma_2)g_5(\theta) \prod_{j=0}^{p} p_j(\beta_j)$$

where $\beta = (\beta_0, \beta_1, \beta_2, \ldots, \beta_p)'$, $g_i(.)$ $(i = 1, 2, \cdots, 5)$ indicates the prior density function which is gamma distribution with known hyper parameters of corresponding argument for baseline parameters and frailty variance; $p_j(.)$ is prior density function for regression coefficient β_j which is normal with known hyperparameters and likelihood function $L(.)$ is the likelihood function of all parameters. Given the distribution $L(.)$ and the priors, all full conditional distributions of the parameters can be calculated. These full conditional distributions are used in a Gibbs sampling procedure. Here we assume that all the parameters are independently distributed. We have full conditional distribution of the parameter λ_1 as,

$$\pi_1(\lambda_1 \mid \gamma_1, \lambda_2, \gamma_2, \theta, \underline{\beta}) \propto L(\lambda_1, \gamma_1, \lambda_2, \gamma_2, \theta, \underline{\beta}) \cdot g_1(\lambda_1)$$
$$\pi_1(\lambda_1 \mid \gamma_1, \lambda_2, \gamma_2, \theta, \underline{\beta}) \approx L(\lambda_1, \gamma_1, \lambda_2, \gamma_2, \theta, \underline{\beta}) \cdot g_1(\lambda_1)$$

Similarly, full conditional distributions for other parameters are given by,

$$\pi_2(\gamma_1 \mid \lambda_1, \lambda_2, \gamma_2, \theta, \underline{\beta}) \approx L(\lambda_1, \gamma_1, \lambda_2, \gamma_2, \theta, \underline{\beta}) \cdot g_2(\gamma_1)$$
$$\pi_3(\lambda_2 \mid \lambda_1, \gamma_1, \gamma_2, \theta, \underline{\beta}) \approx L(\lambda_1, \gamma_1, \lambda_2, \gamma_2, \theta, \underline{\beta}) \cdot g_3(\lambda_2)$$
$$\pi_4(\gamma_2 \mid \lambda_1, \gamma_1, \lambda_2, \theta, \underline{\beta}) \approx L(\lambda_1, \gamma_1, \lambda_2, \gamma_2, \theta, \underline{\beta}) \cdot g_4(\gamma_2)$$
$$\pi_5(\theta \mid \lambda_1, \gamma_1, \lambda_2, \gamma_2, \underline{\beta}) \approx L(\lambda_1, \gamma_1, \lambda_2, \gamma_2, \theta, \underline{\beta}) \cdot g_5(\theta)$$
$$\pi_j'(\beta_j \mid \lambda_1, \gamma_1, \lambda_2, \gamma_2, \theta, \underline{\beta}^j) \approx L(\lambda_1, \gamma_1, \lambda_2, \gamma_2, \theta, \underline{\beta}) \cdot p_j(\beta_j)$$

where $\underline{\beta}^j$ represents a vector of regression coefficients except β_j; $j = 1, 2, \ldots, p$.

To estimate parameters of the model, the Bayesian approach is now popularly used, because the computation of the Bayesian analysis becomes feasible due to advances in computing technology. Several authors have discussed the Bayesian approach for the estimation of parameters of the frailty models. Some of them are, Ibrahim et al. (2001) and references their in, Santos and Achcar (2010). Santos and Achcar (2010) considered parametric models with Weibull and the generalized gamma distribution as the baseline distributions; gamma and the log-normal as frailty distributions. Ibrahim et al. (2001) and references therein considered the Weibull model and piecewise exponential model with gamma frailty. They also considered positive stable frailty models.

To estimate the parameters of the model, we used Metropolis-Hastings algorithm and Gibbs sampler. We monitored the convergence of a Markov chain to a stationary distribution by the Geweke test the (Geweke 1992) and the Gelman–Rubin Statistics Gelman and Rubin (1992). The trace plots, the coupling from the past plots and the sample autocorrelation plots are used to check the behavior of the chain, to decide the burn-in period and the autocorrelation lag, respectively.

Algorithm consists of successively obtaining a sample from the conditional distribution of each of the parameter given all other parameters of the model. These distributions are known as full conditional distributions. In our case, full conditional distributions are not easy to integrate out. Hence, full conditional distributions are obtained by considering that they are proportional to the joint distribution of the parameters of the model. The detail discussion on the simulation study based on Bayesian approach is given in Hanagal and Pandey (2015a) and Hanagal Bhambure (2015).

In order to compare the proposed models we use the Akaike information criteria (AIC), the Bayesian information criteria (BIC) and the Deviance information criteria (DIC). The AIC was introduced by Akaike (1973) and the AIC is defined as,

$$AIC = D(\hat{\boldsymbol{\Theta}}) + 2p$$

where p represents the number of parameters of the model. $D(\hat{\boldsymbol{\Theta}})$ represents an estimate of the deviance evaluated at the posterior mean $\hat{\boldsymbol{\Theta}} = E(\boldsymbol{\Theta} \mid data)$. The deviance is defined by, $D(\boldsymbol{\Theta}) = -2 \cdot logL(\boldsymbol{\Theta})$, where $\boldsymbol{\Theta}$ is a vector of unknown parameters of the model and $L(\boldsymbol{\Theta})$ is the likelihood function of the model.

The BIC was introduced by Schwarz (1978) and the BIC is defined as,

$$BIC = D(\hat{\boldsymbol{\Theta}}) + p \cdot ln(n)$$

where n represents the number of data points.

The DIC, a generalization of AIC was introduced by Spiegelhalter et al. (2002) and is defined as,

$$DIC = D(\hat{\boldsymbol{\Theta}}) + 2 \cdot p_D$$

where p_D is the difference between the posterior mean of the deviance and the deviance of the posterior mean of parameters of interest, that is, $p_D = \overline{D} - D(\hat{\boldsymbol{\Theta}})$, where $\boldsymbol{D} = E(D(\boldsymbol{\Theta}) \mid data)$.

The Bayes factor B_{jk} for a model M_j against M_k for a given data $D = (t_{1j}, t_{2j})$; $(j = 1, 2, 3, \ldots, n)$ is

$$B_{jk} = \frac{P(D|M_j)}{P(D|M_k)}$$

where $P(D|M_k) = \int_S P(D|M_k)\pi(\theta_k|M_k)d\theta_k$; $(k = 1, 2, 3, \ldots, m)$ where θ_k is the vector of unknown parameters of model M_k, $\pi(\theta_k|M_k)$ is the prior density and S is the support of the parameter θ_k. Here m represents the number of models. Raftey (1994), following Jeffreys (1961), proposes the rules of thumb for interpreting twice the logarithm of the Bayes factor. For two models of substantive interest, M_j and

M_k, twice the log of the Bayes factor is approximately equal to the difference in their BIC approximations.

To compute Bayes factor we need to obtain $I_k = P(D|M_k)$. By considering one of the approaches given in Kass and Raftery (1995), we obtain the following MCMC estimate of I_k which is given by,

$$\hat{I}_k = \left\{ \frac{\sum_{i=1}^{N} P(D|\theta^{(i)})^{-1}}{N} \right\}^{-1}$$

which is harmonic mean of the likelihood values. Here N represents the posterior sample size and $\left\{ \theta^{(i)}, i = 1, \ldots, N \right\}$ is the sample from the prior distribution.

9.5   Analysis of Kidney Infection Data

To illustrate the Bayesian estimation procedure we use kidney infection data of McGilchrist and Aisbett (1991). The data related to recurrence times counted from the moment of the catheter insertion until its removal due to infection for 38 kidney patients using portable dialysis equipment. For each patient, the first and the second recurrence times (in days) of infection from the time of insertion of the catheter until it has to be removed owing to infection is recorded. The catheter may have to be removed for reasons other than kidney infection and this is regarded as censoring. So the survival time for a given patient may be the first or the second infection time or the censoring time. After the occurrence or censoring of the first infection sufficient (ten weeks interval) time was allowed for the infection to be cured before the second time the catheter was inserted. So the first and the second recurrence times are taken to be independent apart from the common frailty component. The data consists of five risk variables age, sex, and disease type GN, AN, and PKD where GN, AN, and PKD are short forms of Glomerulo Neptiritis, Acute Neptiritis, and Polycystic Kidney Disease. The kidney infection data is partially presented in Chap. 1.

Table 9.1 p-values of K–S Statistics for goodness of fit test for Kidney Infection data set

Distribution	Recurrence time	
	First	Second
Model I	0.44755	0.70024
Model II	0.33158	0.68668
Model III	0.8341	0.7740
Model IV	0.3669	0.7630
Model V	0.7985	0.7271

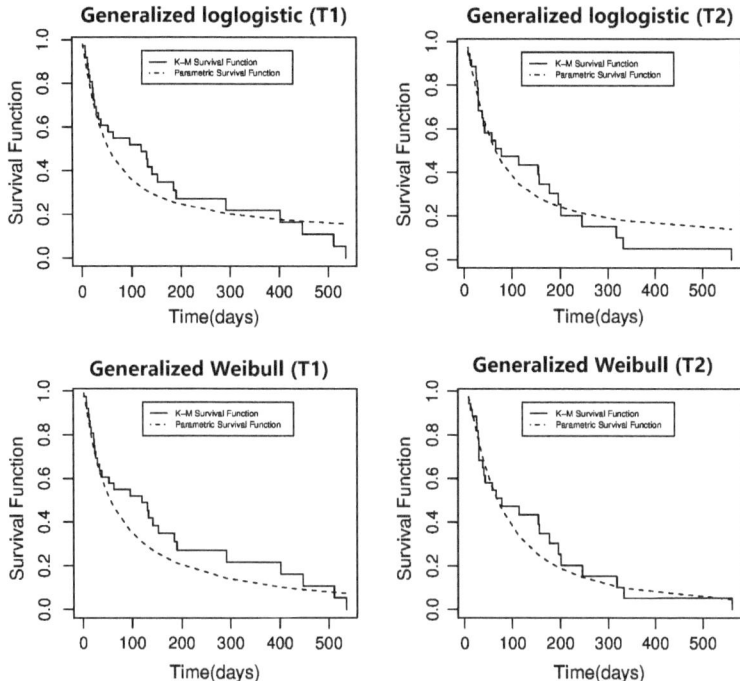

Fig. 9.1 Survival function plots for Kaplan–Meier survival and parametric survival

Let T_1 and T_2 represent the first and the second recurrence time to infection. Five covariates age, sex, and presence or absence of disease type GN, AN, and PKD are represented by X_1, X_2, X_3, X_4, and X_5. First, we check the goodness of fit of the data for the gamma frailty distributions with two baseline distributions and then we apply the Bayesian estimation procedure. To check the goodness of fit of the kidney data set, we consider Kolmogorove–Smirnov (K–S) test for two baseline distributions.

Table 9.1 gives the p-values of goodness of fit test for Model I to Model V. Thus, from p-values of K–S test we can say that there is no statistical evidence to reject the hypothesis that data are from these Models in the marginal case and we assume that they also fit for bivariate case. Figures 9.1 and 9.2 show the marginal survival function of the parametric with nonparametric plots for the five models with frailty and both lines are close to each other.

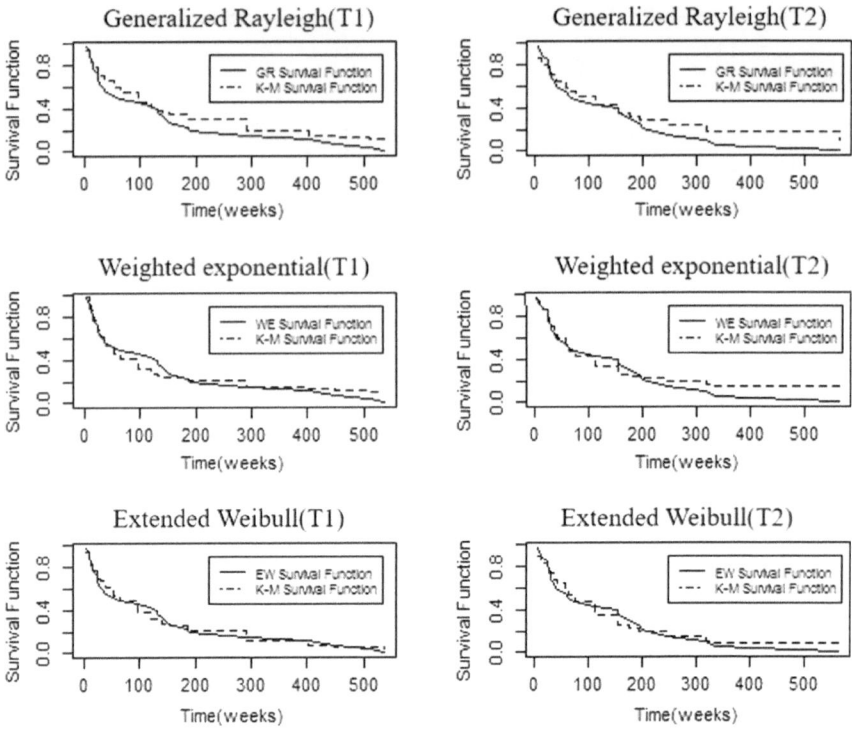

Fig. 9.2 Survival function plots for Kaplan–Meier survival and parametric survival

Here we assume two sets of prior distributions, i.e., uniform prior and gamma prior. We run two parallel chains for all the four models using two sets of prior distributions with the different starting points using the Metropolis-Hastings algorithm and the Gibbs sampler based on normal transition kernels. We iterate both the chains for 1,00,000 times. We got nearly the same estimates of parameters for both the set of prior and hence estimates are not dependent on the different prior distributions. The convergence rate of the Gibbs sampler for both the prior sets is almost the same. Also both the chains show somewhat similar results. So we present here the analysis for only one chain with $G(a_1, a_2)$ as prior to the baseline parameters, for all the ten models.

The trace plots for all the parameters show zigzag pattern which indicates that parameters move and mix more freely (See Fig. 9.3). Thus, it seems that the Markov chain has reached the stationary state. Burn-in period is decided by using coupling from the past plot. However, a sequence of draws after burn-in period may have autocorrelation. Because of the autocorrelation, consecutive draws may not be random, but values at widely separated time points are approximately independent. So, a pseudorandom sample from the posterior distribution can be found by taking values

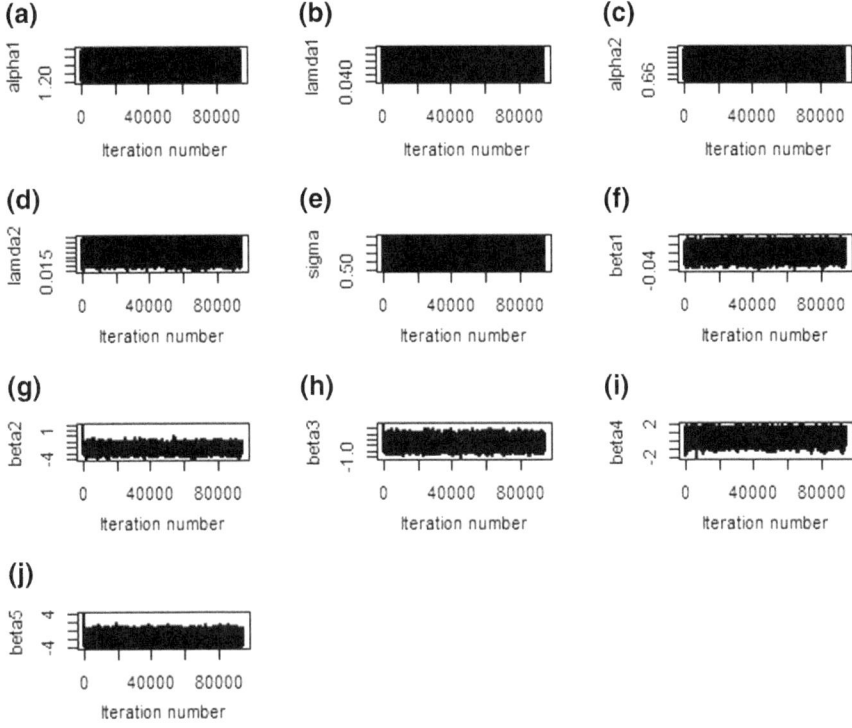

Fig. 9.3   Trace plots of kidney infection data for Model IV

from a single run of the Markov chain at widely spaced time points (autocorrelation lag) after burn-in period. This can be seen in Fig. 9.4. The autocorrelation of the parameters becomes almost negligible after certain lag. ACF plot (see Fig. 9.5) after thinning show that observations are independent. We can also use running mean plots to check how well our chains are mixing. A running mean plot is a plot of the iterations against the mean of the draws up to each iteration. In fact, running mean plots display a time series of the running mean for each parameter in each chain is displayed in Fig. 9.6. These plots should be converging to a value. Running mean plot for each parameter is converging to the posterior mean of the parameter, thus, represents a good mixing of chain. Thus, our diagnostic plots suggest that the MCMC chains are mixing very well. Due to lack of space, we are presenting the trace plots, the coupling from the past plots, the autocorrelation plots after thinning, and the running mean plots for the parameters of Model IV only.

The Gelman–Rubin convergence statistic values are nearly equal to one and the Geweke test statistic values are quite small and the corresponding p-values are large enough to say that the chains attain stationary distribution. The posterior mean and the standard error with 95% credible intervals, the Gelman–Rubin statistics values,

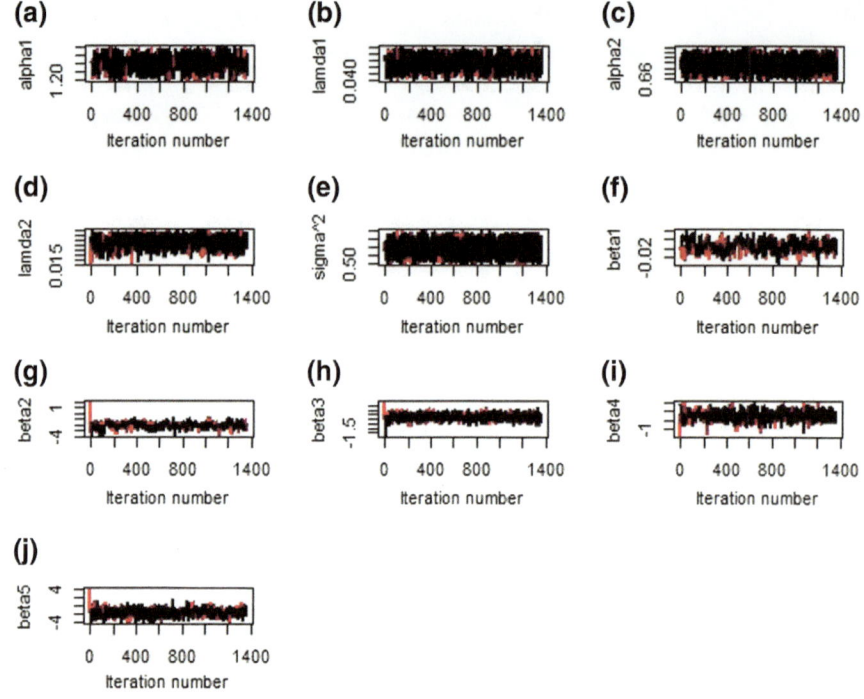

Fig. 9.4 Coupling from the past plot of kidney infection data for Model IV

and the Geweke test values with p-values for Model I to X are presented in Tables 9.2, 9.3, 9.4, 9.5, 9.6, 9.7, 9.8, 9.9, 9.10 and 9.11. The AIC, BIC and DIC values for all four models are given in Table 9.12. The Bayes factors for all models are given in Table 9.13.

The comparison between ten proposed models is done using AIC, BIC, and DIC values given in Table 9.12. The model with the smallest AIC, BIC, and DIC value is Model IV (weighted exponential) distribution with gamma frailty.

We also carry out the Bayesian test based on the Bayes factor to test frailty $\theta = 0$. Table 9.13 gives the Bayes factor values which are high for each test which concludes that the frailty parameter θ is not zero and the frailty is significant and favors to models with frailty.

Some patients are expected to be very prone to infection compared to others with the same covariate value. This is not surprising, as seen in the data set there is a male patient with infection time 8 and 16, and there is also male patient with infection time 152 and 562.

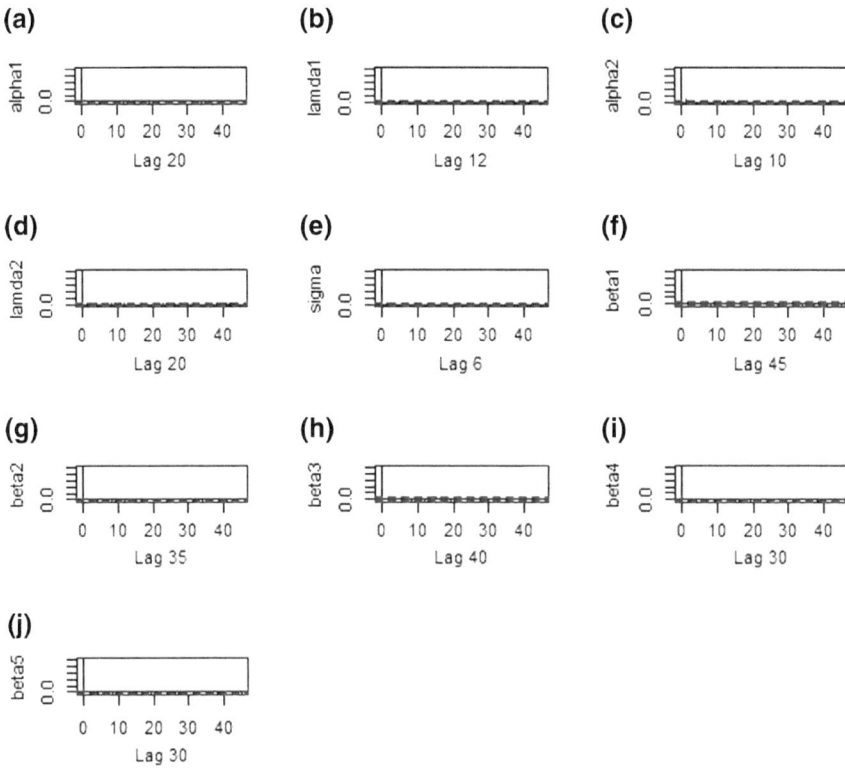

Fig. 9.5 Autocorrelation with thinning number lag of kidney infection data for Model IV

We can observe that the regression coefficients for all the ten models are different. The only credible interval of the regression coefficient β_2 does not contain zero which indicates that the covariate gender is a significant factor for all the models. A negative value of β_2 indicates that female patients have a slightly lower risk for infection than male patients.

Different prior distributions give the same estimates of the parameters. The convergence rate of the Gibbs sampling algorithm does not depend on these choices of the prior distributions in our proposed model for kidney infection data. It is observed that frailty is present and models with frailty fit better than without frailty models.

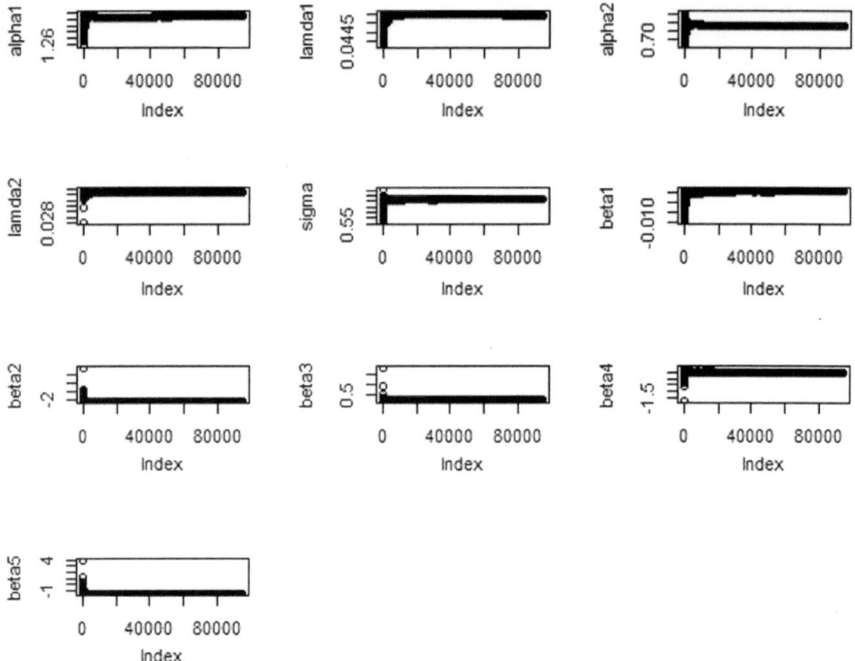

Fig. 9.6 Running mean plots of kidney infection data for Model IV

Table 9.2 Posterior summary for Kidney infarction data set Model I

Parameter	Estimate	Standard error	Lower credible limit	Upper credible Limit	Geweke values	p-values	Gelman and Rubin values
Burn-in period $= 6800$; Autocorrelation lag $= 300$							
α_1	2.3528	0.1563	2.0276	2.7047	0.01339	0.5053	1.0004
λ_1	0.0040	0.0019	0.0011	0.0081	0.01348	0.5053	1.0007
γ_1	1.3506	0.1719	1.0365	1.7077	−0.00827	0.4967	1.0013
α_2	4.0593	0.5330	3.1651	5.0485	−0.00039	0.4998	1.0049
λ_2	0.0017	0.0008	0.0004	0.0036	0.00699	0.5027	1.0027
γ_2	1.2729	0.1194	1.0466	1.4893	−0.00597	0.4976	1.0002
θ	0.4285	0.0594	0.3156	0.5358	0.00292	0.5011	1.0008
β_1	0.0184	0.0095	0.0003	0.0384	0.00269	0.5010	1.0010
β_2	−1.5653	0.4018	−2.3632	−0.7823	−0.00104	0.4995	1.0000
β_3	−0.1593	0.2535	−0.6602	0.3361	−0.01254	0.4949	1.0000
β_4	−0.0963	0.0462	−0.1883	−0.0072	0.01460	0.5058	1.0053
β_5	−1.2407	0.7797	−2.8605	0.2158	−0.00137	0.4994	0.9999

Table 9.3 Posterior summary for Kidney infarction data set Model II

Parameter	Estimate	Standard error	Lower credible limit	Upper credible limit	Geweke values	p-values	Gelman and Rubin values
Burn-in period = 12000; Autocorrelation lag = 180							
α_1	2.5416	0.3068	1.96442	3.17423	0.00674	0.4973	1.0000
λ_1	0.1603	0.0308	0.10757	0.22039	0.00745	0.5029	1.0010
γ_1	0.7672	0.0475	0.67774	0.85804	−0.00944	0.4962	1.0005
α_2	5.0844	0.4871	4.12195	5.94377	0.00080	0.5003	1.0000
λ_2	0.2101	0.0484	0.12505	0.33359	0.00326	0.5013	1.0019
γ_2	0.7087	0.0380	0.63741	0.78077	0.00398	0.5016	0.9999
θ	0.3890	0.1487	0.11149	0.70859	−0.00577	0.4977	1.0000
β_1	0.0019	0.0041	−0.00668	0.00983	−0.01601	0.4936	1.0001
β_2	−1.7487	0.4005	−2.53640	−0.93005	0.00918	0.4936	1.0015
β_3	0.0916	0.1353	−0.19238	0.34828	−0.00389	0.4984	1.0001
β_4	−0.0175	0.0139	−0.04558	0.00966	0.00150	0.5006	1.0050
β_5	0.0270	0.0286	−0.02627	0.08325	−0.01255	0.4949	1.0037

Table 9.4 Posterior summary for kidney infection data for Model III

Burn-in period = 4500

Parameter (values)	Lag	Estimate	SE	Lower credible limit	Upper credible limit	GR values	Geweke values	p-values
α_1	140	0.4638	0.0912	0.2958	0.6677	0.9999	0.0071	0.5028
λ_1	175	0.0079	0.0013	0.0049	0.0099	0.9999	0.0079	0.5031
α_2	60	0.6006	0.1098	0.3912	0.8239	1.0009	0.0054	0.5022
λ_2	350	0.0075	0.0013	0.0048	0.0098	1.0000	0.0024	0.5010
θ	350	0.7189	0.0586	0.5963	0.8438	1.0023	0.0101	0.5040
β_1	180	0.0231	0.0130	−0.0026	0.0496	0.9999	0.0013	0.5005
β_2	140	−1.8263	0.4989	−2.7827	−0.8760	0.9999	−0.0030	0.4988
β_3	80	0.3543	0.5996	−0.8831	1.4974	1.0006	−0.0001	0.4999
β_4	100	0.7420	0.5741	−0.3887	1.8193	1.0000	−0.0022	0.4991
β_5	100	−0.6886	0.9944	−2.5007	1.3070	1.0000	−0.0017	0.4993

Table 9.5 Posterior summary for kidney infection data for Model IV

Burn-in period = 2200

Parameter (values)	Lag	Estimate	SE	Lower credible limit	Upper credible limit	GR values	Geweke values	p-values
α_1	10	1.3020	0.0580	1.2059	1.3958	1.0006	0.0126	0.5050
λ_1	10	0.04537	0.0029	0.0403	0.0498	1.0042	0.0089	0.5035
α_2	10	0.7156	0.0366	0.6536	0.7765	1.0019	−0.0067	0.4973
λ_2	10	0.0367	0.0072	0.0228	0.04899	1.0017	0.0015	0.5006
θ	5	0.5918	0.0551	0.5045	0.6924	1.0009	−0.0033	0.4987
β_1	40	0.0087	0.0134	−0.0171	0.0346	1.0038	−0.0070	0.4972
β_2	40	−1.9827	0.5028	−2.9478	−0.9840	1.0006	0.0057	0.5023
β_3	40	0.0997	0.4342	−0.7502	0.9289	1.0006	0.0050	0.5020
β_4	40	0.5071	0.5497	−0.5957	1.5486	1.0031	0.0023	0.5009
β_5	40	−0.7768	0.9594	−2.7611	1.037	1.0056	0.0030	0.5012

Table 9.6 Posterior summary for kidney infection data for Model V

Burn-in period = 2100

Parameter (values)	Lag	Estimate	SE	Lower credible limit	Upper credible limit	GR values	Geweke values	p-values
γ_1	25	0.4626	0.0207	0.4240	0.4976	1.0010	0.0022	0.5009
α_1	75	13.9997	0.5656	13.0367	14.9393	1.0037	−0.0125	0.4950
λ_1	10	0.0454	0.0350	0.0322	0.0378	1.0034	0.0056	0.5022
γ_2	20	0.4501	0.0162	0.4222	0.4779	1.0001	0.0106	0.5042
α_2	80	9.4735	0.5515	8.5573	10.4263	1.0001	0.0013	0.5005
λ_2	10	0.0249	0.0017	0.0221	0.0278	1.0002	0.0054	0.5022
θ	20	0.8995	0.0172	0.8714	0.9284	1.0051	−0.0025	0.49901
β_1	150	−0.0066	0.0127	−0.03237	0.0181	1.0019	−0.0058	0.4977
β_2	75	−2.0605	0.5203	−3.0389	−1.0045	1.0006	0.0042	0.5012
β_3	100	0.2324	0.6388	−1.0024	1.4798	1.0006	0.00378	0.5015
β_4	140	0.7647	0.6172	−0.4877	1.8692	1.0048	0.0044	0.5017
β_5	100	0.0647	2.0322	−3.6267	3.9915	1.0088	−0.0070	0.4972

Table 9.7 Posterior summary for Kidney infarction data set Model VI

Parameter	Estimate	Standard error	Lower credible limit	Upper credible limit	Geweke values	p values	Gelman and Rubin values
Burn-in period = 6500;		Autocorrelation lag = 200					
α_1	1.56069	0.1592	1.23811	1.86376	0.00244	0.5009	0.9999
λ_1	0.00917	0.0044	0.00189	0.01828	0.00588	0.5023	1.0066
γ_1	1.28285	0.1834	0.96501	1.67353	−0.00184	0.4992	1.0033
α_2	1.28559	0.1448	1.01867	1.53773	−0.00051	0.4997	1.0020
λ_2	0.00425	0.0019	0.00101	0.00828	0.00707	0.5028	1.0004
γ_2	1.44945	0.1601	1.17399	1.77120	−0.00422	0.4983	1.0016
β_1	−0.00081	0.0014	−0.00362	0.00182	0.00250	0.5009	0.9999
β_2	−0.87672	0.2923	−1.43051	−0.26436	0.00061	0.5002	1.0000
β_3	0.17853	0.2649	−0.40278	0.72707	0.00696	0.5027	1.0000
β_4	−0.00889	0.0144	−0.03688	0.01721	−0.01237	0.4950	1.0000
β_5	0.02356	0.0142	−0.00127	0.05098	0.01150	0.5045	0.9999

Table 9.8 Posterior summary for Kidney infarction data set Model VII

Parameter	Estimate	Standard error	Lower credible limit	Upper credible limit	Geweke values	p-values	Gelman and Rubin values
Burn-in period = 12000;		Autocorrelation lag = 180					
α_1	2.4849	0.30943	1.8992	3.0831	−0.00829	0.4967	1.0001
λ_1	0.2031	0.06863	0.0905	0.3589	−0.00614	0.4975	0.9999
γ_1	0.6049	0.07812	0.4601	0.7620	0.01195	0.5047	0.9999
α_2	5.0401	0.50556	4.0999	5.9492	0.00073	0.5003	1.0003
λ_2	0.3222	0.08144	0.1758	0.4942	−0.00887	0.4965	1.0000
γ_2	0.5129	0.06162	0.3882	0.6333	0.01124	0.5045	1.0000
β_1	0.0007	0.00279	−0.0044	0.0063	−0.00968	0.4961	1.0004
β_2	−1.0716	0.31695	−1.6756	−0.4608	−0.01568	0.4937	0.9999
β_3	−0.0159	0.02781	−0.0677	0.0375	0.00845	0.5034	1.0004
β_4	−0.0041	0.00660	−0.0167	0.0078	−0.00533	0.4978	0.9999
β_5	0.0012	0.00185	−0.0021	0.0046	0.00589	0.5024	1.0000

Table 9.9 Posterior summary for kidney infection data for Model VIII

Burn-in period = 1800

Parameter (values)	Lag	Estimate	SE	Lower credible limit	Upper credible limit	GR values	Geweke values	p-values
α_1	20	0.44783	0.0114	0.4307	0.4687	0.9999	−0.0028	0.4989
λ_1	150	0.0056	0.0013	0.0032	0.0081	1.0027	−0.0051	0.4980
α_2	20	0.5981	0.0115	0.5807	0.6187	1.0022	0.0016	0.5006
λ_2	150	0.0052	0.0011	0.0032	0.0078	1.0012	−0.0024	0.4990
β_1	100	0.0209	0.0048	0.0113	0.0290	1.010	−0.0123	0.4951
β_2	125	−1.6336	0.3869	−2.3608	−0.8583	0.9999	0.0097	0.5039
β_3	50	0.0753	0.3922	−0.7066	0.8381	1.0007	0.00817	0.5033
β_4	50	0.7468	0.3850	−0.0309	1.4634	1.005	0.0020	0.5008
β_5	100	−1.7138	0.6110	−2.9308	−0.5483	0.9999	0.0099	0.5040

Table 9.10 Posterior summary for kidney infection data for Model IX

Burn-in period = 2500

Parameter (values)	Lag	Estimate	SE	Lower credible limit	Upper credible limit	GR values	Geweke values	p-values
α_1	150	2.0883	0.1715	1.8139	2.3877	1.0099	0.0103	0.5041
λ_1	20	0.1987	0.0111	0.1809	0.2187	1.0060	−0.0039	0.4984
α_2	45	2.1465	0.08613	2.0070	2.2911	1.0047	−0.0028	0.4989
λ_2	30	0.2511	0.0093	0.2404	0.2745	1.0032	−0.0033	0.4987
β_1	30	−0.0230	0.0047	−0.0297	−0.0126	1.0002	−0.0111	0.4956
β_2	20	−2.6668	0.2457	−3.1526	−2.1901	1.0007	0.0057	0.5023
β_3	10	−0.5081	0.3558	−1.2338	0.1692	1.0004	0.0036	0.50145
β_4	20	0.25078	0.3563	−0.4853	0.9323	1.0000	0.0046	0.5018
β_5	100	−2.3148	0.5143	−3.4059	−1.4092	1.0040	0.0045	0.5018

Table 9.11 Posterior summary for kidney infection data for Model X

Burn-in period = 990

Parameter (values)	Lag	Estimate	SE	Lower credible limit	Upper credible limit	GR values	Geweke values	p-values
γ_1	40	0.3746	0.0284	0.3179	0.4296	1.0010	−0.0088	0.4965
α_1	200	13.514	0.5696	12.4549	14.5708	1.0035	−0.0033	0.4987
λ_1	40	0.0177	0.0046	0.0079	0.0246	1.0027	0.01204	0.5048
γ_2	30	0.3439	0.0281	0.2960	0.4022	0.9998	0.0037	0.5015
α_2	25	9.5023	0.4547	8.6353	10.3926	0.9998	−0.00525	0.4979
λ_2	50	0.0196	0.0028	0.0152	0.0247	1.0061	−0.0028	0.4989
β_1	100	−0.0128	0.01317	−0.0404	0.0117	1.0069	−0.0162	0.4935
β_2	50	−0.9781	0.5554	−2.0634	0.1442	1.00072	0.01032	0.50412
β_3	75	0.2902	0.52673	−0.80951	1.2692	1.0010	0.0099	0.5040
β_4	75	0.6581	0.5587	−0.5198	1.6766	1.0076	0.0083	0.5033
β_5	30	−0.2049	1.5308	−3.2786	2.7443	1.0028	0.0042	0.5017

Table 9.12 Comparison of AIC, BIC, DIC

Models	AIC	BIC	DIC
Model I	696.9474	708.9749	678.1421
Model II	685.439	703.0278	672.4216
Model III	684.6523	701.0281	669.5283
Model IV	678.5526	691.2909	666.6380
Model V	696.8703	716.5214	686.7336
Model VI	696.9474	714.9608	683.9278
Model VII	690.2814	708.2949	678.103
Model VIII	891.5817	706.3200	689.5056
Model IX	706.7480	721.4863	706.7039
Model X	701.2239	719.2374	751.7975

Table 9.13 Bayesian tests based on Bayes factor values

Numerator model against denominator model	$2log(B_{jk})$	Range	Evidence against model in denominator
Model I against Model VI	3.73	2–6	Moderate
Model II against Model VII	11.72	>10	Very strong
Model III against Model VIII	257.6379	>10	Very strong
Model IV against Model IX	92.0560	>10	Very strong
Model V against Model X	823.345	>10	Very strong

$B_{jk} = \frac{M_j}{M_k}$

References

Arnold, B.C., Beaver, R.J.: The skew Cauchy distribution. Stat. Probab. Lett. **49**, 285–290 (2000)
Bennett, S.: Log-logistic regression model for survival data. Appl. Stat. **32**(2), 165–171 (1983)
Burr, I.W.: Cumulative frequency distribution. Ann. Math. Stat. **13**, 215–232 (1942)
Clayton, D.G.: A model for association in bivariate life tables and its application in epidemiological studies of familial tendency in chronic disease incidence. Biometrika **65**, 141–151 (1978)
Cox, D.R., Snell, E.J.: Analysis of Binary Data. Chapman and Hall, New York (1989)
El-Saidi, M.A., Singh, K.P., Bartolucci, A.A.: A note on a characterization of the generalized log-logistic distribution. Environmetrics **1**(4), 337–342 (1990)
Gelman, A., Rubin, D.B.: A single series from the Gibbs sampler provides a false sense of security. In: Bernardo, J.M., Berger, J.O., Dawid, A.P., Smith, A.F.M., (eds.), Bayesian Statistics, vol. 4, pp. 625–632. Oxford University Press, Oxford (1992)
Geweke, J.: Evaluating the Accuracy of Sampling-Based Approaches to the Calculation of Posterior Moments. In: Bernardo, J.M., Berger, J., Dawid, A.P., Smith, A.F.M. (eds.) Bayesian Statistics, vol. 4, pp. 169–193. Oxford University Press, Oxford (1992)
Gupta, R.D., Kundu, D.: A new class of weighted exponential distributions, statistics. J. Theor. Appl. Stat. **43**(6), 621–634 (2009)
Hanagal, D.D.: A positive stable frailty regression model in bivariate survival data. J. Indian. Soc. Probab. Stat. **19**, 35–44 (2005)

Hanagal, D.D.: A gamma frailty regression model in bivariate survival data. IAPQR Trans. **31**, 73–83 (2006)

Hanagal, D.D.: Positive stable frailty regression models in mixture distributions. In: Proceedings of 3rd International Conference on Reliability and Safety Engineering, 17–19, December, 2007, held at Indian Institute of Technology, Udaipur, India, pp. 350–356 (2007a)

Hanagal, D.D.: Gamma frailty regression models in mixture distributions. Econ. Qual. Control. **22**(2), 295–302 (2007b)

Hanagal,D.D.: Modeling heterogeneity for bivariate survival data by the lognormal distribution. Stat. Probab. Lett. **78**(9), 1101–1109 (2008)

Hanagal, D.D.: Correlated compound Poisoon frailty model for the bivariate survival data. Int. J. Stat. Manag. Syst. **5**, 127–140 (2010)

Hanagal, D.D.: Modeling Survival Data Using Frailty Models. Chapman and Hall, New York (2011)

Hanagal, D.D.: Frailty models in public health. In: Rao, A.S.R.S., Pyne S., Rao, C.R. (eds.) Handbook of Statistics. Disease Modelling and Public Health, vol. 37(B), pp. 209–247. Elsevier, Amsterdam (2017)

Hanagal, D.D., Bhambure, S.M.: Analysis of kidney infection data using positive stable frailty models. Adv. Reliab. **1**, 21–39 (2014)

Hanagal, D.D., Bhambure, S.M.: Comparison of shared gamma frailty models using Bayesian approach. Model Assist. Stat. Appl. **10**, 25–41 (2015)

Hanagal, D.D., Bhambure, S.M.: Modeling bivariate survival data using shared inverse Gaussian frailty model. Commun. Stat. Theory Methods **45**(17), 4969–4987 (2016)

Hanagal, D.D., Dabade, A.D.: Modeling hetrogeneity in bivariate survival data by compound Poisson distribution using Bayesian approach. Int. J. Stat. Manag. Syst. **7**(1–2), 36–84 (2012)

Hanagal, D.D., Dabade, A.D.: Modeling of inverse Gaussian frailty model for bivariate survival data. Commun. Stat. Theory Methods **42**(20), 3744–3769 (2013a)

Hanagal, D.D., Dabade, A.D.: Bayesian estimation of parameters and comparison of shared gamma frailty models. Commun. Stat. Simul. Comput. **42**(4), 910–931 (2013b)

Hanagal, D.D., Dabade, A.D.: Compound negative binomial shared frailty models for bivariate survival data. Stat. Probab. Lett. **83**, 2507–2515 (2013c)

Hanagal, D.D., Dabade, A.D.: A comparative study of shared frailty models for bivariate survival data with generalized exponential baseline distribution. J. Data Sci. **11**, 109–142 (2013d)

Hanagal, D.D., Dabade, A.D.: Comparisons of frailty models for kidney infection data under Weibull baseline distribution. Int. J. Math. Model. Numer. Optim. **5**(4), 342–373 (2014)

Hanagal, D.D., Dabade, A.D.: Comparisons of frailty models for kidney infection data under exponential power baseline distribution. Commun. Stat. Theory Methods **44**(23), 5091–5108 (2015)

Hanagal, D.D., Kamble, A.T.: Bayesian estimation in shared gamma frailty models. Int. J. Stat. Reliab. Eng. **1**(2), 88–112 (2014a)

Hanagal, D.D., Kamble, A.T.: Bayesian estimation in shared inverse Gaussian frailty models. Int. J. Stat. **1**, 9–20 (2014b)

Hanagal, D.D., Kamble, A.T.: Bayesian estimation in shared positive stable frailty models. J. Data Sci. **13**, 615–640 (2014c)

Hanagal, D.D., Kamble, A.T.: Bayesian estimation in shared compound Poisson frailty models. J. Reliab. Stat. Stud. **8**(1), 159–180 (2015)

Hanagal, D.D., Kamble, A.T.: Bayesian estimation in shared compound negative binomial frailty models. Res. Rev. J. Stat. Math. Sci. **2**(1), 53–67 (2016)

Hanagal, D.D., Pandey, A.: Inverse Gaussian shared frailty for modeling kidney infection data. Adv. Reliab. **1**, 1–14 (2014)

Hanagal, D.D., Pandey, A.: Gamma frailty models for bivariate survival data. J. Stat. Comput. Simul. **85**(15), 3172–3189 (2015a)

Hanagal, D.D., Pandey, A.: Gamma frailty model based on reversed hazard rate. Commun. Stat. Theory Methods **45**(7), 2071–2088 (2015b)

Hanagal, D.D., Pandey, A.: Gamma shared frailty model based on reversed hazard rate. Commun. Stat., Theory Methods **45**(7), 2071–2088 (2016)

Hanagal, D.D., Pandey, A.: Shared frailty models based on reversed hazard rate for modified inverse Weibull distribution as a baseline distribution. Commun. Stat., Theory Methods. **46**(1), 234–246 (2017)

Hanagal, D.D., Pandey, A., Sankaran, P.G.: Shared frailty model based on reversed hazard rate for left censoring data. Commun. Stat. Simul. Comput. **46**(1), 230–243 (2017a)

Hanagal, D.D., Pandey, A., Ganguly, A.: Correlated gamma frailty models for bivariate survival data. Commun. Stat. Simul. Comput. **46**(5), 3627–3644. (2017b)

Ibrahim, J.G., Chen, M.H., Sinha, D.: Bayesian Survival Analysis. Springer, New York (2001)

Jeffreys, H.: Theory of Probability, 3rd edn. Oxford University Press, Oxford (1961)

Jones, M.C.: Families of distributions arising from distributions of order statistics. Test **13**, 1–43 (2004)

Kass, R.E., Raftery, A.E.: Bayes factor. J. Am. Stat. Assoc. **90**(430), 773–795 (1995)

Kheiri, S., Kimber, A., Meshkani, M.R.: Bayesian analysis of an inverse Gaussian correlated frailty model. Comput. Stat. Data Anal. **51**, 5317–5326 (2007)

McGilchrist, C.A., Aisbett, C.W.: Regression with frailty in survival analysis. Biometrics **47**, 461–466 (1991)

Mudholkar, G.S., Srivastava, D.K.: Exponentiated Weibull family for analyzing bathtub failure data. IEEE Trans. Reliab. **42**, 299–302 (1993)

Mudholkar, G.S., Srivastava, D.K., Freimer, M.: The exponential Weibull family: a re-analysis of the bus-motor-failure data. Technometrics **37**, 436–445 (1995)

Mudholkar, G.S., Srivastava, D.K., Kollia, G.D.: A generalization of the Weibull distribution with application to the analysis of survival data. J. Am. Stat. Assoc. **91**(436), 1575–1583 (1996)

Nelsen, R.B.: An Introduction to Copulas, 2nd edn. Springer, New York (2006)

O'Quigley, J., Struthers, L.: Survival models based upon the logistic and loglogistic distributions. Comput. Programs Biomed. Res. **15**, 3–12 (1982)

Raftey, A.E.: Approximate Bayes factors and accounting for model uncertainty in generalized linear models. Biometrika **83**(2), 251–266 (1994)

Santos, C.A., Achcar, J.A.: A Bayesian analysis for multivariate survival data in the presence of covariates. J. Stat. Theory Appl. **9**, 233–253 (2010)

Schwarz, G.: Estimating the dimension of a model. Ann. Stat. **6**(2), 461–464 (1978)

Spiegelhalter, D.J., Best, N.G., Carlin, B.P., Van der Linde, A.: Bayesian measure of model complexity and fit (with discussion). J. R. Stat. Soc. B **64**, 583–639 (2002)

Surles, J.G., Padgett, W.J.: Inference for reliability and stress-strength for a scaled Burr Type X distribution. Lifetime Data Anal. **7**, 187–200 (2001)

Surles, J.G., Padgett, W.J.: Some properties of a scaled Burr type X distribution. J. Stat. Plan. Inference **18**(1), 271–280 (2004)

Xie, M., Tang, Y., Goh, T.N.: A modified Weibull extension with bathtub-shaped failure rate function. Reliab. Eng. Syst. Saf. **76**(3), 279–285 (2002)

Chapter 10
Shared Gamma Frailty Models Based on Reversed Hazard

10.1 Introduction

The models derived in previous chapter and reference sited in are based on the assumption that a common random effect acts multiplicatively on the hazard rate function. In many practical situations, reversed hazard rate (RHR) is more appropriate to analyze the survival data. Reversed hazard rate was proposed as a dual to the hazard rate by Barrow et al. (1963). Shake and Shantung (1994) and Block et al. (1998) provided a general definition of reversed hazard rate (RHR) as

$$m(t) = \lim_{\triangle t \to 0} P(t - \triangle t < T \le t | T \le t) / \triangle t, \quad t > 0. \tag{10.1}$$

The reversed hazard rate specifies the instantaneous rate of death or failure at time t, given that it failed before time t. Thus, in a small interval, $m(t) \triangle t$ is the approximate probability of failure in the interval, given failure before the end of the interval $(t - \triangle t, t]$. In lifetime data analysis, the concepts of reversed hazard rate has potential application when the time elapsed since failure is a quantity of interest in order to predict the actual time of failure. The reversed hazard rate is more useful in estimating reliability function when the data are left censored or right truncated. Reversed hazard rate plays a vital role in the analysis of parallel systems, in reliability and survival analysis. In case of parallel system of identical independently distributed components, the hazard rate of the system life is not proportional to the hazard rate of each component. However, the reversed hazard rates are proportional. The more details of reversed hazard rate of a distribution can be seen in Barrow et al. (1963), Shake and Shantung (1994), Block et al. (1998) and Sengupta and Nanda (1999).

The reversed hazard rate has been found to be useful for estimation of the survival function for left-censored lifetimes (see Kalbfliesh and Lawless 1989). For example, in certain systems or situations, sometimes the failure is prevented through numerous safety measures (see Gleeja 2008). Andersen et al. (1993), Lawless (2003) have discussed the use of reversed hazard rate for the analysis of left-censored or right-

© Springer Nature Singapore Pte Ltd. 2019
D. D. Hanagal, *Modeling Survival Data Using Frailty Models*,
Industrial and Applied Mathematics, https://doi.org/10.1007/978-981-15-1181-3_10

truncated data. Sankaran and Gleeja (2011) introduced a class of semiparametric frailty models in terms of reversed hazard rates, which is useful for the analysis of left-censored data. Hanagal and Bhambure (2014, 2017a, b) analyzed Australian twin data using shared gamma and inverse Gaussian frailty models based on reversed hazard rates. Hanagal and Pandey (2014, 2015a, b, c, d, e, 2016a, b, 2017a) developed shared gamma and inverse Gaussian frailty models based on reversed hazard rates to analyze Australian twin data using different baseline distributions.

Duffy et al. (1990) considered Australian twin data which consist of information about the age at appendectomy of monozygotic (MZ) and dizygotic (DZ) twins. There were some pairs with missing age at onset and those are the left-censored observations. Duffy et al. (1990) excluded these left-censored observations in the analysis. It is, therefore, appropriate to model common random effect by including those left-censored observations, which can be done by developing frailty models using RHR. Accordingly, Sankaran and Gleeja (2011) introduced frailty as a common random effect that acts multiplicatively on reversed hazard rates, which is useful for the analysis of left-censored data. In this chapter, parametric shared frailty model with gamma frailty using reversed hazard rate is developed. We use generalized log-logistic type I, generalized log-logistic type II distributions, and modified inverse Weibull distribution as baseline distributions and we compare these models with the Australian twin data and suggest a better model.

10.2   General Shared Frailty Models

The shared frailty model is relevant to event time of related individuals, similar organs, and repeated measurements. For example, the failure time of paired organs like kidneys, lungs, eyes, ears, dental implants, etc. is considered as event times. In this model, individuals from a group share common risks. For the shared frailty model, it is assumed that survival times are conditionally independent, for a given shared frailty. The shared frailty means the dependence between the survival times is only due to unobservable covariates or frailty. When there is no variability in the distribution of frailty variable Z, then Z has a degenerate distribution and when the distribution of Z is not degenerate, there is a positive dependence.

Suppose n individuals are observed for the study and let the bivariate random vector (T_{1j}, T_{2j}) represent the first and the second lifetimes of the jth individual $(j = 1, 2, 3, \ldots, n)$. Also, suppose that $\mathbf{X_0}$, $\mathbf{X_1}$, and $\mathbf{X_2}$ are the observed covariates, where $\mathbf{X_0}$ is the common covariate, $\mathbf{X_1}$ and $\mathbf{X_2}$ are the covariates corresponding to T_{1j} and T_{2j}, respectively. Let a vector $\mathbf{X}_{lj} = (X_{1lj}, \ldots, X_{k_l lj})$, $(l = 0, 1, 2)$ for the jth individual where X_{alj} $(a = 1, 2, 3, \ldots, k_l)$ represents the value of the ath observed covariate for the jth individual. We assume that the first and the second survival times for each individual share the same value of the covariates. Let Z_j be shared frailty for the jth individual. Assuming that the frailties are acting multiplicatively on the baseline reversed hazard rate and both the survival times of individuals are conditionally independent for a given frailty, the conditional reversed hazard rate for the jth individual at the ith $(i = 1, 2)$ survival time t_{ij} for a given frailty $Z_j = z_j$

has the following form:

$$m(t_{ij} \mid z_j, \mathbf{X}_j) = z_j m_0(t_{ij}) e^{\mathbf{X}_{0j}\beta_0 + \mathbf{X}_{ij}\beta_i}, \quad i = 1, 2,$$

where $m_0(t_{ij})$ is the baseline reversed hazard at time t_{ij} and β is a vector of order k of regression coefficients. The conditional cumulative reversed hazard rate for the jth individual at ith lifetime t_{ij} for a given frailty $Z_j = z_j$ is

$$M(t_{ij} \mid z_j, \mathbf{X}_j) = z_j M_0(t_{ij}) \eta_{0j} \eta_{ij},$$

where $\eta_{0j} = e^{\mathbf{X}_{0j}\beta_0}$, $\eta_{ij} = e^{\mathbf{X}_{ij}\beta_i}$, $i = 1, 2$ and $M_0(t_{ij})$ is the cumulative baseline reversed hazard rate at time t_{ij}. The conditional distribution function for the jth individual at the ith lifetime t_{ij} for a given frailty $Z_j = z_j$ is

$$F(t_{ij} \mid z_j, \mathbf{X}_j) = e^{-M(t_{ij} \mid z_j, \mathbf{X}_j)} = e^{-z_j M_0(t_{ij}) \eta_{0j} \eta_{ij}}.$$

Under the assumption of independence, the bivariate conditional distribution function for a given frailty $Z_j = z_j$ at time t_{1j} and t_{2j} is

$$F(t_{1j}, t_{2j} \mid z_j, \mathbf{X}_j) = F(t_{1j} \mid z_j, \mathbf{X}_j) F(t_{2j} \mid z_j, \mathbf{X}_j)$$
$$\times e^{-z_j(M_{01}(t_{1j})\eta_{1j} + M_{02}(t_{2j})\eta_{2j})\eta_{0j}},$$

where $M_{01}(t_{1j})$ and $M_{01}(t_{2j})$ are cumulative baseline reversed hazard rates at times $t_{1j} > 0$ and $t_{2j} > 0$, respectively.

The unconditional bivariate distribution function can be obtained by integrating over the frailty variable Z_j having the probability density function $f_Z(z_j)$ for the jth individual.

$$\begin{aligned}
F(t_{1j}, t_{2j} \mid \mathbf{X}_j) &= \int_{Z_j} F(t_{1j}, t_{2j} \mid z_j) f_Z(z_j) dz_j \\
&= \int_{Z_j} e^{-z_j(M_{01}(t_{1j})\eta_{1j} + M_{02}(t_{2j})\eta_{2j})\eta_{0j}} f_Z(z_j) dz_j \\
&= L_{Z_j}[(M_{01}(t_{1j})\eta_{1j} + M_{02}(t_{2j})\eta_{2j})\eta_{0j}], \quad (10.2)
\end{aligned}$$

where $L_{Z_j}(.)$ is the Laplace transform of the frailty variable of Z_j for the jth individual. Here onward, we represent $F(t_{1j}, t_{2j} \mid \mathbf{X}_j)$ as $F(t_{1j}, t_{2j})$.

Duffy et al. (1990) considered Australian twin data which consist of information about the age at appendectomy of monozygotic (MZ) and dizygotic (DZ) twins. There were some pairs with missing age at onset and those are the left-censored observations. Duffy et al. (1990) excluded these left-censored observations in the analysis. It is, therefore, appropriate to model common random effect by including those left-censored observations, which can be done by developing frailty models using RHR. Accordingly, Sankaran and Gleeja (2011) introduced frailty as a common random effect that acts multiplicatively on reversed hazard rates, which is useful for the analysis of left-censored data. Hanagal and Pandey (2014, 2015a, b, 2016a, b) and Hanagal et al. (2017) analyzed Australian twin data using gamma and inverse Gaussian frailty models using reversed hazard rate. Hanagal and Bhambure (2014, 2016) analyzed Australian twin data using shared inverse Gaussian frailty based on reversed hazard rate. Hanagal and Bhambure (2017a, b) developed shared positive stable frailty and gamma frailty models with exponentiated Gumbel, generalized Rayleigh, and generalized inverse Rayleigh as the baseline distributions based on reversed hazard rate.

10.3 Shared Gamma Frailty Model Based on Reversed Hazard Rate

Sankaran and Gleeja (2006, 2008) introduced a measure of association based on the reversed hazard rate in a similar manner as was introduced by Clayton (1978) based on the hazard rate. In case of gamma frailty, the measure of association given by Sankaran and Gleeja (2006) is also constant. Assume that a common continuous random variable Z follows a gamma distribution. For identifiability, we assume Z has expected value equal to one.

When Z follows gamma distribution with single parameter θ as discussed in Chap. 5, the bivariate distribution function can be written incorporating gamma frailty for the random variable Z as follows:

$$F(t_{1j}, t_{2j}) = [1 + \theta\eta_{0j}((M_{01}(t_{1j})\eta_{1j} + M_{02}(t_{2j})\eta_{2j}))]^{-\frac{1}{\theta}}, \qquad (10.3)$$

where $M_{01}(t_{1j})$ and $M_{02}(t_{2j})$ are the cumulative baseline reversed hazard functions of the lifetimes T_{1j} and T_{2j}, respectively.

The bivariate distribution in the presence of covariates, when the frailty variable is degenerate, is given by

$$F(t_{1j}, t_{2j}) = e^{-\left(\eta_{0j}((M_{01}(t_{1j})\eta_{1j} + M_{02}(t_{2j})\eta_{2j}))\right)}. \qquad (10.4)$$

10.4 Baseline Distributions

10.4.1 Generalized Log-Logistic Type I Distribution

Now rearranging the parameters of Eq. (9.3), the cumulative distribution function of the generalized log-logistic distribution type I is

$$F(t) = \left(\frac{(\lambda t)^{\gamma}}{1 + (\lambda t)^{\gamma}}\right)^{\alpha}.$$

The corresponding reversed hazard rate and cumulative reversed hazard rate are, respectively, given as follows:

$$m(t) = \frac{\alpha\gamma}{t(1 + (\lambda t)^\gamma)},$$

$$M(t) = \alpha ln \left(\frac{1 + (\lambda t)^\gamma}{(\lambda t)^\gamma} \right).$$

When $\alpha = 1$, this distribution reduces to log-logistic distribution. The reversed hazard rate of the generalized log-logistic type I distribution is decreasing function of $t > 0$.

10.4.2 Generalized Log-Logistic Type II Distribution

Now rearranging the parameters of Eq. (9.4), the cumulative distribution function of the generalized log-logistic distribution type II is

$$F(t) = 1 - (1 + (\lambda t)^\gamma)^{-\alpha}.$$

The corresponding reversed hazard rate and cumulative reversed hazard rate are, respectively, given as follows:

$$m(t) = \frac{\alpha\gamma\lambda(\lambda t)^{-1+\gamma}(1 + (\lambda t)^\gamma)^{-1-\alpha}}{1 - (1 + (\lambda t)^\gamma)^{-\alpha}},$$

$$M(t) = -ln(1 - (1 + (\lambda t)^\gamma)^{-\alpha}).$$

When $\alpha = 1$, this distribution reduces to log-logistic distribution.

10.4.3 Exponentiated Gumbel Distribution

In literature, exponentiated family of distributions is defined in two ways. The exponentiated Gumbel (EG) distribution was introduced by Nadarajah (2006). Kakade et al. (2008) introduced exponentiated Gumbel (EG) distribution using another format. The class of exponentiated Gumbel distributions has a shape and a scale parameter. Some of its application areas in climate modeling include global warming problem, flood frequency analysis, offshore modeling, rainfall modeling, and wind speed modeling.

A continuous random variable T is said to follow the exponentiated Gumbel distribution if its cumulative distribution function is

$$F(t) = \left(exp\left[-e^{-\lambda t}\right]\right)^{\alpha}; \; -\infty < t < \infty, \alpha > 0, \lambda > 0,$$

where α and λ are, respectively, the shape and the scale parameters of the distribution. The reverse hazard rate and cumulative reverse hazard rate are, respectively,

$$m(t) = \alpha \lambda e^{-\lambda t}; \; -\infty < t < \infty, \alpha > 0, \lambda > 0,$$

$$M(t) = -\log\left(exp\left[-e^{-\lambda t}\right]\right)^{\alpha}; \; -\infty < t < \infty, \alpha > 0, \lambda > 0.$$

10.4.4 Modified Inverse Weibull Distribution

The modified inverse Weibull distribution is more convenient for computational point of view for left-censored data. The cumulative distribution function, the cumulative reversed hazard rate, and the reversed hazard rate of the modified inverse Weibull are, respectively, given as follows:

$$F(t) = exp\left(-\alpha t^{-\lambda} e^{-\gamma t}\right), \, t > 0, \alpha > 0, \lambda > 0, \gamma > 0,$$

$$M(t) = \alpha t^{-\lambda} e^{-\gamma t},$$

$$m(t) = \alpha e^{-\gamma t} t^{-1-\lambda} (\lambda + \gamma t).$$

When $\gamma = 0$, this distribution reduces to the inverse Weibull distribution. The reversed hazard rate of the modified inverse Weibull distribution is decreasing function of $t > 0$. For more details, see Kumar and Singh (2011).

10.4.5 Generalized Inverse Rayleigh Distribution

Burr (1942) introduced 12 different forms of cumulative distribution functions for modeling lifetime data. Recently, Surles and Padgett (2001) (see also Surles and Padgett 2005) introduced the two-parameter Burr type X distribution and named it as the generalized Rayleigh distribution. Note that the two-parameter generalized Rayleigh distribution is a particular case of the generalized Weibull distribution, originally proposed by Mudholkar and Srivastava (1993) (see also Mudholkar et al. 1995). The generalized inverse Rayleigh distribution is obtained by making transformation $Y = 1/X$ where X is the generalized Rayleigh distribution. The generalized inverse Rayleigh distribution has a shape and a scale parameter.

If a continuous random variable T follows the two-parameter generalized inverse Rayleigh distribution, then the cumulative distribution function, reversed hazard rate, and cumulative reversed hazard rate are, respectively,

$$F(t) = \begin{cases} \left(1 - (1 - e^{-\frac{\lambda}{t^2}})^{\alpha}\right) & ; \ t > 0, \alpha > 0, \lambda > 0 \\ 0 & ; \ otherwise, \end{cases}$$

$$m(t) = \begin{cases} \dfrac{2\alpha\lambda e^{-\frac{\lambda}{t^2}}\left(1 - e^{-\frac{\lambda}{t^2}}\right)^{\alpha-1}}{\left(1 - \left(1 - e^{-\frac{\lambda}{t^2}}\right)^{\alpha}\right)t^3} & ; \ t > 0, \alpha > 0, \lambda > 0 \\ 0 & ; \ otherwise, \end{cases}$$

$$M(t) = \begin{cases} -\log\left(1 - (1 - e^{-\frac{\lambda}{t^2}})^{\alpha}\right) & ; \ t > 0, \alpha > 0, \lambda > 0 \\ 0 & ; \ otherwise, \end{cases}$$

where α and λ are, respectively, the shape and the scale parameters.

10.5 Gamma Frailty Models Based on Reversed Hazard with Baseline Distributions

Substituting the cumulative reversed hazard function for the generalized log-logistic type I, type II baseline distributions, exponentiated Gumbel, modified inverse Weibull, and generalized inverse Rayleigh distributions in Eqs. (10.3) and (10.4), we get the unconditional bivariate distribution functions at time $t_{1j} > 0$ and $t_{2j} > 0$ as

$$F(t_{1j}, t_{2j}) = \left[1 + \theta\eta_{0j}\left\{\eta_{1j}\alpha_1\left(\ln\left(\frac{1 + (\lambda_1 t_1)^{\gamma_1}}{(\lambda_1 t_1)^{\gamma_1}}\right)\right) + \eta_{2j}\alpha_2\left(\ln\left(\frac{1 + (\lambda_2 t_2)^{\gamma_2}}{(\lambda_2 t_2)^{\gamma_2}}\right)\right)\right\}\right]^{-\frac{1}{\theta}} \quad (10.5)$$

for the case of the generalized log-logistic type I distribution with frailty,

$$F(t_{1j}, t_{2j}) = \left[1 - \theta\eta_{0j}\left\{\eta_{1j}ln(1 - (1 + (\lambda_1 t_{1j})^{\gamma_1})^{-\alpha_1}) + \eta_{2j}ln(1 - (1 + (\lambda_2 t_{2j})^{\gamma_2})^{-\alpha_2})\right\}\right]^{-\frac{1}{\theta}} \quad (10.6)$$

for the case of the generalized log-logistic type II distribution with frailty,

$$F(t_{1j}, t_{2j}) = \left[1 + \theta\eta_{0j}\left\{\eta_{1j}\alpha_1 t_{1j}^{-\lambda_1}e^{-\gamma_1 t_1} + \eta_{2j}\alpha_2 t_{2j}^{-\lambda_2}e^{-\gamma_2 t_2}\right\}\right]^{-\frac{1}{\theta}} \quad (10.7)$$

for the case of the modified inverse Weibull distribution with frailty,

$$F(t_{1j}, t_{2j}) = [1 - \theta\eta_{0j}((\log\left(exp\left[-e^{-\lambda_1 t_{1j}}\right]\right)^{\alpha_1} \eta_{1j} + \log\left(exp\left[-e^{-\lambda_2 t_{2j}}\right]\right)^{\alpha_2} \eta_{2j}))]^{-\frac{1}{\theta}},$$
$$\tag{10.8}$$

for the case of the exponentiated Gumbel distribution with frailty,

$$F(t_{1j}, t_{2j}) = \left[1 - \theta\eta_{0j}\left(\log\left(1 - (1 - e^{-\frac{\lambda_1}{t_{1j}^2}})^{\alpha_1}\right)\eta_{1j} + \log\left(1 - (1 - e^{-\frac{\lambda_2}{t_{2j}^2}})^{\alpha_2}\right)\eta_{2j}\right)\right]^{-\frac{1}{\theta}} \tag{10.9}$$

for the case of the generalized inverse Rayleigh distribution with frailty,

$$F(t_{1j}, t_{2j}) = e^{\left(-\eta_{0j}\left\{\eta_{1j}\alpha_1\left(ln\left(\frac{1+(\lambda_1 t_1)^{\gamma_1}}{(\lambda_1 t_1)^{\gamma_1}}\right)\right)+\eta_{2j}\alpha_2\left(ln\left(\frac{1+(\lambda_2 t_2)^{\gamma_2}}{(\lambda_2 t_2)^{\gamma_2}}\right)\right)\right\}\right)} \tag{10.10}$$

for the case of the generalized log-logistic type I distribution without frailty,

$$F(t_{1j}, t_{2j}) = e^{\eta_{0j}\left\{\eta_{1j}ln(1-(1+(\lambda_1 t_{1j})^{\gamma_1})^{-\alpha_1})+\eta_{2j}ln(1-(1+(\lambda_2 t_{2j})^{\gamma_2})^{-\alpha_2})\right\}} \tag{10.11}$$

for the case of the generalized log-logistic type II distribution without frailty,

$$F(t_{1j}, t_{2j}) = e^{\left(-\eta_{0j}\left\{\eta_{1j}\alpha_1 t_{1j}^{-\lambda_1}e^{-\gamma_1 t_1}+\eta_{2j}\alpha_2 t_{2j}^{-\lambda_2}e^{-\gamma_2 t_2}\right\}\right)} \tag{10.12}$$

for the case of the modified inverse Weibull distribution without frailty,

$$F(t_{1j}, t_{2j}) = e^{\eta_{0j}\left(\log\left(exp\left[-e^{-\lambda_1 t_{1j}}\right]\right)^{\alpha_1}\eta_{1j}+\log\left(exp\left[-e^{-\lambda_2 t_{2j}}\right]\right)^{\alpha_2}\eta_{2j}\right)} \tag{10.13}$$

for the case of the exponentiated Gumbel distribution without frailty,
and

$$F(t_{1j}, t_{2j}) = e^{\eta_{0j}\left(\log\left(1-(1-e^{-\frac{\lambda_1}{t_{1j}^2}})^{\alpha_1}\right)\eta_{1j}+\log\left(1-(1-e^{-\frac{\lambda_2}{t_{2j}^2}})^{\alpha_2}\right)\eta_{2j}\right)} \tag{10.14}$$

for the case of the generalized inverse Rayleigh distribution without frailty.

Here onward, we call Eqs. (10.5)–(10.14), as Model RH-I, Model RH-II, Model RH-III, Model RH-IV, Model RH-V, Model RH-VI, Model RH-VII, Model RH-VIII, Model RH-IX, and Model RH-X, respectively. Model RH-I, Model RH-II, Model RH-III, Model RH-IV, and Model RH-V are models with frailty and Model RH-VI, Model RH-VII, Model RH-VIII, Model RH-IX, and Model RH-X are models without frailty.

10.6 Likelihood Specification and Bayesian Estimation of Parameters

Suppose there are n individuals under study, whose first and second observed failure times are represented by (t_{1j}, t_{2j}). Let c_{1j} and c_{2j} be the observed censoring times for the jth individual ($j = 1, 2, 3, \ldots, n$) for the first and the second recurrence times, respectively. We use the left censoring scheme. Also, we assume independence between the censoring scheme and the lifetimes of individuals.

The contribution of the bivariate lifetime random variable of the jth individual in likelihood function is given by

$$L_j(t_{1j}, t_{2j}) = \begin{cases} f_1(t_{1j}, t_{2j}), & t_{1j} > c_{1j}, t_{2j} > c_{2j}, \\ f_2(t_{1j}, c_{2j}), & t_{1j} > c_{1j}, t_{2j} < c_{2j}, \\ f_3(c_{1j}, t_{2j}), & t_{1j} < c_{1j}, t_{2j} > c_{2j}, \\ f_4(c_{1j}, c_{2j}), & t_{1j} < c_{1j}, t_{2j} < c_{2j}, \end{cases}$$

and likelihood function is

$$L(\underline{\psi}, \underline{\beta}, \theta) = \prod_{j=1}^{n_1} f_1(t_{1j}, t_{2j}) \prod_{j=1}^{n_2} f_2(t_{1j}, c_{2j}) \prod_{j=1}^{n_3} f_3(c_{1j}, t_{2j}) \prod_{j=1}^{n_4} f_4(c_{1j}, c_{2j}), \quad (10.15)$$

where θ, $\underline{\psi}$, and $\underline{\beta}$ are, respectively, the frailty parameter, the vector of baseline parameters, and the vector of regression coefficients. The counts n_1, n_2, n_3, and n_4 be the number of individuals for which the first and the second failure times (t_{1j}, t_{2j}) lie in the ranges $t_{1j} > c_{1j}, t_{2j} > c_{2j}$; $t_{1j} > c_{1j}, t_{2j} < c_{2j}$; $t_{1j} < c_{1j}, t_{2j} > c_{2j}$; and $t_{1j} < c_{1j}, t_{2j} < c_{2j}$, respectively, and let for gamma frailty,

$$f_1(t_{1j}, t_{2j}) = \frac{\partial^2 F(t_{1j}, t_{2j})}{\partial t_{1j} \partial t_{2j}}$$
$$= (1 + \theta) m_{01}(t_{1j}) m_{02}(t_{2j}) F(t_{1j}, t_{2j})^{(1+2\theta)} \eta_{0j}^2 \eta_{1j} \eta_{2j},$$
$$f_2(t_{1j}, c_{2j}) = \frac{\partial F(t_{1j}, c_{2j})}{\partial t_{1j}} = m_{01}(t_{1j}) F(t_{1j}, c_{2j})^{(\theta+1)} \eta_{0j} \eta_{1j},$$
$$f_3(c_{1j}, t_{2j}) = \frac{\partial F(c_{1j}, t_{2j})}{\partial t_{2j}} = m_{02}(t_{2j}) F(c_{1j}, t_{2j})^{(\theta+1)} \eta_{0j} \eta_{2j}, \text{ and}$$
$$f_4(c_{1j}, c_{2j}) = F(c_{1j}, c_{2j}).$$

Substituting the reversed hazard functions $m_{01}(t_{1j})$, $m_{02}(t_{2j})$, the distribution function $F(t_{1j}, t_{2j})$, and the cumulative reversed hazard functions $M_{01}(t_{1j})$ and $M_{02}(t_{2j})$ for the generalized log-logistic distribution type I and type II, modified inverse Weibull, exponentiated Gumbel, and generalized inverse Rayleigh distributions, we get the likelihood function given by Eq. (10.15). Similarly, we get the likelihood function for without frailty model.

Table 10.1 p-values of K–S statistics for goodness-of-fit test for Australian twin data set

Model	T_1 p-value	T_2 p-value
Model RH-I	0.44452	0.57118
Model RH-II	0.94333	0.9403
Model RH-III	0.47994	0.5507
Model RH-IV	0.1195	0.2744
Model RH-V	0.3402	0.1413

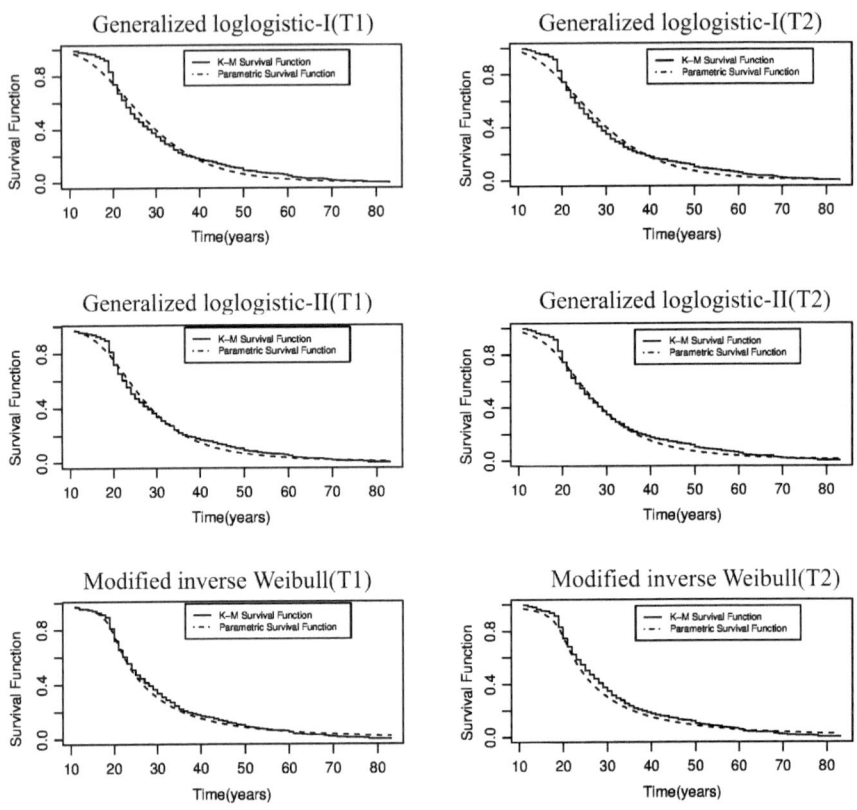

Fig. 10.1 Survival function plots for (K–M survival and parametric survival)

Unfortunately, for the maximum likelihood estimators (MLEs), there is problem of convergence of the estimates in the Newton–Raphson iterative procedure because we are estimating parameters simultaneously. As the method of maximum likelihood fails to estimate the parameters due to convergence problem, we use Bayesian approach. The detailed discussion on the simulation study based on Bayesian approach is given in Hanagal and Pandey (2014, 2017a) and Hanagal Bhambure (2017b).

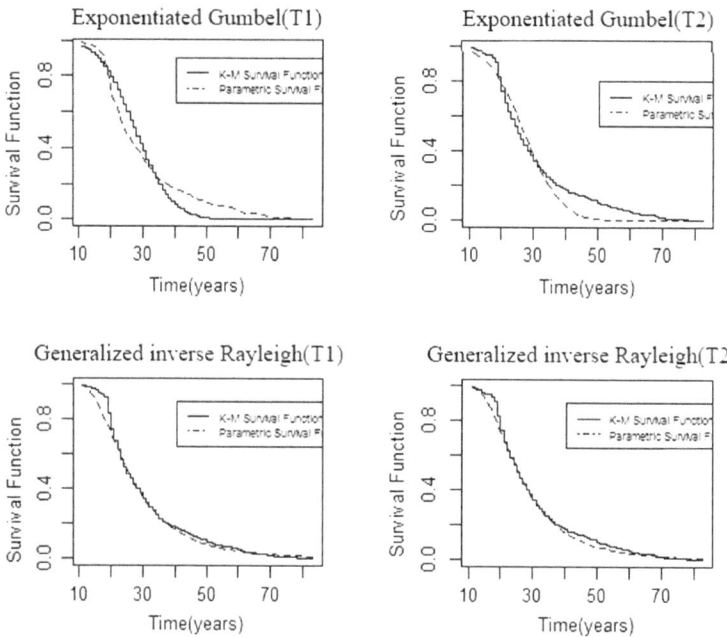

Fig. 10.2 Survival function plots for (K–M survival and parametric survival)

10.7 Australian Twin Data

Now we apply all six models to the Australian twin data given in Duffy et al. (1990). The data consist of six zygote categories. We consider the subset of the data with zygote category 4. The data consist of male gender only and consist of 350 pair of twins with 9 and 11 censored in twin 1 and twin 2, respectively. An individual having age at onset less than 11 is considered as left-censored observation. The data have information on the age at appendectomy of twins. The genetic factor or environmental factor involved in the risk of appendectomy is the frailty variable. Here there is a common covariate age for both T_1 and T_2 and one covariate each for T_1, T_2, i.e., presence or absence of appendectomy. To check goodness of fit of Australian twin data set, we obtain Kolmogorov–Smirnov (K–S) statistics and their p-values for T_1 and T_2 separately. The Australian twin data are partially presented in Chap. 1.

For all the models, p-values of K–S statistics are provided in Table 10.1. These p-values of K–S test are quite high. We can say that there is no statistical evidence to reject the hypothesis that data are from these models for marginal distributions and assume that they also fit for bivariate case. Figures 10.1 and 10.2 show the parametric plot with semiparametric plot of Models RH-1 to RH-V.

We run two parallel chains for all models using two sets of prior distributions with the different starting points using the Metropolis–Hastings algorithm and the Gibbs sampler based on normal transition kernels. We iterate both the chains for 1,00,000

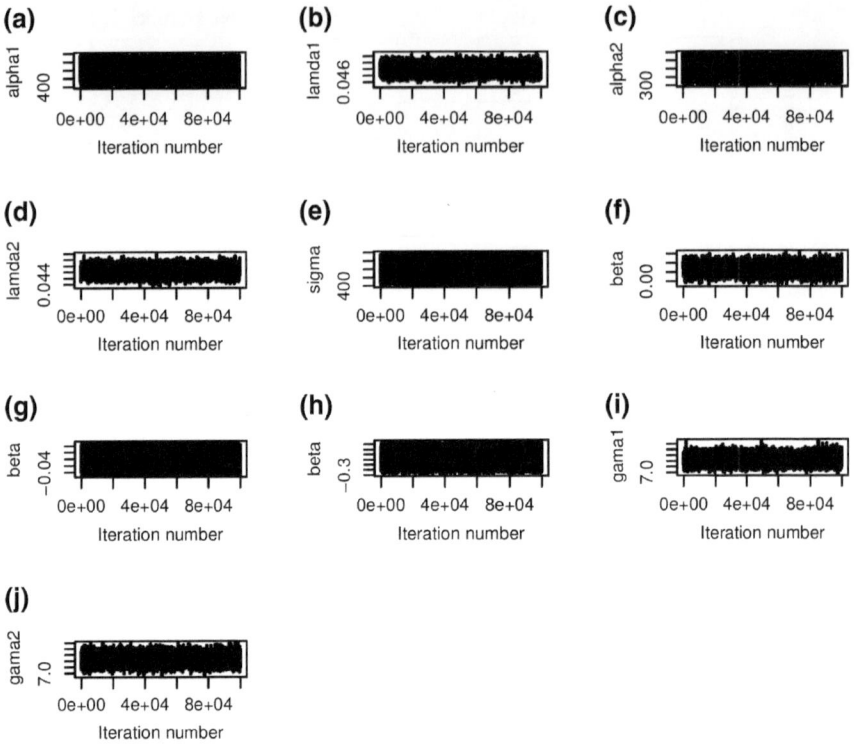

Fig. 10.3 Trace plots for Australian twin data set (Model RH-II)

times. We got nearly same estimates of parameters for both the set of priors, so estimates are not dependent on the different prior distributions. Convergence rates of Gibbs sampler for both the prior sets are almost the same. Also, both the chains show somewhat similar results, so we present here the analysis for only one chain with $G(1, 0.0001)$ as prior for the baseline parameters and $G(0.0001, 0.0001)$ as the prior for the frailty parameter θ. Due to lack of space, we are presenting diagnostic plots (the trace plots, the coupling from the past plots, autocorrelation plots, and the autocorrelation plots after thinning) only for Model RH-II in Figs. 10.3, 10.4, 10.5, and 10.6.

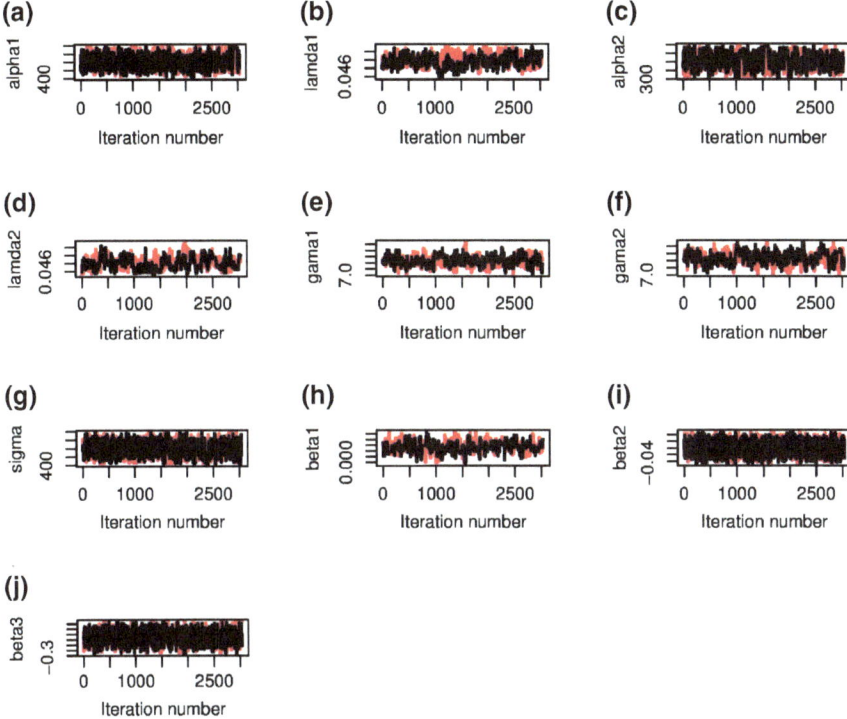

Fig. 10.4 Coupling from the past plots for Australian twin data set (Model RH-II)

The posterior mean and standard error with 95% credible intervals for the baseline parameters, the frailty parameter, and the regression coefficients are presented in Tables 10.2, 10.3, 10.4, 10.5, 10.6, 10.7, 10.8, 10.9, 10.10, and 10.11.

The posterior summaries of the Model RH-I to Model RH-X are given in Tables 10.2, 10.3, 10.4, 10.5, 10.6, 10.7, 10.8, 10.9, 10.10, and 10.11. Tables 10.2, 10.3, 10.4, 10.5, 10.6, 10.7, 10.8, 10.9, 10.10, and 10.11 present the estimates, the credible intervals, the Geweke test, and the Gelman–Rubin statistics for all the parameters of the Model RH-I to Model RH-X, respectively.

The Gelman–Rubin convergence statistic values are nearly equal to one and the Geweke test statistic values are quite small and the corresponding p-values are large enough to say that the chains attain stationary distribution. The posterior mean and the standard error with 95% credible intervals, the Gelman–Rubin statistics values, and the Geweke test values with p-values for Model RH-I to Model RH-X are presented in Tables 10.2, 10.3, 10.4, 10.5, 10.6, 10.7, 10.8, 10.9, 10.10, and 10.11. For Model RH-I, Model RH-II, Model RH-III, Model RH-IV, and Model RH-V, the estimates of

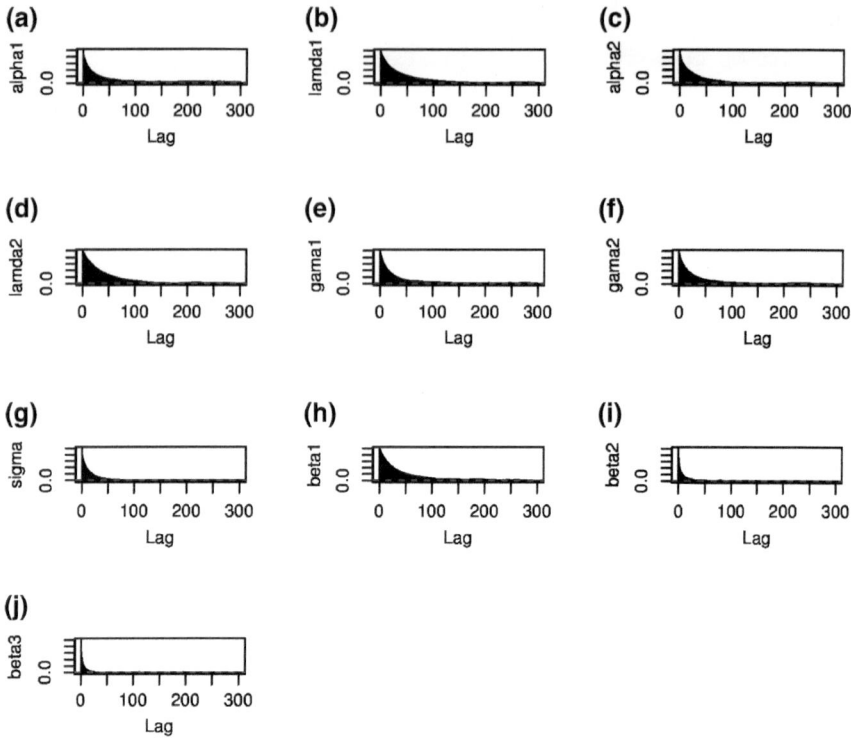

Fig. 10.5 Autocorrelation plots for Australian twin data set (Model RH-II)

the shared frailty parameter θ are, respectively, 1.5069, 495.0658, 0.37803, 0.0123, and 0.2498. This shows that there is a heterogeneity between the pairs of twins. To compare ten models, we first use AIC, BIC, and DIC values which are given in Table 10.12 and Bayes factors in Table 10.13. From Tables 10.12 and 10.13, we observe that with frailty models fit better than without frailty models based on AIC, BIC, DIC, and Bayes factor. This shows that Model RH-II is better than all other models based on reversed hazard. A Bayesian test based on Bayes factor for testing $\theta = 0$ against $\theta > 0$ and which supports the alternative hypothesis, i.e., models with frailty fit better.

The credible interval of the regression coefficient β_0 of the covariate age does not contain zero for the Model RH-I, Model RH-II, Model RH-III, Model RH-VI, and Model RH-VIII, and hence age is significant factor in these models only. The credible intervals of the regression coefficients β_1 and β_2 do not contain zero for the Model

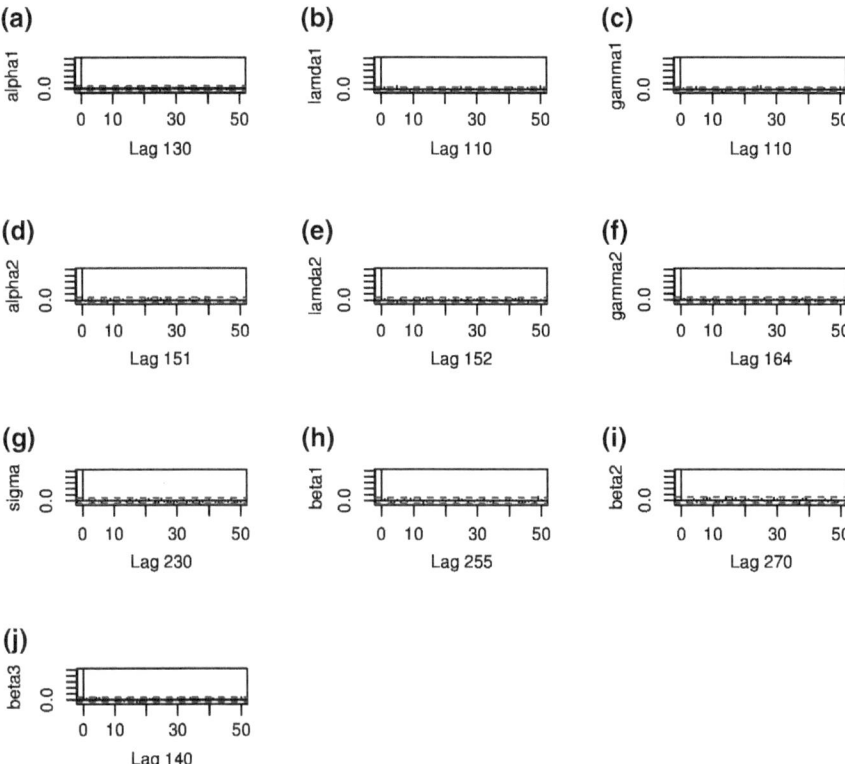

Fig. 10.6 Autocorrelation plots after thinning for Australian twin data set (Model RH-II)

RH-V, and hence β_1 and β_2 are significant only in Model RH-V. The convergence rate of the Gibbs sampling algorithm does not depend on these choices of the prior distributions in our proposed model for Australian twin data. The Geweke test values are near to zero and the corresponding p-values are quite high and the Gelman–Rubin statistics for all the parameters of all six models based on data are very close to one.

The AIC, BIC, and DIC values for Model RH-II are least among all six models. Bayes factors show that models with frailty (Model RH-I, Model RH-II, Model RH-III, Model RH-IV, and Model RH-V) are better than the models without frailty (Model RH-VI, Model RH-VII, Model RH-VIII, Model RH-IX, and Model RH-X) and Model RH-II is the best and the frailty is significant.

Table 10.2 Posterior summary for Australian twin data set Model RH-I

Parameter	Estimate	Standard error	Lower credible limit	Upper credible limit	Geweke values	p-values	Gelman and Rubin values
Burn-in period = 2800;		Autocorrelation lag = 300					
α_1	10.1756	0.6104	9.09167	11.16265	−0.00573	0.4977	1.0071
λ_1	0.0658	0.0029	0.05986	0.07149	−0.00392	0.4984	1.0049
γ_1	4.9199	0.1942	4.57526	5.27052	0.00928	0.5037	1.0016
α_2	8.9601	0.5449	8.00492	9.91093	−0.00537	0.4978	1.0009
λ_2	0.0648	0.0032	0.05927	0.07122	0.00116	0.5004	1.0015
γ_2	4.8083	0.2593	4.33849	5.30615	0.00018	0.5000	1.0019
θ	1.5069	0.1958	1.12593	1.88339	0.00140	0.5005	0.9999
β_0	0.0268	0.0077	0.01354	0.04242	0.00207	0.5008	0.9999
β_1	0.0006	0.0334	−0.06036	0.07216	0.01348	0.5053	1.0032
β_2	0.0714	0.1379	−0.21991	0.30209	0.00745	0.5029	1.0002

Table 10.3 Posterior summary for Australian twin data set Model RH-II

Parameter	Estimate	Standard error	Lower credible limit	Upper credible limit	Geweke values	p-values	Gelman and Rubin values
Burn-in period = 3000;		Autocorrelation lag = 300					
α_1	503.8080	50.4847	407.0884	596.2543	−0.00179	0.4992	1.01
λ_1	0.0498 .	0.0015	0.0470	0.0526	0.00629	0.5025	1.00
γ_1	8.0760	0.3469	7.4897	8.7622	−0.00669	0.4973	1.01
α_2	400.3714	48.7989	312.1472	486.2848	−0.00617	0.4975	1.00
λ_2	0.0480	0.0015	0.0451	0.0510	0.00040	0.5001	1.01
γ_2	8.1338	0.3632	7.3948	8.8684	−0.00989	0.4960	1.00
θ	495.0658	48.4160	410.165	588.7990	−0.00485	0.4980	1.00
β_0	0.0136	0.0049	0.0048	0.0239	−0.00625	0.4975	1.02
β_1	−0.0012	0.0241	−0.0460	0.0416	0.00567	0.4975	1.00
β_2	0.0597	0.1338	−0.1891	0.2905	−0.00105	0.4995	1.00

Table 10.4 Posterior summary for Australian twin data set Model RH-III

Parameter	Estimate	Standard error	Lower credible limit	Upper credible limit	Geweke values	p-values	Gelman and Rubin values
Burn-in period = 5800;		Autocorrelation lag = 200					
α_1	19.67384	0.5502	18.75981	20.62422	−0.00031	0.4998	1.0001
λ_1	0.07043	0.0056	0.06069	0.07949	0.00031	0.5001	1.0006
γ_1	0.11820	0.0040	0.11025	0.12614	−0.00669	0.4973	1.0032
α_2	17.56482	0.5639	16.63352	18.51358	−0.00617	0.4975	1.0038
λ_2	0.06652	0.0057	0.05608	0.07660	0.00040	0.5001	1.0007
γ_2	0.11523	0.0044	0.10624	0.12358	−0.00989	0.4960	1.0012
θ	0.37803	0.0831	0.22329	0.55351	−0.00485	0.4980	1.0029
β_0	0.00973	0.0036	0.00269	0.01677	−0.00625	0.4975	1.0049
β_1	−0.02188	0.0767	−0.14433	0.13373	0.00567	0.4975	1.0011
β_2	0.08516	0.1398	−0.22952	0.32082	−0.00105	0.4995	0.9999

Table 10.5 Posterior summary for Australian twin data for Model RH-IV

Burn-in period = 1965

Parameter (values)	Lag	Estimate	SE	Lower credible limit	Upper credible limit	GR values	Geweke values	p-values
α_1	80	6.4117	0.0491	6.3112	6.4780	1.0037	−0.0148	0.4940
λ_1	100	0.08393	0.0022	0.0795	0.0885	1.0000	0.0008	0.5003
α_2	100	8.8046	0.0523	8.7086	8.8930	1.0005	−0.0106	0.4957
λ_2	80	0.0943	0.0023	0.0896	0.0989	1.0024	−0.0065	0.4974
θ	80	0.0123	0.0049	0.0052	0.0229	1.0025	−0.0059	0.4976
β_0	20	0.00008	0.0006	−0.00009	0.00009	0.9999	−0.0043	0.4982
β_1	10	0.0002	0.0050	−0.0090	0.0091	1.0091	−0.0023	0.4990
β_2	10	0.0001	0.0051	−0.0090	0.0093	1.0083	−0.0041	0.4983

Table 10.6 Posterior summary for Australian twin data for Model RH-V

Burn-in period = 2100

Parameter (values)	Lag	Estimate	SE	Lower credible limit	Upper credible limit	GR values	Geweke values	p-values
α_1	100	1.9287	0.0511	1.8163	1.9975	1.0093	−0.0152	0.4939
λ_1	70	825.5704	5.5945	815.4421	834.5583	1.0012	−0.0013	0.4994
α_2	50	1.7198	0.0502	1.6179	1.7951	1.0003	−0.0052	0.4979
λ_2	90	726.872	5.4160	715.9279	734.6729	0.9999	−0.0045	0.4981
θ	30	0.2498	0.0044	0.2425	0.2575	1.0083	−0.0061	0.4975
β_0	20	0.00006	0.0006	−0.00009	0.00009	0.9998	0.0085	0.5034
β_1	5	0.2494	0.0020	0.2461	0.2528	1.0001	−0.0012	0.4995
β_2	5	0.2500	0.0028	0.2452	0.2547	1.0014	0.0018	0.5007

Table 10.7 Posterior summary for Australian twin data set Model RH-VI

Parameter	Estimate	Standard error	Lower credible limit	Upper credible limit	Geweke values	p-values	Gelman and Rubin values
Burn-in period = 2800;		Autocorrelation lag = 300					
α_1	1.4806	0.2172	1.08298	1.87900	−0.00716	0.4971	1.0091
λ_1	0.0475	0.0031	0.04162	0.05341	−0.00838	0.4966	1.0008
γ_1	1.3022	0.1518	3.29435	3.93994	0.00624	0.5024	1.0017
α_2	0.0456	0.0026	1.00322	1.56740	−0.00976	0.4961	1.0096
λ_2	3.6265	0.1957	0.04062	0.05151	−0.00932	0.4962	1.0088
γ_2	3.6135	0.1680	3.25814	3.99208	0.01088	0.5043	1.0018
β_0	0.0059	0.0026	0.00068	0.01158	−0.00174	0.4993	1.0005
β_1	8.9e-06	0.0024	−0.00437	0.00442	−0.00050	0.4997	1.0054
β_2	0.0592	0.1285	−0.20118	0.29163	−7.76e-05	0.4999	1.0134

Table 10.8 Posterior summary for Australian twin data set Model RH-VII

Parameter	Estimate	Standard error	Lower credible limit	Upper credible limit	Geweke values	p-values	Gelman and Rubin values
Burn-in period = 2800;		Autocorrelation lag = 300					
α_1	0.6047	0.1027	0.4205	0.8341	0.01169	0.5047	1.00
λ_1	0.0475	0.0026	0.0428	0.0526	−0.00679	0.4972	1.03
γ_1	5.1896	0.5964	4.1191	6.4377	−0.01175	0.4953	1.00
α_2	0.6736	0.0885	0.5048	0.8412	0.01642	0.5065	1.00
λ_2	0.0463	0.0029	0.0406	0.0524	−0.00860	0.4965	1.00
γ_2	4.7336	0.4456	3.9453	5.7410	−0.01335	0.4946	1.01
β_0	0.0042	0.0041	−0.0041	0.0119	0.00415	0.5016	1.00
β_1	−0.0013	0.0239	−0.0441	0.0452	0.01221	0.5048	1.00
β_2	0.0481	0.1225	−0.1985	0.2838	−0.00571	0.4977	1.01

Table 10.9 Posterior summary for Australian twin data set Model RH-VIII

Parameter	Estimate	Standard error	Lower credible limit	Upper credible limit	Geweke values	p-values	Gelman and Rubin values
Burn-in period = 2800;		Autocorrelation lag = 190					
α_1	11.44908	0.5554	10.47060	12.34491	−0.00330	0.4986	1.0075
λ_1	0.06949	0.0112	0.04948	0.08727	0.01716	0.5068	1.0043
γ_1	0.10227	0.0036	0.09499	0.10941	−0.00179	0.4992	1.0065
α_2	10.43929	0.5275	9.44735	11.34131	−0.00460	0.4981	1.0008
λ_2	0.07101	0.0106	0.05109	0.08880	−0.00714	0.4971	1.0031
γ_2	0.09919	0.0038	0.09192	0.10693	9.27e-05	0.5001	0.9999
β_0	0.00575	0.0020	0.00152	0.00950	0.003835	0.5015	1.0000
β_1	−0.01649	0.0715	−0.14075	0.12942	−0.007237	0.4971	1.0008
β_2	0.06323	0.1238	−0.17651	0.29295	0.004567	0.5018	1.0000

Table 10.10 Posterior summary for Australian twin data for Model RH-IX

Burn-in period = 1480

Parameter (values)	Lag	Estimate	SE	Lower credible limit	Upper credible limit	GR values	Geweke values	p-values
α_1	50	5.0270	0.0434	4.9194	5.0782	1.0028	0.0065	0.5026
λ_1	10	0.0767	0.0022	0.0723	0.0812	1.0017	0.0045	0.5018
α_2	60	8.5052	0.0527	8.4075	8.5936	1.0091	0.0057	0.5023
λ_2	5	0.0939	0.0024	0.0892	0.0989	0.9998	−0.0021	0.4991
β_0	30	−0.00007	0.00005	−0.00009	0.00009	1.0032	0.0050	0.5020
β_1	40	0.00030	0.0049	−0.0089	0.0092	0.9998	−0.0088	0.4964
β_2	40	0.0002	0.0050	−0.0090	0.0092	1.0048	0.0103	0.5041

Table 10.11 Posterior summary for Australian twin data for Model RH-X

Burn-in period = 960

Parameter (values)	Lag	Estimate	SE	Lower credible limit	Upper credible limit	GR values	Geweke values	p-values
α_1	70	1.9161	0.0536	1.8112	1.9973	0.9997	0.0006	0.5002
λ_1	80	798.4733	5.5537	790.378	809.2554	1.0031	−0.0056	0.4977
α_2	50	1.7109	0.0518	1.6104	1.7934	1.0059	−0.00006	0.4999
λ_2	80	699.644	5.6643	690.6249	709.464	1.0099	−0.0024	0.4990
β_0	90	−0.0000007	0.00006	−0.00009	0.00010	1.0038	0.0176	0.5070
β_1	60	−0.00037	0.0057	−0.0094	0.0093	1.0006	0.0107	0.5042
β_2	80	−0.00027	0.0056	−0.0094	0.0094	1.0022	−0.0013	0.4994

Table 10.12 AIC, BIC, and DIC comparison

Model	AIC	BIC	DIC
Model RH-I	5367.552	5413.980	5357.351
Model RH-II	5247.973	5292.201	5241.062
Model RH-III	5367.552	5413.980	5357.351
Model RH-IV	5424.76	5455.625	5413.346
Model RH-V	5351.437	5382.301	5336.626
Model RH-VI	5355.809	5396.766	5351.894
Model RH-VII	5781.328	5901.931	5935.093
Model RH-VIII	5384.161	5426.847	5375.313
Model RH-IX	5453.923	5480.929	5444.396
Model RH-X	5403.255	5430.26	5390.599

Table 10.13 Bayes factor values and decision for models fitted to Australian twin data set

Numerator model against denominator model	$2log(B_{jk})$	Range	Evidence against model in denominator
Model RH-I against Model RH-VI	110.25	>10	Very strong
Model RH-II against Model RH-VII	1515.59	>10	Very strong
Model RH-III against Model RH-VIII	11.34	>10	Very strong
Model RH-IV against Model RH-IX	33.0837	>10	Very strong
Model RH-V against Model RH-X	53.5692	>10	Very strong

$$B_{jk} = \frac{M_j}{M_k}$$

References

Andersen, P.K., Borgan, O., Gill, R.D., Keiding, N.: Statistical Models Based on Counting Processes. Springer, New York (1993)

Barlow, R.E., Marshal, A.W., Proschan, F.: Properties of the probability distribution with monotone hazard rate. Ann. Math. Stat. **34**, 375–389 (1963)

Block, H.W., Savits, T.H., Singh, H.: On the reversed hazard rate function. Probab. Eng. Inf. Sci. **12**, 69–90 (1998)

Burr, I.W.: Cumulative frequency distribution. Ann. Math. Stat. **13**, 215–232 (1942)

Clayton, D.G.: A model for association in bivariate life tables and its application in epidemiological studies of familial tendency in chronic disease incidence. Biometrika **65**, 141–151 (1978)

Duffy, D.L., Martin, N.G., Mathews, J.D.: Appendectomy in Australian twins. Aust. J. Hum. Genet. **47**(3), 590–592 (1990)

Gleeja, V.L.: Department modelling and analysis of bivariate lifetime data using reversed hazard rates. Ph.D. thesis, Cochin University of Science and Technology, India (2008)

Hanagal, D.D., Bhambure, S.M.: Shared inverse Gaussian frailty model based on reversed hazard rate for modeling Australian twin data. J. Indian Soc. Probab. Stat. **15**, 9–37 (2014)

Hanagal, D.D., Bhambure, S.M.: Modeling bivariate survival data using shared inverse Gaussian frailty model. Commun. Stat. Theory Methods **45**(17), 4969–4987 (2016)

Hanagal, D.D., Bhambure, S.M.: Modeling Australian twin data using shared positive stable frailty models based on reversed hazard rate. Commun. Stat. Theory Methods **46**(8), 3754–3771 (2017a)

Hanagal, D.D., Bhambure, S.M.: Shared gamma frailty models based on reversed hazard rate for modeling Australian twin data. Commun. Stat. Theory Methods **46**(12), 5812–5826 (2017b)

Hanagal, D.D., Pandey, A.: Gamma shared frailty model based on reversed hazard rate for bivariate survival data. Stat. Probab. Lett. **88**, 190–196 (2014)

Hanagal, D.D., Pandey, A.: Gamma frailty model based on reversed hazard rate. Commun. Stat.: Theory Methods **45**(7), 2071–2088 (2015a)

Hanagal, D.D., Pandey, A.: Shared frailty models based on reversed hazard rate for modeling Australian twin data. Indian Assoc. Prod. Qual. Reliab. Trans. **40**(1), 61–93 (2015b)

Hanagal, D.D., Pandey, A.: Modeling bivariate survival data based on reversed hazard rate. Int. J. Math. Model. Numer. Optim. **6**(1), 72–199 (2015c)

Hanagal, D.D., Pandey, A.: Shared frailty models based on reversed hazard rate for modeling Australian twin data. Indian Assoc. Prod. Qual. Reliab. Trans. **40**(1), 61–93 (2015d)

Hanagal, D.D., Pandey, A.: Inverse Gaussian shared frailty models with generalized exponential and generalized inverted exponential as baseline distributions. J. Data Sci. **13**(2), 569–602 (2015e)

Hanagal, D.D., Pandey, A.: Inverse Gaussian shared frailty models based on reversed hazard rate. Model Assist. Stat. Appl. **11**, 137–151 (2016a)

Hanagal, D.D., Pandey, A.: Gamma shared frailty model based on reversed hazard rate. Commun. Stat.: Theory Methods **45**(7), 2071–2088 (2016b)

Hanagal, D.D., Pandey, A.: Shared frailty models based on reversed hazard rate for modified inverse Weibull distribution as a baseline distribution. Commun. Stat. Theory Methods **46**(1), 234–246 (2017a)

Hanagal, D.D., Pandey, A.: Shared inverse Gaussian frailty models based on additive hazards. Commun. Stat. Theory Methods **46**(22), 11143–11162 (2017b)

Hanagal, D.D., Pandey, A., Sankaran, P.G.: Shared frailty model based on reversed hazard rate for left censoring data. Commun. Stat.: Simul. Comput. **46**(1), 230–243 (2017)

Kakade, C.S., Shirke, D.T., Kundu, D.: Inference for P(Y<X) in exponentiated Gumbel distribution. J. Stat. Appl. **3**(2), 121–133 (2008)

Kalbfliesh, J.D., Lawless, J.F.: Inference based on retrospective ascertainment: an analysis of the data on transmission-related AIDS. J. Am. Stat. Assoc. **84**, 360–372 (1989)

Kumar, D., Singh, A.: Recurrence relations for single and product moments of lower record values from modified-inverse Weibull distribution. Gen. Math. Notes **3**(1), 26–31 (2011)

Lawless, J.F.: Statistical Models and Methods for Lifetime Data, 2nd edn. Wiley, New York (2003)

Mudholkar, G.S., Srivastava, D.K.: Exponentiated Weibull family for analyzing bathtub failure data. IEEE Trans. Reliab. **42**, 299–302 (1993)

Mudholkar, G.S., Srivastava, D.K., Freimer, M.: The exponential Weibull family: a re-analysis of the bus-motor-failure data. Technometrics **37**, 436–445 (1995)

Nadarajah, S.: The exponential Gumbel distribution with climate application. Environmetrics. **17**(1), 13–23 (2006)

Sankaran, P.G., Gleeja, V.L.: On bivariate reversed hazard rates. J. Jpn. Stat. Soc. **10**, 181–198 (2006)

Sankaran, P.G., Gleeja, V.L.: Proportional reversed hazard and frailty models. Metrika **68**, 333–342 (2008)

Sankaran, P.G., Gleeja, V.L.: On proportional reversed hazards frailty models. Metron **69**(2), 151–173 (2011)

Sengupta, A., Nanda, A.K.: Log concave and concave distributions in reliability. Nav. Res. Logist. **46**, 419–433 (1999)

Shaked, M., Shantikumar, J.G.: Stochastic Orders and Their Applications. Academic, New York (1994)

Surles, J.G., Padgett, W.J.: Inference for reliability and stress-strength for a scaled Burr type X distribution. Lifetime Data Anal. **7**, 187–200 (2001)

Surles, J.G., Padgett, W.J.: Some properties of a scaled Burr type X distribution. J. Stat. Plan. Inference **128**(1), 271–280 (2005)

Chapter 11
Comparison of Gamma and Inverse Gaussian Frailty Models

11.1 Introduction

In this chapter, we compare the gamma frailty and inverse Gaussian frailty models with three different baseline distributions, namely, Gompertz, log-logistic, and bivariate exponential of Marshall and Olkin (1967). We also analyze three data sets, namely, acute leukemia data, litters of rat data, and diabetic retinopathy data with six proposed models based on gamma and inverse Gaussian frailty models. Hanagal and Sharma (2012a, b, c) proposed shared gamma frailty models with log-logistic baseline distribution and analyze the litters of rat data (tumorigenesis data). Hanagal and Sharma (2013b) developed inverse Gaussian frailty models with Gompertz baseline distribution to analyze litters of rat data. Hanagal and Sharma (2013a, 2015a) proposed shared gamma and inverse Gaussian frailty models with log-logistic baseline distribution to analyze acute leukemia data. Hanagal and Sharma (2015b) analyzed diabetic retinopathy data using shared gamma and inverse Gaussian frailty models for the multiplicative model with bivariate exponential distribution as the baseline distribution. The gamma share frailty model has been discussed in detail in Chap. 9 with five baseline distributions. Now we briefly summarize the inverse Gaussian frailty model. An alternative to gamma frailty distribution is inverse Gaussian frailty distribution. The inverse Gaussian frailty distribution has been discussed in detail in Chap. 5, Sect. 5.3. From Sect. 5.3 and under the restriction, $mu = 1$, the density function and the Laplace transformation of the inverse Gaussian distribution are given by

$$f_Z(z) = \begin{cases} \left[\dfrac{1}{2\pi\theta}\right]^{\frac{1}{2}} z^{-\frac{3}{2}} e^{\frac{(z-1)^2}{2z\theta}} & ; \ z > 0, \theta > 0 \\ 0 & ; \ otherwise, \end{cases}$$

© Springer Nature Singapore Pte Ltd. 2019
D. D. Hanagal, *Modeling Survival Data Using Frailty Models*,
Industrial and Applied Mathematics, https://doi.org/10.1007/978-981-15-1181-3_11

and the Laplace transform is

$$L_Z(s) = exp\left[\frac{1 - (1 + 2\theta s)^{\frac{1}{2}}}{\theta}\right],$$

with variance of Z as θ. The frailty variable Z is degenerate at $Z = 1$ when θ tends to zero.

11.2 Baseline Distributions

11.2.1 Gompertz Distribution

Gompertz model, used most frequently by medical researchers and biologists in modeling the mortality ratio data, was formulated by Gompertz (1825). Gompertz distribution is a growth model and has been used in relation with tumor development. Ahuja and Nash (1979) showed that Gompertz distribution, with a simple conversion, related to some distributions in the Pearson distributions family. Osman (1987) used a Gompertz distribution with two parameters, worked on the features of the distribution, and offered that it should be used in modeling the life span data analyzing the survival ratio in heterogenic masses. It has been widely used, especially in actuarial and biological applications and in demography.

The Gompertz baseline hazard function corresponds to

$$h(t) = \lambda \exp(\gamma t)$$

and the cumulative hazard function is

$$H(t) = \lambda \gamma^{-1}(\exp(\gamma t) - 1)$$

with $\lambda > 0, \gamma \in R$. For $\gamma = 0$, the baseline hazard rate reduces to the exponential hazard. The corresponding survival function is

$$S(t) = \exp[-\lambda \gamma^{-1}(\exp(\gamma t) - 1)]$$

We note that for $\gamma > 0$, $S(t)$ goes to zero for $t \to \infty$. With $\gamma < 0$, $S(t)$ goes to $0 < \exp(\lambda \gamma^{-1}) < 1$ for $t \to \infty$. Therefore, the event never occurs for a proportion $\exp(\lambda \gamma^{-1})$ of the population. We therefore consider the case $\gamma > 0$.

Here, the two-parameter Gompertz distribution is considered. Let us assume that the independent random variables T_1 and T_2 have Gompertz distribution with parameters λ_1, γ_1 and λ_2, γ_2, respectively. In short, we say $Gomp(\lambda_j, \gamma_j)$, $(j = 1, 2)$.

11.2.2 Log-Logistic Distribution

The log-logistic distribution has a fairly flexible functional form, it is one of the parametric survival time models in which the hazard rate may be decreasing, increasing,
as well as hump-shaped, that is, it initially increases and then decreases. If the mortality ratio in a life analysis slowly decreases after it reaches to a maximum point
over a finite period, it is suitable to use a non-monotonic failure rate distribution
model on the survival data. An example of this is given by Langlands et al. (1979) in
a study of the curability of breast cancer data, where peak mortality occurred after
about 3 years.

   In cases where one comes across to censored data, using log-logistic distribution is
mathematically more advantageous than other distributions. According to the study
of Gupta et al. (1999), the log-logistic distribution is proved to be suitable in analyzing
survival data conducted by Cox (1970), Cox and Oakes (1984), Bennett (1983) and
O'Quigley and Struthers (1982). Gupta et al. (1999) used log-logistic distribution in
survival analysis on lung cancer data in their studies. In their research, they estimated
the point where the mortality ratio reached maximum level. They estimated the
parameters of the distribution using the maximum likelihood estimate and bootstrap
methods and they observed the proximity of the results. Log-logistic analysis is used
as a parametric model in survival analysis for events whose rate increases initially and
decreases later, for example, mortality from cancer following diagnosis or treatment.
It has a fairly flexible functional form with two parameters, denoted by $\log L(\gamma, \lambda)$.

   The distribution imposes the following functional forms on the density, survival,
hazard, and cumulative hazard function:

probability density function
$$f(t) = \frac{\left(\frac{\gamma}{\lambda}\right)\left(\frac{t}{\lambda}\right)^{\gamma-1}}{[1+\left(\frac{t}{\lambda}\right)^{\gamma}]^2} \quad (\gamma > 0, \lambda > 0),$$

survival function
$$S(t) = \left[1 + \left(\frac{t}{\lambda}\right)^{\gamma}\right]^{-1},$$

hazard function
$$h(t) = \frac{\left(\frac{\gamma}{\lambda}\right)\left(\frac{t}{\lambda}\right)^{\gamma-1}}{1+\left(\frac{t}{\lambda}\right)^{\gamma}},$$

cumulative hazard function
$$H(t) = \ln\left[1 + \left(\frac{t}{\lambda}\right)^{\gamma}\right].$$

The fact that the cumulative distribution function can be written in closed form is
particularly useful for analysis of survival data with censoring (Bennett 1983). The
log-logistic distribution is very similar in shape to the lognormal distribution, but is
more suitable for use in the analysis of survival data. This is because of its greater
mathematical tractability when dealing with the censored observations which occur
frequently in such data. The contribution made by a right-censored observation to the

likelihood is equal to the value of the survivor function at the time of censoring. This
can be evaluated explicitly for the log-logistic distribution, but not for the lognormal.

Here, the two-parameter log-logistic distribution is considered. Let us assume
that the independent random variables T_1 and T_2 have log-logistic distribution with
parameters γ_1, λ_1 and γ_2, λ_2, respectively. In short, we say $LLD(\gamma_j, \lambda_j), (j = 1, 2)$.

11.2.3 Bivariate Exponential Distribution

Marshall and Olkin (M–O) Marshall and Olkin (1967) proposed bivariate exponential
(BVE) distribution for failure time distribution of paired components in which two
components can fail simultaneously. This model holds two properties, a lack of
memory property (LMP) and exponential marginals. In this case, there is a positive
probability due to simultaneous failures of two components in a parallel system with
two components. It is not absolutely continuous with respect to Lebesgue measure
in R^2 but contains a singular component with respect to Lebesgue measure in R^1.

Properties of this Marshall–Olkin model are described in detail in Barlow and
Proschan (1975). It has been applied in reliability theory (Harris 1968) where it may
be used to model the time to failure of paired components such as aircraft engines or
the time to the registration of events on adjacent Geiger counters and may be used
in survival analysis to model the time to failure of paired organs such as eyes, lungs,
kidneys, etc. Hence, Marshall–Olkin bivariate exponential (MOBVE) distribution
can be used quite effectively to analyze such bivariate data set.

Marshall and Olkin (1967) proposed a bivariate extension of the exponential
distribution as a model for failure time distribution of a system where the lifetimes
(T_1, T_2) of the two components (A, B) may depend on each other and the lifetime of
main system may also depend on the lifetimes of both components. The cumulative
hazard function and corresponding survival function of the lifetimes (T_1, T_2) of the
two components are given by

$$H(t_1, t_2) = \lambda_1 t_1 + \lambda_2 t_2 + \lambda_3 t_{(2)}; \qquad t_1, t_2 > 0$$

and

$$\begin{aligned} S(t_1, t_2) &= P(T_1 > t_1, T_2 > t_2) \\ &= \exp[-\lambda_1 t_1 - \lambda_2 t_2 - \lambda_3 t_{(2)}]; \qquad t_1, t_2 > 0, \end{aligned}$$

where $t_{(2)} = max(t_1, t_2)$; $\lambda_1, \lambda_2, \lambda_3 > 0$ are scale parameters.

The corresponding density function can be defined by

$$f(t_1, t_2) = \begin{cases} \lambda_1(\lambda_2 + \lambda_3) \exp[-\lambda_1 t_1 - (\lambda_2 + \lambda_3)t_2] \;; 0 < t_1 < t_2 \\ (\lambda_1 + \lambda_3)\lambda_2 \exp[-(\lambda_1 + \lambda_3)t_1 - \lambda_2 t_2] \;; 0 < t_2 < t_1 \\ \lambda_3 \exp(-\lambda t) \qquad\qquad\qquad\qquad ; t_1 = t = t_2. \end{cases}$$

The bivariate exponential (BVE) model has some important properties, which are as follows:

1. Both marginal distributions of BVE are univariate exponential. More specifically speaking, we can state that

$$(T_1, T_2) \sim BVE(\lambda_1, \lambda_2, \lambda_3) \Longrightarrow T_1 \sim Exp(\lambda_1 + \lambda_3)$$
$$T_2 \sim Exp(\lambda_2 + \lambda_3)$$
$$T_{(1)} = min(T_1, T_2) \sim Exp(\lambda_1 + \lambda_2 + \lambda_3),$$

where $(\lambda_1 + \lambda_3)$, $(\lambda_2 + \lambda_3)$, and $(\lambda_1 + \lambda_2 + \lambda_3)$ are the scale parameters of T_1, T_2, and $T_{(1)}$, respectively.

2. This BVE model is not absolutely continuous with respect to Lebesgue measure in R^2, as it has a singularity on the diagonal $T_1 = T_2$.
3. The parameter λ_3 reflects the dependence between the two variables (T_1, T_2) with $\lambda_3 = 0$ implying that T_1 and T_2 are independent.
4. The probability of simultaneous failures, that is,

$$P(T_1 = T_2) = \frac{\lambda_3}{\lambda_1 + \lambda_2 + \lambda_3}$$

is positive and also the correlation between T_1 and T_2.

5. The probabilities in the remaining two regions are as follows:

$$P(T_1 < T_2) = \frac{\lambda_1}{\lambda_1 + \lambda_2 + \lambda_3} \quad and$$

$$P(T_1 > T_2) = \frac{\lambda_2}{\lambda_1 + \lambda_2 + \lambda_3}.$$

Hanagal and Kale (1991, 1992) proposed tests for λ_3, symmetry, and independence based on MLEs in bivariate exponential of Marshall and Olkin (1967). Hanagal (1992, 1997) developed estimation of parameters and proposed test for independence and symmetry in bivariate exponential of Marshall and Olkin (1967) based on censored samples. Hanagal (1995) proposed test for reliability of a component in bivariate exponential of Marshall and Olkin (1967). Hanagal (1996) proposed the method of selection of a better component in two-component system which follows a bivariate exponential of Marshall and Olkin (1967).

11.3 Frailty Models with Gompertz and Log-Logistic Baseline

The unconditional bivariate survival function at time $t_{1j} > 0$ and $t_{2j} > 0$ can be obtained by integrating over the frailty variable Z_j having the probability function $f_Z(z_j)$, for the jth individual.

$$S(t_{1j}, t_{2j}) = \int_{Z_j} S(t_{1j}, t_{2j} \mid z_j) f_Z(z_j) dz_j$$

$$= \int_{Z_j} e^{-z_j(H_{01}(t_{1j}) + H_{02}(t_{2j}))\eta_j} f_Z(z_j) dz_j$$

$$= L_{Z_j}[(H_{01}(t_{1j}) + H_{02}(t_{2j}))\eta_j],$$

where $\eta_j = e^{X_j\beta}$, $L_{Z_j}(.)$ is the Laplace transform of the frailty variable of Z_j for the jth individual and $H_{01}(t_{1j})$ and $H_{02}(t_{2j})$ are the cumulative baseline hazard rate at time $t_{1j} > 0$ and $t_{2j} > 0$. Now Z follows either gamma and/or inverse Gaussian distribution with single parameter θ as discussed in Chap. 5, and the above bivariate survival function can be written incorporating gamma and inverse Gaussian frailty for the random variable Z as follows. The unconditional bivariate distribution function of lifetimes T_1 and T_2 with gamma inverse Gaussian frailty is

$$S(t_{1j}, t_{2j}) = [1 + \theta\eta_j\{(H_{01}(t_{1j}) + H_{02}(t_{2j}))\}]^{-\frac{1}{\theta}} \tag{11.1}$$

for the gamma frailty.

$$S(t_{1j}, t_{2j}) = exp\left[\frac{1 - (1 + 2\theta\eta_j(H_{01}(t_{1j}) + H_{02}(t_{2j})))^{\frac{1}{2}}}{\theta}\right] \tag{11.2}$$

for the inverse Gaussian frailty and where $H_{01}(t_1)$ and $H_{02}(t_2)$ are the cumulative baseline hazard functions of the lifetimes T_1 and T_2, respectively.

According to different assumptions on the baseline distributions, we get different shared frailty models.

Substituting cumulative hazard function for the Gompertz and log-logistic baseline distributions in Eqs. (11.1) and (11.2), we get the unconditional bivariate survival functions at time $t_{1j} > 0$ and $t_{2j} > 0$ as

$$S_\theta(t_{1j}, t_{2j}) = [1 + \theta\eta_j\{\lambda_1\gamma_1^{-1}(exp(\gamma_1 t_{1j}) - 1) + \lambda_2\gamma_2^{-1}(exp(\gamma_2 t_{2j}) - 1)\}]^{-1/\theta} \tag{11.3}$$

for the case of the Gompertz baseline distribution with gamma frailty.

$$S_\theta(t_{1j}, t_{2j}) = \left[1 + \theta\left\{ln\left(1 + \left(\frac{t_{1j}}{\lambda_1}\right)^{\gamma_1}\right) + ln\left(1 + \left(\frac{t_{2j}}{\lambda_2}\right)^{\gamma_2}\right)\right\}\eta_j\right]^{-1/\theta} \tag{11.4}$$

for the case of the log-logistic baseline distribution with gamma frailty.

$$S_\theta(t_{1j}, t_{2j}) = exp\left[\frac{1 - (1 + 2\theta\eta_j\{\lambda_1\gamma_1^{-1}(exp(\gamma_1 t_{1j}) - 1) + \lambda_2\gamma_2^{-1}(exp(\gamma_2 t_{2j}) - 1)\})^{1/2}}{\theta}\right] \tag{11.5}$$

for the case of the Gompertz baseline distribution with inverse Gaussian frailty.

$$S_\theta(t_{1j}, t_{2j}) = \exp\left[\frac{1 - \left(1 + 2\theta\left\{ln\left(1 + \left(\frac{t_{l1}}{\lambda_1}\right)^{\gamma_1}\right) + ln\left(1 + \left(\frac{t_{l2}}{\lambda_2}\right)^{\gamma_2}\right)\right\}\eta_j\right)^{1/2}}{\theta}\right] \quad (11.6)$$

for the case of the log-logistic baseline distribution with inverse Gaussian frailty.

Here onward, we call Eqs. (11.3)–(11.6), as Model G-I, Model G-II, Model IG-I, and Model IG-II, respectively. Model G-I and Model G-II are the models with gamma frailty and Model IG-I to Model IG-II are the models with inverse Gaussian frailty.

11.4 Likelihood Specification and Bayesian Estimation of Parameters

Suppose there are n individuals under study, whose first and second observed failure times are represented by (t_{1j}, t_{2j}). Let c_{1j} and c_{2j} be the observed censoring times for the jth individual ($j = 1, 2, 3, \ldots, n$) for first and second recurrence times, respectively. We also assume the independence between censoring scheme and lifetimes of individuals.

The contribution of bivariate lifetime random variable of the jth individual in likelihood function is given by

$$L_j(t_{1j}, t_{2j}) = \begin{cases} f_1(t_{1j}, t_{2j}), & t_{1j} < c_{1j}, t_{2j} < c_{2j}, \\ f_2(t_{1j}, c_{2j}), & t_{1j} < c_{1j}, t_{2j} > c_{2j}, \\ f_3(c_{1j}, t_{2j}), & t_{1j} > c_{1j}, t_{2j} < c_{2j}, \\ f_4(c_{1j}, c_{2j}), & t_{1j} > c_{1j}, t_{2j} > c_{2j}. \end{cases}$$

and the likelihood function is

$$L(\psi, \beta, \theta) = \prod_{j=1}^{n_1} f_1(t_{1j}, t_{2j}) \prod_{j=1}^{n_2} f_2(t_{1j}, c_{2j}) \prod_{j=1}^{n_3} f_3(c_{1j}, t_{2j}) \prod_{j=1}^{n_4} f_4(c_{1j}, c_{2j}),$$

where θ, ψ, and β are, respectively, the frailty parameter, the vector of baseline parameters, and the vector of regression coefficients.

The counts n_1, n_2, n_3, and n_4 are the numbers of individuals for which first and the second failure times (t_{1j}, t_{2j}) lie in the ranges $t_{1j} < c_{1j}, t_{2j} < c_{2j}$; $t_{1j} < c_{1j}, t_{2j} > c_{2j}$; $t_{1j} > c_{1j}, t_{2j} < c_{2j}$; and $t_{1j} > c_{1j}, t_{2j} > c_{2j}$, respectively, and

$$f_1(t_{1j}, t_{2j}) = \frac{\partial^2 S(t_{1j}, t_{2j})}{\partial t_{1j} \partial t_{2j}},$$

$$f_2(t_{1j}, c_{2j}) = -\frac{\partial S(t_{1j}, c_{2j})}{\partial t_{1j}},$$

$$f_3(c_{1j}, t_{2j}) = -\frac{\partial S(c_{1j}, t_{2j})}{\partial t_{2j}}, and$$

$$f_4(c_{1j}, c_{2j}) = S(c_{1j}, c_{2j}).$$

The functions, f_1, f_2, f_3, and f_4 are evaluated in the four models.
For Model G-I,

$$f_1 = (1 + \theta)\lambda_1\lambda_2 \exp(2x_i'\beta) \exp(\gamma_1 t_{i1} + \gamma_2 t_{i2})S^{(1+2\theta)}(t_{1j}, t_{2j})$$
$$f_2 = \lambda_1 \eta_j \exp(\gamma_1 t_{i1})S^{(1+\theta)}(t_{1j}, c_{2j})$$
$$f_3 = \lambda_2 \eta_j \exp(\gamma_2 t_{2j})S^{(1+\theta)}(c_{1j}, t_{2j})$$
$$f_4 = S(c_{1i}, c_{2i}),$$

where $S(., .)$ is given by Eq. (11.3).
For Model G-II, we have

$$f_1 = \frac{(1 + \theta)\gamma_1\gamma_2 t_{1j}^{\gamma_1-1} t_{2j}^{\gamma_2-1}\eta_j^2}{\lambda_1^{\gamma_1}\lambda_2^{\gamma_2}[1 + (t_{1j}/\lambda_1)^{\gamma_1}][1 + (t_{2j}/\lambda_2)^{\gamma_2}]}S^{(1+2\theta)}(t_{1j}, t_{2j})$$

$$f_2 = \frac{\gamma_1 t_{1j}^{\gamma_1-1}\eta_j}{\lambda_1^{\gamma_1}[1 + (t_{1j}/\lambda_1)^{\gamma_1}]}S^{(1+\theta)}(t_{1j}, c_{2j})$$

$$f_3 = \frac{\gamma_2 t_{2j}^{\gamma_2-1}\eta_j}{\lambda_2^{\gamma_2}[1 + (t_{2j}/\lambda_2)^{\gamma_2}]}S^{(1+\theta)}(c_{1j}, t_{2j})$$

$$f_4 = S(c_{1j}, c_{2j}),$$

where $S_\theta(., .)$ is given by Eq. (11.4).
For Model IG-I, we have

$$f_1 = \frac{\lambda_1\lambda_2 \exp(\gamma_1 t_{1j} + \gamma_2 t_{2j})S(t_{1j}, t_{2j})\phi_2(t_{1j}, t_{2j})}{\left[\phi_1(t_{1j}, t_{2j})\right]^{\frac{3}{2}}}\eta_j^2$$

$$f_2 = \frac{\lambda_1 \exp(\gamma_1 t_{1j})S(t_{1j}, c_{2j})}{\left[\phi_1(t_{1j}, c_{2j})\right]^{\frac{1}{2}}}\eta_j$$

$$f_3 = \frac{\lambda_2 \exp(\gamma_2 t_{2j})S(c_{1j}, t_{2j})}{\left[\phi_1(c_{1j}, t_{2j})\right]^{\frac{1}{2}}}\eta_j$$

$$f_4 = S(c_{1j}, c_{2j}),$$

where $S_\theta(.,.)$ is given by Eq.(11.5) and $\phi_1(a_j, b_j) = 1 + 2\theta\{\lambda_1\gamma_1^{-1}(\exp(\gamma_1 a_j - 1)) + \lambda_2\gamma_2^{-1}(\exp(\gamma_2 b_j - 1))\}\eta_j$; $\phi_2(a_j, b_j) = \theta + [\phi_1(a_j, b_j)]^{\frac{1}{2}}$.

For Model IG-II, we have

$$f_1 = \frac{\gamma_1\gamma_2 t_{1j}^{\gamma_1-1} t_{2j}^{\gamma_2-1} \phi_4(t_{1j}, t_{2j}) S(t_{1j}, t_{2j})\eta_j^2}{\lambda_1^{\gamma_1}\lambda_2^{\gamma_2}[1 + (t_{1j}/\lambda_1)^{\gamma_1}][1 + (t_{2j}/\lambda_2)^{\gamma_2}] \left[\phi_3(t_{1j}, t_{2j})\right]^{\frac{3}{2}}}$$

$$f_2 = \frac{\gamma_1 t_{1j}^{\gamma_1-1} S(t_{1j}, c_{2j})\eta_j}{\lambda_1^{\gamma_1}[1 + (t_{1j}/\lambda_1)^{\gamma_1}] \left[\phi_3(t_{1j}, c_{2j})\right]^{\frac{1}{2}}}$$

$$f_3 = \frac{\gamma_2 t_{2j}^{\gamma_2-1} S(c_{1j}, t_{2j})\eta_j}{\lambda_2^{\gamma_2}[1 + (t_{2j}/\lambda_2)^{\gamma_2}] \left[\phi_3(c_{1j}, t_{2j})\right]^{\frac{1}{2}}}$$

$$f_4 = S(c_{1j}, c_{2j}),$$

where $S(.,.)$ is given by Eq.(11.6) and $\phi_3(a_j, b_j) = 1 + 2\theta\left\{ln\left(1 + \left(\frac{a_j}{\lambda_1}\right)^{\gamma_1}\right) + ln\left(1 + \left(\frac{b_j}{\lambda_2}\right)^{\gamma_2}\right)\right\}\eta_j$; $\phi_4(a_j, b_j) = \theta + [\phi_3(a_j, b_j)]^{\frac{1}{2}}$.

Unfortunately, computing the maximum likelihood estimators (MLEs) involves solving high-dimensional optimization problem. As the method of maximum likelihood fails to estimate the parameters due to convergence problem in the iterative procedure, we use the Bayesian approach.

11.5 Analysis of Acute Leukemia Data

We illustrate the proposed model with one well-known example. The proposed methods are applied to the data set of acute leukemia remission times of patients, given by Freireich et al. (1963). The data are reported in Hougaard (2000). We examine the effect of a clinical trial of a drug 6-mercaptopurine (6-MP) versus a placebo in 42 children with acute leukemia.

Here we demonstrate the method using the well-known leukemia data, consisting of 21 pairs matched of leukemia patients, analyzed by Cox (1972), Hougaard (2000), Ibrahim et al. (2001), Spiegelhalter et al. (2002), among others. The leukemia remission times data were first given by Freireich et al. (1963).

The random variable of interest consists of remission times (in weeks) of the patients assigned to treatment with a 6-MP drug or a placebo during remission maintenance therapy. After having been judged to be in a state of partial or complete remission for the primary treatment with prednisone, a patient was paired with a second patient in the same state. One randomly chosen patient in each pair received the maintenance treatment 6-MP and the other a placebo. It was assumed that deaths at a given time always preceded censoring at the same time, and other ties were broken by randomization. Success (failure) was defined to occur in the ith pair if the time from remission to relapse or censoring for the patient on 6-MP (placebo) exceeded the time to relapse for the patient on placebo (6-MP). The trial was stopped once the number of successes or failures had reached significance. Out of 21 patients in treatment group, 9 failed during the study period and 12 were censored. In contrast, none of the data is censored in placebo group, that is, all 21 patients in the placebo group went out of remission during the study period. The data set contains a single covariate x with value 0 or 1 indicating remission status (0=partial, 1=complete). The acute leukemia data are partially presented in Chap. 1.

In the analysis, we have used the R program. Given the model assumptions, this program performs the Gibbs sampler by simulating from the full conditional distributions. The Bayesian estimators were obtained through the implementation of the Metropolis–Hastings algorithm within Gibbs sampling scheme based on normal transition kernels. We implemented 95,000 iterations of the algorithm and described the first 3,500 and 3,000 iterations as a burn in for Model I and Model II, respectively. To generate the Gibbs posterior samples, we choose to use two parallel chains. The chains should start from over-dispersed initial values to ensure good convergence of parameter space.

We have taken the independent prior as $\lambda_i \sim \Gamma(10^{-4}, 10^{-4})$, $\gamma_i \sim \Gamma(1, 10^{-4})$, $\beta \sim N(0, 10^5)$, and $\theta \sim \Gamma(10^{-4}, 10^{-4})$ for both models. Here, results for chain I and chain II are similar, so we present result for only one chain (i.e., chain I).

To check goodness of fit of acute leukemia data set, we consider Kolmogorov–Smirnov (K–S) test for two baseline distributions. Table 11.1 gives the p-values of K–S statistics for all the four models.

Table 11.1 gives the p-values of goodness-of-fit test for Model I to Model IV. Thus, from p-values of K–S test, we can say that there is no statistical evidence to reject the hypothesis that data are from these models in the marginal case and we assume that they also fit for bivariate case. Due to lack of space, we show the graph of parametric and nonparametric survival functions of gamma frailty model with Gompertz baseline distribution in Fig. 11.1. These graphs show that the survival curves are very close to each other.

In the analysis, we have used the R program. Given the model assumptions, this program performs the Gibbs sampler by simulating from the full conditional distributions. A widely used prior for frailty parameter θ is gamma distribution with mean one and large variance, $\Gamma(\phi, \phi)$, say with a small choice of ϕ and the prior for regression parameter β is normal with mean zero and large variance, say σ^2. Similar types of prior distributions are used in Ibrahim et al. (2001), Sahu et al. (1997), and Santos and Achcar (2010). So, in our study, also, we use same prior for

Table 11.1 p-values of K–S statistics for goodness-of-fit test for acute leukemia data set

Distribution	Recurrence time	
	First	Second
Model G-I	0.9465	0.9004
Model G-II	0.9358	0.8968
Model IG-I	0.9341	0.9540
Model IG-II	0.9669	0.9630

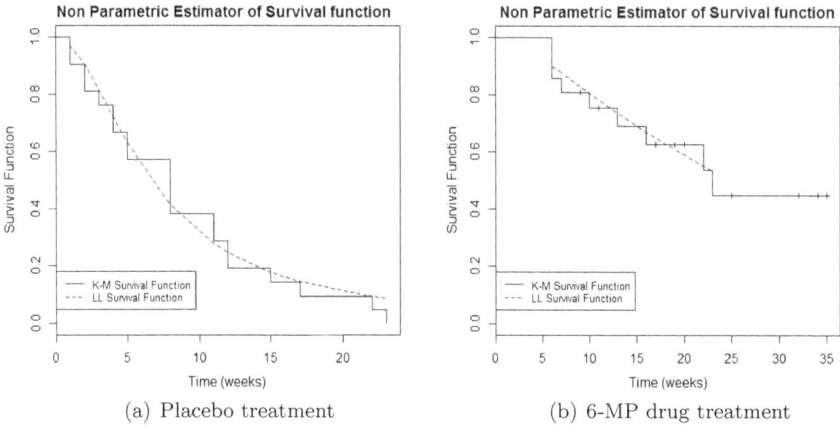

Fig. 11.1 Comparison of nonparametric survival function with Gompertz survival function for acute leukemia data

θ and β's. Since we do not have any prior information about baseline parameters, λ_1, γ_1, λ_2, and γ_2, prior distributions are assumed to be informative. For baseline parameters λ_1, λ_2, γ_1, and γ_2, the prior is $\Gamma(a, b)$, for the frailty parameter θ, the prior is $\Gamma(\phi, \phi)$, and for regression coefficients β_i, $(i = 1, \ldots, 5)$, the prior is $N(0, \sigma^2)$. Here $\Gamma(a, b)$ is gamma distribution with shape parameter a and scale parameter b. All the hyperparameters ϕ, a, b, and σ^2 are known. We set hyperparameters as $\phi = 0.0001$, $a = 1$; $b = 0.0001$, and $\sigma^2 = 10^5$.

To estimate the parameters, we run two parallel Markov chains with the different starting points using Metropolis–Hastings algorithm within Gibbs sampling. We iterate both the chains for 95,000 times and discard 2,500 observations as burn in. As in the simulation, here also, results for chain I and chain II are similar, so we present result for only one chain (i.e., chain I).

Figure 11.2 shows the trace plot, coupling from past plot and sample autocorrelation plot for the parameter β for chain I and Model G-1 only. For other parameters, graphs have similar pattern, and so due to lack of space, we are not presenting graphs for other parameters. Trace plots for all the parameters show zigzag pattern which indicates that parameters move more freely. Thus, it seems that the Markov chain has reached the stationary state. However, a sequence of draws after burn-in period may have autocorrelation. Because of autocorrelation, consecutive draws may not be random, but values at widely separated time points are approximately independent. So, a pseudorandom sample from the posterior distribution can be found by taking values from a single run of the Markov chain at widely spaced time points (autocorrelation lag) after burn-in period. Simulated values of parameters have autocorrelation of lag k (see Tables 11.2, 11.3, 11.4, and 11.5), so every kth iteration is selected as sample to thin the chain and discarding the rest. The autocorrelation of parameters becomes almost negligible after the defined lag, given in Tables 11.2, 11.3, 11.4, and 11.5.

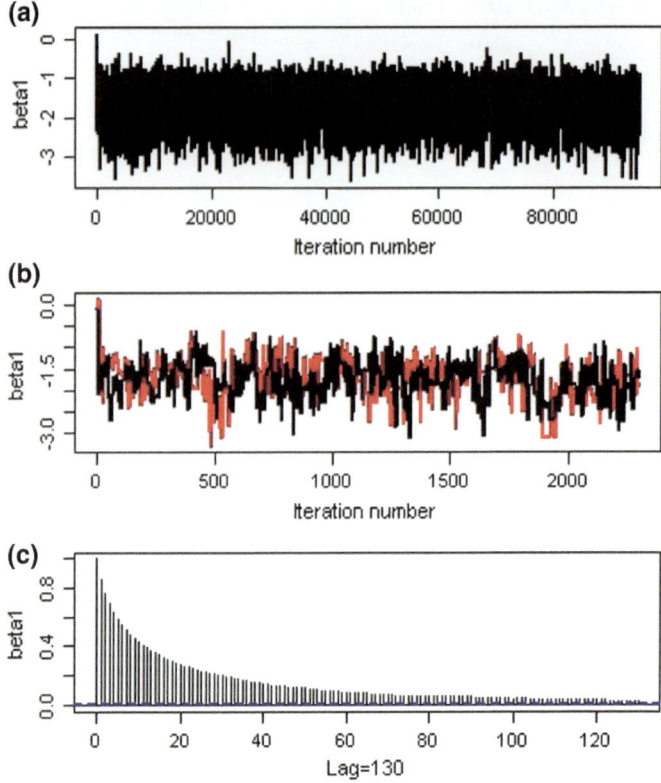

Fig. 11.2 a Trace plot, **b** Coupling from past plot and **c** Sample autocorrelation plot for the parameter β for acute leukemia data

Figure 11.3 shows autocorrelations plot with thinning number lag, histogram, running mean plot, and posterior density for the parameter β only in acute leukemia data. We can also use running mean plots to check how well our chains are mixing. A running mean plot is a plot of the iterations against the mean of the draws up to each iteration. In fact, running mean plots display a time series of the running mean for each parameter in each chain, as shown in Fig. 11.3 for β only, not for all parameters due to lack of space. These plots should be converging to a value. Running mean plot for each parameter is converging to the posterior mean of the parameter, and thus represents a good mixing of chain. Thus, our diagnostic plots suggest that the MCMC chains are mixing very well.

Monitoring convergence of the chains has been done via the Brooks and Gelman (1998) convergence diagnostic. Hence, once convergence has been achieved, 91,000 observations are taken from each chain after the burn-in period. Gelman–Rubin convergence statistic values and Geweke test statistic values with corresponding p-values for all the parameters are given in Tables 11.2, 11.3, 11.4, and 11.5. On inspection of the Brooks and Gelmans diagnostic, we find the BGR (Brooks and

Table 11.2 Posterior summary for acute leukemia data set for gamma frailty with Gompertz baseline

Par	BGR	Geweke test		A.Lag	Estimate	S.E.	Credible lower limit	Interval upper limit
		Test-stat	p-value					
λ_1	1.0012	0.0189	0.5076	300	0.0393	0.0154	0.0143	0.0739
λ_2	1.0516	−0.0114	0.4954	100	0.0138	0.0084	0.0026	0.0344
γ_1	1.0037	−0.0287	0.4885	250	0.1214	0.0447	0.0440	0.2154
γ_2	1.0087	0.0005	0.5002	200	0.0383	0.0262	0.0028	0.0971
θ	1.0013	−0.0223	0.4911	250	0.3536	0.2793	0.0548	1.1282
β	1.0513	0.0113	0.5045	150	0.3417	0.4772	−0.5689	1.3067

Table 11.3 Posterior summary for acute leukemia data set for gamma frailty with log-logistic baseline

Par	BGR	Geweke test		A.Lag	Estimate	S.E.	Credible lower limit	Interval upper limit
		Test-stat	p-value					
λ_1	1.0092	0.0008	0.5003	35	0.0598	0.0091	0.0359	0.0696
λ_2	1.0000	0.0102	0.5041	20	0.0507	0.0143	0.0182	0.0693
γ_1	1.0095	0.0028	0.5011	130	1.1902	0.4950	0.5393	2.4534
γ_2	1.0084	0.0013	0.5005	120	0.5274	0.2644	0.2070	1.2034
θ	1.0157	−0.0001	0.5000	180	0.4942	0.2878	0.5984	1.1658
β	1.0098	−0.0031	0.4988	130	−1.7664	0.4719	−2.6988	−0.8938

Table 11.4 Posterior summary for acute leukemia data set for inverse Gaussian frailty with Gompertz baseline

Par	BGR	Geweke test		A.Lag	Estimate	S.E.	Credible lower limit	Interval upper limit
		Test-stat	p-value					
λ_1	1.0039	0.0015	0.5006	100	0.0683	0.0282	0.0219	0.1269
λ_2	1.0045	−0.0095	0.4962	60	0.0175	0.0111	0.0042	0.0476
γ_1	1.0023	−0.0145	0.4942	80	0.0835	0.0301	0.0277	0.1373
γ_2	0.9999	−0.00073	0.4997	50	0.0379	0.0242	0.0022	0.0931
θ	1.00009	−0.0065	0.4974	130	0.4034	0.3235	0.0534	1.1784
β	1.0026	0.0099	0.5039	120	0.1091	0.4657	−0.7368	1.0439

Gelman Ratio) convergent to one, this shows that the convergence for the coefficient of regression β, the variance of frailty θ, and other parameters have been obtained. Also, the Geweke test statistic values are quite small and corresponding p-values are large enough to say the chains attain stationary distribution.

Table 11.5 Posterior summary for acute leukemia data set for inverse Gaussian frailty with log-logistic baseline

Par	BGR	Geweke test		A.Lag	Estimate	S.E.	Credible lower limit	Interval upper limit
		Test-stat	p-value					
λ_1	270	1.0364	0.0132	0.5052	0.0865	0.0125	0.0486	0.0994
λ_2	200	1.0013	−0.0006	0.4997	0.0742	0.0202	0.0267	0.0995
γ_1	170	1.0005	−0.0012	0.4994	1.1201	0.3741	0.5721	1.9686
γ_2	100	1.0036	−0.0118	0.4952	0.4967	0.1937	0.2219	0.9625
θ	100	1.0161	−0.0084	0.49661	0.6751	0.3601	0.0811	1.4088
β_1	60	1.0035	0.0009	0.5003	−1.5277	0.4254	−2.4354	−0.7401

The Table 11.2, 11.3, 11.4, and 11.5 present posterior summary along with Gelman–Rubin convergence statistic values and Geweke test statistic values with corresponding p-values for Model I to Model IV, respectively. Monitoring convergence of the chains has been done via the Brooks and Gelman (1998) convergence diagnostic. Hence, once convergence has been achieved, from each chain after the burn-in period. On inspection of the Brooks and Gelmans diagnostic, we find the Brooks and Gelman ratio (BGR) convergent to one, and this shows that the convergence for the coefficient of regression β, the variance of frailty θ, and other parameters have been obtained. Also, the Geweke test statistic values are quite small and corresponding p-values are large enough to say the chains attain stationary distribution.

The autocorrelation of parameters becomes almost negligible after the defined lag, given in Tables 11.2 and 11.5 for all the models. There is not much difference in the posterior estimates of baseline parameters, presented in Tables 11.2, 11.3, 11.4, and 11.5 for all the models. On the average, λ_1 is greater than λ_2 for all the four models. This is attributed to the effectiveness of 6-MP drug. Thus, it is concluded that 6-MP patients have significantly less risk of leukemia relapse than placebo group patients. The posterior estimate of $\theta = 0.3536$ for Model G-I, $\theta = 0.4942$ for Model G-II, $\theta = 0.4034$ for Model IG-I, and $\theta = 0.6751$ for Model IG-II show that there exists significant heterogeneity in population of patients even though each patient shares the same value of the covariate. The regression coefficient β is not significant in Model G-I and Model IG-I while in Model G-II and Model IG-II the regression coefficient β is significant which is very clear from the credible intervals. Credible intervals of β in Model G-II and Model IG-II do not contain zero. Thus, patients have significant effect due to a partial or complete remission of their leukemia for Model G-II and Model IG-II. In other words, we can say that there is risk of acute leukemia relapse for both partial or complete remission patients in log-logistic baseline distribution with gamma and inverse Gaussian frailty models.

To compare both models, we first use AIC, BIC, and DIC values which are given in Table 11.6. As it is clear from the table, the AIC, BIC, and DIC values for Model G-I and Model IG-I are very small as compared to Model G-II and Model IG-II, and hence Model G-I and Model IG-I are better than other two models. To take decision

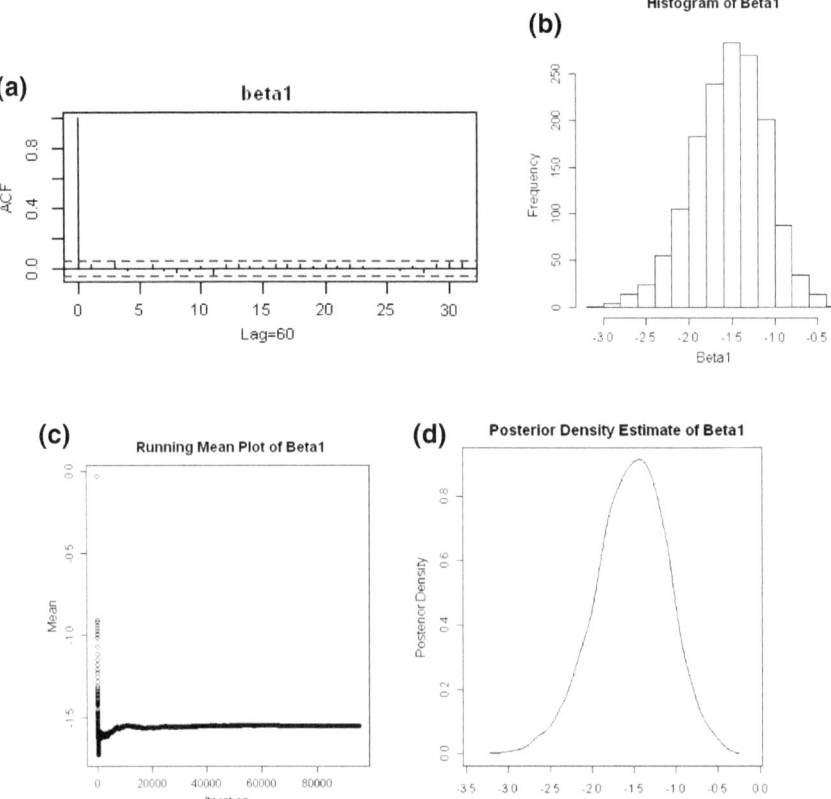

Fig. 11.3 Graphs of **a** Autocorrelations with thinning number lag (given below the figure), **b** Histogram, **c** Running mean plots, and **d** Posterior density plots for the parameter β for acute leukemia data for Model G1

Table 11.6 AIC, BIC, and DIC values for acute leukemia data set

Model	AIC	BIC	DIC
Model G-I	228.8574	235.1246	224.8326
Model G-II	319.0666	327.8147	316.1176
Model IG-I	228.3047	234.5718	223.9149
Model IG-II	319.6527	329.5828	314.9786

about better model between Model G-I and Model IG-I, we use Bayes factor. From Table 11.7, which represents Bayes factor for models, we can observe that between Model G-I and Model IG-I, there is positive evidence against Model IG-I. So, we conclude that the gamma frailty with Gompertz baseline distribution (Model IG-I) is better than the inverse Gaussian frailty with Gompertz baseline distribution (Model G-I) for modeling acute leukemia data.

Table 11.7 Bayes factor values for acute leukemia data set

Nr model against Dr model	Bayes factor	Range	Evidence against model in Dr
Model G-I vs Model IG-I	2.1088	2–6	Moderate
Model G-II vs Model IG-II	2.1775	2–6	Moderate

Table 11.8 p-values for Kolmogorov–Smirnov test statistic for litter-matched tumorigenesis data set

Distribution	Recurrence time	
	First	Second
Model G-I	0.9804	0.9753
Model G-II	0.9865	0.9779
Model IG-I	0.9838	0.9796
Model IG-II	0.9821	0.9652

11.6   Analysis of Litters of Rat Data

In this section, the method is applied to the animal tumorigenesis data described by Mantel et al. (1977). The experiment involved 50 male and 50 female litters, which consist of three rats within each litter. One rat in each litter was treated with putative carcinogen and the other two served as control animals. The data recorded are the time to tumor appearance. Censoring was induced by death from other causes, as well as by the end of study after 104 weeks. The sample of male rats was heavily censored, because there were only two male rats that developed tumors. The litters of rat data are partially presented in Chap. 1. Therefore, we restrict our analysis to the subset of the data concerning the female rats. Since three rats within each litter are from the same parents, therefore, they share common genes, pre-birth genetic behavior, environmental exposures, or carcinogenic exposures. These common genetic factors and shared carcinogenic exposures induce association in the times to tumor appearance between litter mates. Our main motive of this study is an attempt to control genetic factors. Here, the random litter effect itself is of prime interest in the analysis. So, we consider only controlled rats within each litter.

We now fit the proposed shared frailty models to the female rats' tumor time data. We have considered a statistical test also, viz., Kolmogorov–Smirnov (K–S) test for testing goodness-of-fit hypotheses to all the four models. Test procedure is developed for testing goodness of fit with data subjected to random right censoring. Here, we assume that survival times of individuals are conditionally independent so we apply K–S test to the survival times of both the rats separately. The p-values of K–S test for both baseline distributions are presented in Table 11.8 which are very large approximately close to 1. Thus, from the p-values of K–S test (see Table 11.8), we can say that there is no statistical evidence to reject the hypothesis that data are from Gompertz distribution and log-logistic distribution.

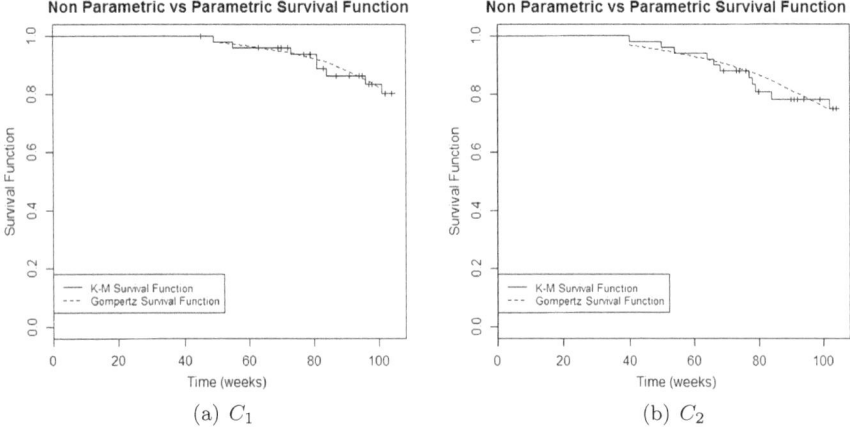

Fig. 11.4 Comparison of nonparametric survival function with Gompertz survival function for litter-matched tumorigenesis data (Model IG-I)

Figure 11.4 plots the Kaplan–Meier estimates and hypothesized theoretical distribution $S_0(t)$ for inverse Gaussian frailty with Gompertz baseline (Model IG-I) which demonstrates a close agreement between the two, i.e., nonparametric and parametric survival curves.

In the analysis, we have used the R program. Given the model assumptions, this program performs the Gibbs sampler by simulating from the full conditional distributions. A widely used prior for frailty parameter θ is gamma distribution with mean one and large variance, say $\Gamma(\phi, \phi)$, with a small choice of ϕ and the prior for regression parameter β is normal with mean zero and large variance, say σ^2. Similar types of prior distributions are used in Ibrahim et al. (2001), Sahu et al. (1997) and Santos and Achcar (2010). So, in our study, also, we use same prior for frailty parameters θ. Since we do not have any prior information about baseline parameters, $\lambda_1, \gamma_1, \lambda_2$, and γ_2, prior distributions of these parameters are assumed to be flat. We consider two different sets of prior distributions for baseline parameters, one is $\Gamma(a, b)$ and another is $U(c, d)$. All the hyperparameters ϕ, a, b, c, and d are known. Here $\Gamma(a, b)$ is gamma distribution with shape parameter a and scale parameter b and $U(c, d)$ represents uniform distribution over the interval c to d. We set hyperparameters as $\phi = 0.00001$, $a = 1$; $b = 0.0001$, $c = 0$, and $d = 100$.

We run two parallel chains for both models using two sets of prior distributions with the different starting points using Metropolis–Hastings algorithm within Gibbs sampler based on normal transition kernels. We implemented 95,000 iterations of the algorithm. To diminish the effect of the starting distribution, we generally discard the early iterations of each sequence and focus attention on the remaining. We described the first 2,700 and 6,500 iterations as a burn in for Model I and Model II, respectively. There is no effect of prior distributions on posterior summaries because estimates of parameters are nearly same. Here, results for chain I and chain II are similar so we present results for only one chain (i.e., chain I) with $\Gamma(a, b)$ as prior for

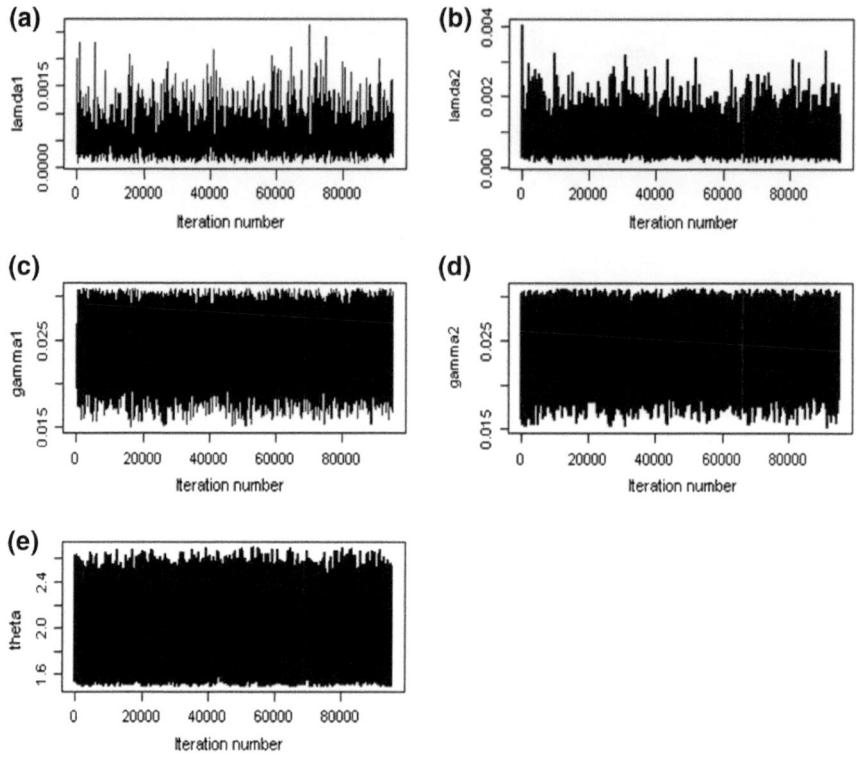

Fig. 11.5 Posterior for Model IG-I: time series plots of the posterior samples for litter-matched tumorigenesis data

baseline parameters. Trace plots for all the parameters show zigzag pattern which indicates that parameters move and mix more freely. Thus, it seems that the Markov chain has reached the stationary state. However, a sequence of draws after burn-in period may have autocorrelation. Because of autocorrelation, consecutive draws may not be random, but values at widely separated time points are approximately independent. So, a pseudorandom sample from the posterior distribution can be found by taking values from a single run of the Markov chain at widely spaced time points (autocorrelation lag) after burn-in period. Graphs for time series (or trace) plot and sample autocorrelation plot with thinning (i.e., after considering lag shown in figures) for the parameters are shown in Figs. 11.5 and 11.6 for Model IG-I only. Simulated values of parameters have autocorrelation of lag k value given below each plot in Fig. 11.7, so every kth iteration is selected as sample to thin the chain and discarding the rest. The autocorrelation of parameters becomes almost negligible after the defined lag, given in figures.

We can also use running mean plots to check how well our chains are mixing. A running mean plot is a plot of the iterations against the mean of the draws up to each iteration. In fact, running mean plots display a time series of the running mean for

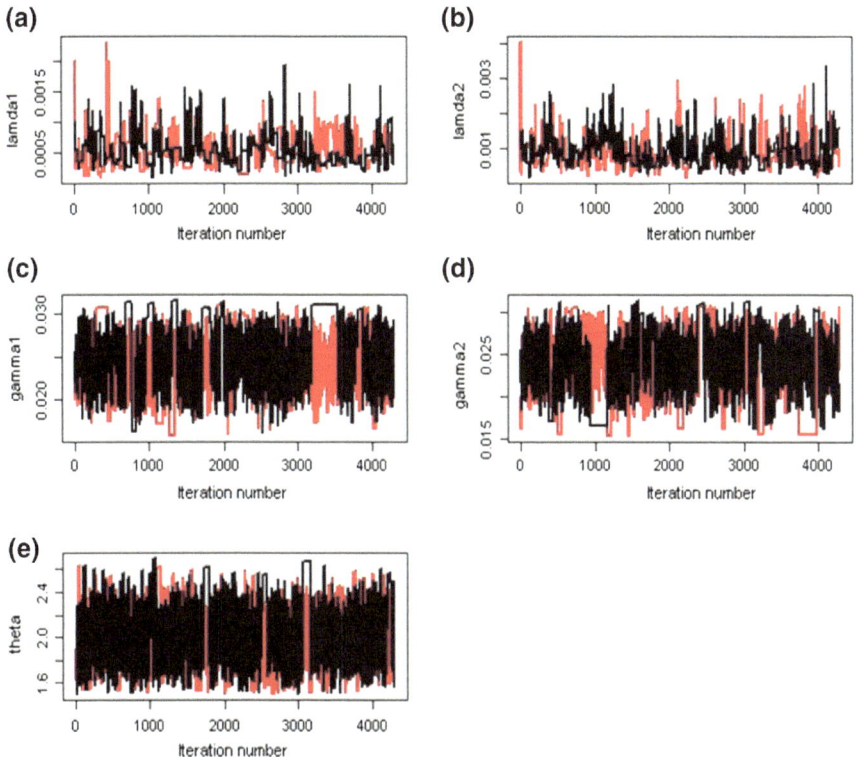

Fig. 11.6 Posterior for Model IG-I: coupling from past plots of the posterior samples for litter-matched tumorigenesis data

each parameter in each chain, as shown in Fig. 11.8 for Model IG-I only. Due to lack of space, we present the graphs of all these plots for Model IG-I only. These plots should be converging to a value. Running mean plot for each parameter is converging to the posterior mean of the parameter, and thus represents a good mixing of chain. Thus, our diagnostic plots suggest that the MCMC chains are mixing very well.

Tables 11.9, 11.10, 11.11, and 11.12 present the posterior mean, standard deviation, and 95% credible intervals for all baseline parameters, frailty variance along with Gelman–Rubin convergence statistic values, and Geweke test statistic values with corresponding p-values for all the four models. Monitoring convergence of the chains has been done via the Brooks and Gelman (1998) convergence diagnostic. On inspection of the Brooks and Gelman's diagnostic, we find the Brooks and Gelman ratio (BGR) convergent to one, and this shows that the convergence for variance of frailty θ and other parameters have been obtained. Also, the Geweke test statistic values are quite small and corresponding p-values are large enough to say the chains attain stationary distribution.

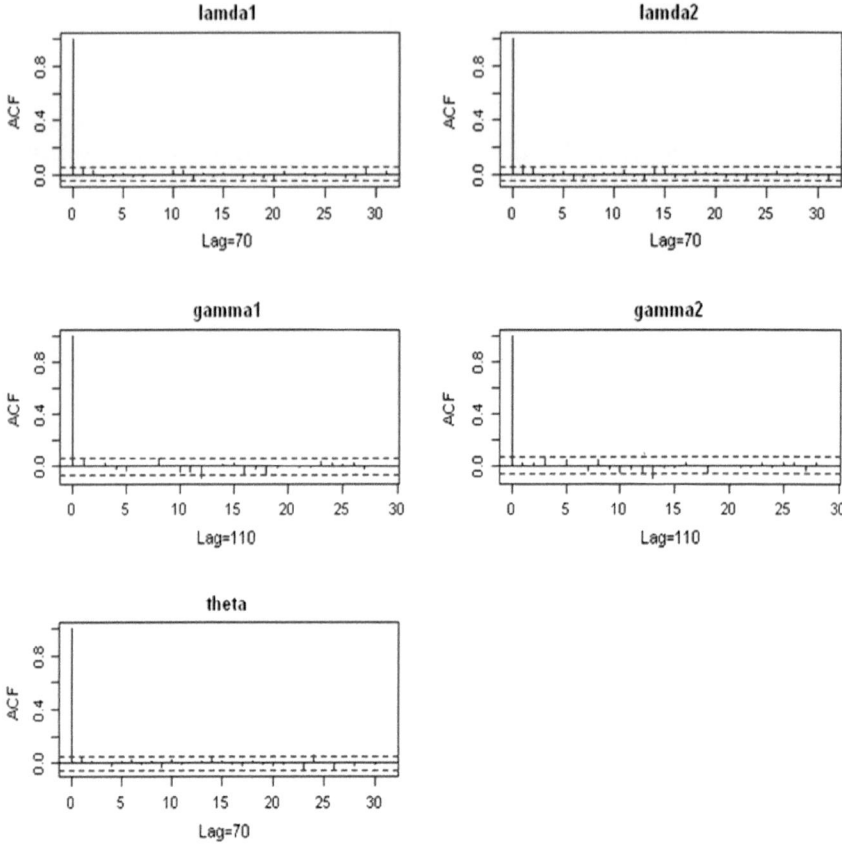

Fig. 11.7 Plots of autocorrelations with thinning number lag (given below the figure) of the posterior samples for litter-matched tumorigenesis data for Model IG-I

There is little difference between the posterior estimates of baseline parameters γ_1, γ_2 and frailty parameter θ for Model I and Model II, presented in Tables 11.9, 11.10, 11.11, and 11.12. The posterior estimate of dispersion of random effects, i.e., $\theta = 1.0028$, $\theta = 1.0027$, 1.0377, and 1.0001 for Model G-1, G-II, IG-1, and IG-II, respectively, shows that there exists highly significant heterogeneity in population of rats. Thus, there is a dependence within the litter.

To compare both models, we first use AIC, BIC, and DIC values which are given in Table 11.13. As it is clear from Table 11.13, the differences of AIC, BIC, and DIC values between gamma frailty and inverse Gaussian frailty are significant, so AIC, BIC, and DIC values are worthy to take decision between the gamma and inverse Gaussian frailties. According to these information criteria, gamma frailty models are preferred. To take strong decision about better model between Model G-I and Model G-II, we can use Bayes factor also. Table 11.14 represents Bayes factor for models and we can observe that there is very strong positive evidence for Model IG-I against

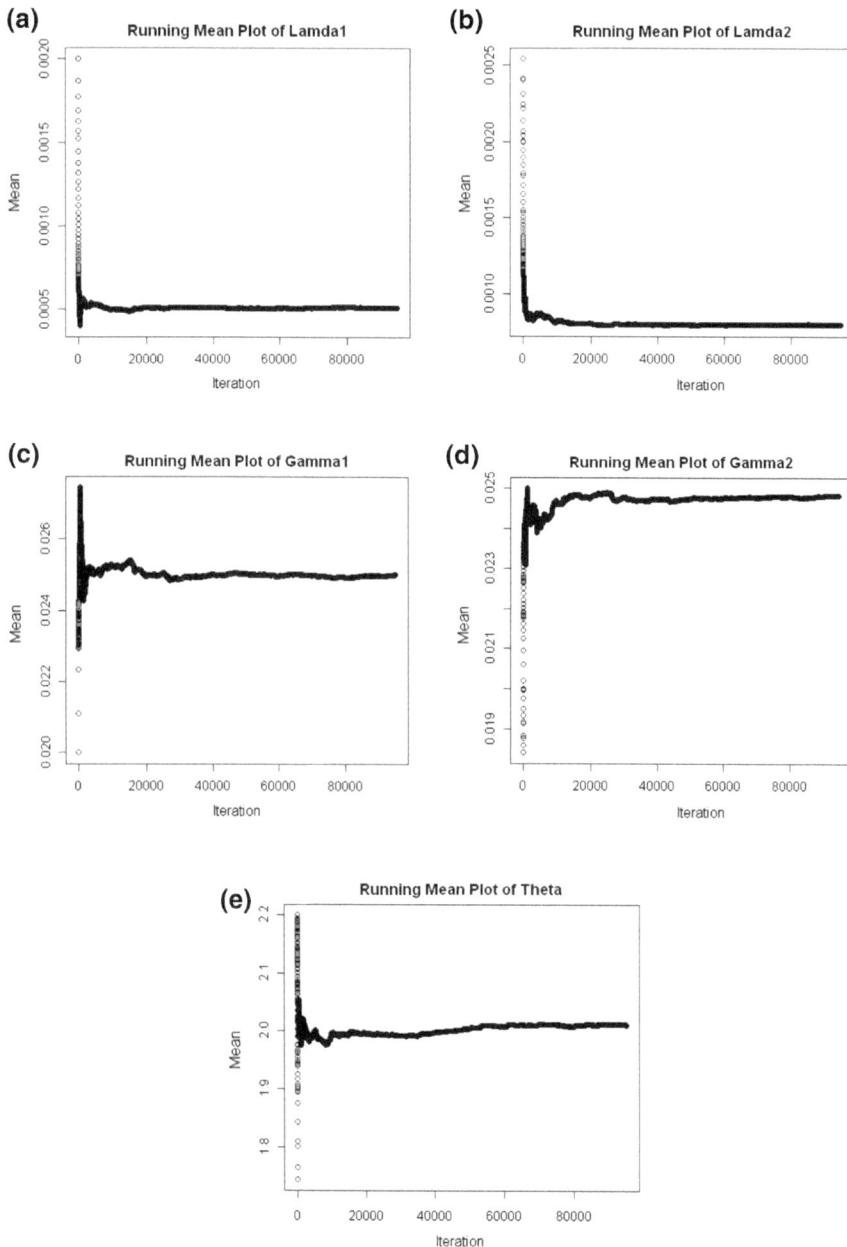

Fig. 11.8 Graphs of running mean plots for litter-matched tumorigenesis data for Model IG-I

Table 11.9 Posterior summary for litter-matched tumorigenesis data set for Model G-I

Par	BGR	Geweke test		Estimate	S.E.	Credible lower limit	Interval upper limit
		Test-stat	p-value				
λ_1	1.0016	0.0141	0.5056	0.0006	0.0003	0.0002	0.0014
λ_2	1.0007	−0.0137	0.4945	0.0009	0.0004	0.0003	0.0020
γ_1	1.0005	−0.0107	0.4956	0.0244	0.0046	0.0156	0.0316
γ_2	1.0012	0.0128	0.5051	0.0242	0.0043	0.0160	0.0315
θ	1.0028	0.0041	0.5016	1.9875	0.3127	1.5209	2.6236

Table 11.10 Posterior summary for litter-matched tumorigenesis data set for Model G-II

Par	BGR	Geweke test		Estimate	S.E.	Credible lower limit	Interval upper limit
		Test-stat	p-value				
λ_1	1.00004	−0.0011	0.4995	0.0054	0.0027	0.0005	0.0098
λ_2	1.0005	−0.0043	0.4982	0.0055	0.0028	0.0004	0.0098
γ_1	1.0026	−0.0112	0.4955	0.0272	0.0031	0.0181	0.0298
γ_2	1.0039	−0.0036	0.4985	0.0279	0.0027	0.0197	0.0299
θ	1.0027	−0.0059	0.4976	2.2057	0.3287	1.5373	2.6709

Table 11.11 Posterior summary for litter-matched tumorigenesis data set for Model IG-I

Par	BGR	Geweke test		Estimate	S.E.	Credible lower limit	Interval upper limit
		Test-stat	p-value				
λ_1	1.1623	0.0059	0.5023	0.0005	0.0002	0.0001	0.0011
λ_2	1.0895	0.0079	0.5031	0.0007	0.0003	0.0003	0.0016
γ_1	1.0168	−0.0060	0.4975	0.0250	0.0042	0.0159	0.0308
γ_2	1.0123	−0.0105	0.4957	0.0248	0.0039	0.0165	0.0306
θ	1.0377	−0.0041	0.4983	1.9958	0.3182	1.5183	2.6637

all other models. Thus, inverse Gaussian frailty model with Gompertz as baseline distribution (Model IG-I) is better model as compared to other three models for modeling tumorigenesis data.

Therneau and Grambsch (2000) analyzed this data using gamma and Gaussian frailty models. They observed the estimate of the variance of the random effect is highest when Gaussian frailty with AIC method is used. Hanagal (2011) also considered the same data for Weibull distribution as the baseline model to analyze and test for no frailty in frailty models. From the Gaussian and gamma frailty models, he observed from the R output that frailty variable (litter) is very highly significantly related to the recurrence time. Now we test for no frailty in shared frailty models.

Table 11.12 Posterior summary for litter-matched tumorigenesis data set for Model IG-II

Par	BGR	Geweke test		Estimate	S.E.	Credible lower limit	Interval upper limit
		Test-stat	p-value				
λ_1	1.0058	0.00581	0.5023	0.0056	0.0027	0.00061	0.0097
λ_2	1.0063	0.0128	0.5051	0.0055	0.0027	0.00056	0.0098
γ_1	1.0053	−0.0077	0.4969	0.0271	0.0032	0.0185	0.0308
γ_2	1.0014	−0.0041	0.4984	0.0279	0.0024	0.0217	0.0308
θ	1.0001	0.0041	0.5016	2.2532	0.3098	1.6081	2.6673

Table 11.13 AIC, BIC, and DIC values for litter-matched tumorigenesis data set

Models	AIC	BIC	DIC
G-I	267.649	279.114	261.457
G-II	451.564	461.772	442.860
IG-I	266.398	278.219	260.920
IG-II	452.302	462.444	443.466

Table 11.14 Bayes factor values and decision for comparison of shared frailty models fitted to litter-matched tumorigenesis data set

Nr model against Dr model	$2log_e(B_{jk})$	Range	Evidence against model in Dr
IG-I vs G-I	10.21189	≥10	Very strong
IG-I vs G-II	194.868	≥10	Very strong
IG-I vs IG-II	193.6946	≥10	Very strong
G-I vs G-II	183.6793	≥10	Very strong
G-I vs IG-II	183.3847	≥10	Very strong
IG-II vs G-II	1.173384	0–2	Poor

Table 11.15 Bayes factor values and decision to test of significance for frailty in litter-matched tumorigenesis data set

Nr model	Dr model	$2log_e(B_{jk})$	Range	Evidence against model in Dr
G-I	Baseline	6.363487	6–10	Strong
G-II	Baseline	43.38789	≥10	Very strong
IG-I	Baseline	2.4439	2–6	Moderate
IG-II	Baseline	43.2899	≥10	Very strong

To test significance of frailty, we compared two models, one with shared frailty as model M_1 and another without frailty as model M_0, so we use Bayes factor for this comparison. But this is not the case for Model II. From Table 11.15, it is cleared that there is significant difference between the values of information criterion of model with frailty and model without frailty and even these values are minimum for Gompertz baseline models. Also, Bayes factor value (see Table 11.15) is positive and there is very strong evidence against the without frailty models. Thus, it is observed from the results that frailty variable, i.e., litter effect is very highly significantly related to the recurrence time of rats.

11.7 Frailty Models with Bivariate Exponential Baseline

The conditional survival function of BVE with fixed covariates and given frailty $(Z = z)$ is given by (from Section 5.2.3)

$$S(t_{1j}, t_{2j} \mid Z_j = z_j) = \exp[-z_j H(t_{1j}, t_{2j})]$$
$$= \exp\left[-z_j \eta_j \left\{\lambda_1 t_{1j} + \lambda_2 t_{2j} + \lambda_3 t_{(2)j}\right\}\right],$$

where Z_j $(j = 1, 2, \ldots, n)$ follows gamma distribution and inverse Gaussian distributions.

The bivariate survivor function for jth patient at time $t_{1j} > 0$ and $t_{2j} > 0$, after integrating out Z_i, can be easily expressed by means of the Laplace transform of the frailty distribution, evaluated at the total integrated conditional hazard. Thus, we get the unconditional bivariate survival functions based on gamma frailty and inverse Gaussian frailty as

$$S(t_{1j}, t_{2j}) = \left[1 + \theta\{H_0(t_{1j}, t_{2j})\}\eta_j\right]^{-1/\theta}$$
$$= \left[1 + \theta\{\lambda_1 t_{1j} + \lambda_2 t_{2j} + \lambda_3 t_{(2)j}\}\eta_j\right]^{-1/\theta} \qquad (11.7)$$

and

$$S(t_{1j}, t_{2j}) = \exp\left\{\frac{1 - \left[1 + 2\theta H_0(t_{1j}, t_{2j})\eta_j\right]^{\frac{1}{2}}}{\theta}\right\}$$
$$= \exp\left[\frac{1 - \left(1 + 2\theta\{\lambda_1 t_{1j} + \lambda_2 t_{2j} + \lambda_3 t_{(2)j}\}\eta_j\right)^{1/2}}{\theta}\right]. \qquad (11.8)$$

Here onward, we call Eqs. (11.7) and (11.8) as Model G-III and Model IG-III, respectively. Thus, Model G-III is the shared gamma frailty model under Marshall–Olkin bivariate exponential baseline hazard and Model IG-III is the shared inverse Gaussian frailty model under the same Marshall–Olkin bivariate exponential baseline hazard. Equation (11.7) is the bivariate Burr distribution.

The unconditional bivariate survival functions of Model G-III and Model IG-III given in Eqs. (11.7) and (11.8) have two types of dependencies, one is due to simultaneous failures and the other is due to frailty. The parameters $\lambda_3 = 0$ and $\theta = 0$ in Eqs. (11.7) and (11.8) lead to independence of the lifetimes of the two components.

Suppose there are n individuals under study, whose first and second observed failure times are represented by (t_{1j}, t_{2j}). Let c_{1j} and c_{2j} be the observed censoring times for the jth individual ($j = 1, 2, 3, \ldots, n$) for first and second failure times, respectively. We also assume the independence between censoring scheme and lifetimes of individuals.

The contribution of bivariate lifetime random variable of the jth individual in likelihood function is given by

$$L_j(t_{1j}, t_{2j}) = \begin{cases} f_1(t_{1j}, t_{2j}), & t_{1j} < c_{1j}, t_{2j} < c_{2j}, t_{1j} < t_{2j} \\ f_2(t_{1j}, t_{2j}), & t_{1j} < c_{1j}, t_{2j} < c_{2j}, t_{1j} > t_{2j} \\ f_3(t_{1j}, t_{2j}), & t_{1j} < c_{1j}, t_{2j} < c_{2j}, t_{1j} = t_{2j} \\ f_4(t_{1j}, c_{2j}), & t_{1j} < c_{1j}, t_{2j} > c_{2j}, \\ f_5(c_{1j}, t_{2j}), & t_{1j} > c_{1j}, t_{2j} < c_{2j}, \\ f_6(c_{1j}, c_{2j}), & t_{1j} > c_{1j}, t_{2j} > c_{2j}, \end{cases}$$

and the likelihood function is

$$L(\psi, \beta, \theta) = \prod_{j=1}^{n_1} f_1(t_{1j}, t_{2j}) \prod_{j=1}^{n_2} f_2(t_{1j}, t_{2j}) \prod_{j=1}^{n_3} f_3(t_{1j}, t_{2j})$$

$$\times \prod_{j=1}^{n_4} f_4(t_{1j}, c_{2j}) \prod_{j=1}^{n_5} f_5(c_{1j}, t_{2j}) \prod_{j=1}^{n_6} f_6(c_{1j}, c_{2j}),$$

where θ, ψ, and β are, respectively, the frailty parameter, the vector of baseline parameters, and the vector of regression coefficients.

The counts $n_1, n_2, n_3, n_4, n_5,$ and n_6 are the number of individuals for which first and the second failure times (t_{1j}, t_{2j}) lie in the ranges $t_{1j} < c_{1j}, t_{2j} < c_{2j}, t_{1j} < t_{2j}$, $t_{1j} < c_{1j}, t_{2j} < c_{2j}, t_{1j} > t_{2j}$, $t_{1j} < c_{1j}, t_{2j} < c_{2j}, t_{1j} = t_{2j}$, $t_{1j} < c_{1j}, t_{2j} > c_{2j}$; $t_{1j} > c_{1j}, t_{2j} < c_{2j}$ and $t_{1j} > c_{1j}, t_{2j} > c_{2j}$, respectively, and the functions, $f_1, f_2,$ $f_3, f_4, f_5,$ and f_6, are evaluated in the two frailty models.

For gamma frailty model,

$$f_1(t_{1j}, t_{2j}) = (1+\theta)\lambda_1(\lambda_2 + \lambda_3)\eta_j^2 S^{(1+2\theta)}(t_{1j}, t_{2j}), \quad 0 < t_{1j} < c_{1j}, t_{2j} < c_{2j}, t_{1j} < t_{2j},$$

$$f_2(t_{1j}, t_{2j}) = (1+\theta)(\lambda_1 + \lambda_3)\lambda_2\eta_j^2 S^{(1+2\theta)}(t_{1j}, t_{2j}), \quad 0 < t_{1j} < c_{1j}, t_{2j} < c_{2j}, t_{1j} > t_{2j},$$

$$f_3(t_{1j}, t_{2j}) = \lambda_3\eta_j S^{(1+\theta)}(t_j, t_j), \quad 0 < t_{1j} < c_{1j}, t_{2j} < c_{2j}, t_{1j} = t_{2j},$$

$$f_4(t_{1j}, c_{2i}) = \lambda_1\eta_j S^{(1+\theta)}(t_{1j}, c_{2j}), \quad 0 < t_{1j} < c_{1j}, c_{2j} < t_{2j},$$

$$f_5(c_{1j}, t_{2j}) = \lambda_2\eta_j S^{(1+\theta)}(c_{1j}, t_{2j}), \quad 0 < t_{2j} < c_{2j}, c_{1j} < t_{1j},$$

$$f_6(c_{1j}, c_{2j}) = S(c_{1j}, c_{2j}), \quad c_{1j} < t_{1j}, c_{2j} < t_{2j},$$

and $S(.,.)$ is given by Eq. (11.7).

For inverse Gaussian frailty model,

$$f_1(t_{1j}, t_{2j}) = \frac{\lambda_1(\lambda_2 + \lambda_3)\phi_2(t_{1j}, t_{2j})S(t_{1j}, t_{2j})\eta_j^2}{[\phi_1(t_{1j}, t_{2j})]^{\frac{3}{2}}}, \quad 0 < t_{1j} < c_{1j}, t_{2j} < c_{2j}, t_{1j} < t_{2j},$$

$$f_2(t_{1j}, t_{2j}) = \frac{(\lambda_1 + \lambda_3)\lambda_2\phi_2(t_{1j}, t_{2j})S(t_{1j}, t_{2j})\eta_j^2}{[\phi_1(t_{1j}, t_{2j})]^{\frac{3}{2}}}, \quad 0 < t_{1j} < c_{1j}, t_{2j} < c_{2j}, t_{1j} > t_{2j},$$

$$f_3(t_{1j}, t_{2j}) = \frac{\lambda_3 S(t_j, t_i)\eta_j}{[\phi_1(t_j, t_j)]^{\frac{1}{2}}}, \quad 0 < t_{1j} < c_{1j}, t_{2j} < c_{2j}, t_{1j} = t_{2j},$$

$$f_4(t_{1j}, c_{2i}) = \frac{\lambda_1 S(t_{1j}, c_{2j})\eta_j}{[\phi_1(t_{1j}, c_{2j})]^{\frac{1}{2}}}, \quad 0 < t_{1j} < c_{1j}, c_{2j} < t_{2j},$$

$$f_5(c_{1j}, t_{2j}) = \frac{\lambda_2 S(c_{1j}, t_{2j})\eta_j}{[\phi_1(c_{1j}, t_{2j})]^{\frac{1}{2}}}, \quad 0 < t_{2j} < c_{2j}, c_{1j} < t_{1j}, and$$

$$f_6(c_{1j}, c_{2j}) = S(c_{1j}, c_{2j}), \quad c_{1j} < t_{1j}, c_{2j} < t_{2j},$$

where $\phi_1(a_j, b_j) = [1 + 2\theta H(a_j, b_j)\eta_j]$; $\phi_2(a_j, b_j) = \theta + [\phi_1(a_j, b_j)]^{\frac{1}{2}}$; and $S(.,.)$ is given by Eq. (11.8).

Here f_1 and f_2 are the pdf with respect to Lebesgue measure in R^2 and f_3, f_4 and f_5 are the pdf with respect to Lebesgue measure in R^1 in their respective regions I_1, I_2, I_3, I_4, and I_5. We use Bayesian estimation strategies for the estimation of the parameters and model selection criteria.

11.8   Analysis of Diabetic Retinopathy Data

We now fit the proposed shared frailty models, Model G-III (given in Eq. (11.7)) and Model IG-III (given in Eq. (11.8)), to the diabetic retinopathy time data, with two covariates in the analysis, one is laser type (0-xenon, 1-argon) and the second is type of diabetes (0-juvenile,1-adult) denoted by X_1 and X_2, respectively. The diabetic retinopathy data set is partially presented in Chap. 1. Therneau and Grambsch (2000) analyzed this data using gamma and Gaussian frailty models.

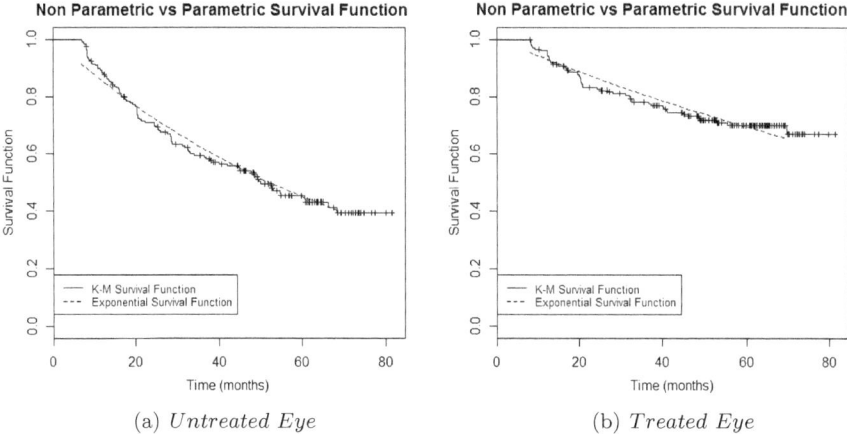

Fig. 11.9 Comparison of nonparametric survival function with exponential survival function for diabetic retinopathy data

First, we check goodness of fit of the data for baseline distribution and then apply the Bayesian estimation procedure to both shared frailty models. In the analysis of this study, we have used the R package. To check goodness of fit of data set, first, we consider graphical procedure to check appropriateness of the model.

Figure 11.9a, b which plots the Kaplan–Meier estimates and hypothesized theoretical distribution $S(t)$ for proposed model demonstrates a close agreement between the two, i.e., nonparametric and parametric survival curves for baseline exponential distribution. Thus, from Fig. 11.9 also, we can conclude that data are from bivariate exponential distribution of Marshall and Olkin (1967).

We classify the survival times into eight and six groups for untreated and treated eyes, respectively. Tables 11.16 and 11.17 give the classification for untreated and treated eyes, respectively. We have considered Kolmogorov–Smirnov (K–S) test to test goodness of fit of the marginal exponential of (T_1, T_2) separately. The K–S test statistic is based on the empirical distribution function. Test procedure is developed for testing goodness of fit with grouped data which are subjected to random right censoring. The p-values of K–S test for baseline distribution are presented in Table 11.18.

The p-values of K–S test are very large approximately close to 1. Thus, from goodness-of-fit graphs and p-values of K–S test (Table 11.18), we can say that there is no statistical evidence to reject the hypothesis that data are from exponential distribution.

In particular, we have used the R program for analysis purpose. Given the model assumptions, this program performs the Gibbs sampler by simulating from the full conditional distributions. A widely used prior for frailty parameter θ is gamma distribution with mean one and large variance, $\Gamma(\phi, \phi)$, say with a small choice of ϕ and the prior for regression parameter β is normal with mean zero and large vari-

Table 11.16 Classification of survival times for untreated eye of diabetic retinopathy data set

Class interval	Censoring	Death	Risk
[5, 10)	3	17	197
[10, 15)	2	15	177
[15, 20)	2	13	160
[20, 25)	1	14	145
[25, 30)	3	11	130
[30, 40)	7	11	116
[40, 50)	23	10	98
[50, 85)	55	10	65

Table 11.17 Classification of survival times for treated eye of diabetic retinopathy data set

Class interval	Censoring	Death	Risk
[5, 10)	2	7	197
[10, 15)	4	11	188
[15, 20)	5	7	173
[20, 25)	1	8	161
[25, 40)	15	10	152
[40, 85)	116	11	127

Table 11.18 p-values of Kolmogorov–Smirnov test statistic for diabetic retinopathy data set

Model	Untreated eye	Treated eye
G-III	0.9831	0.9928
IG-III	0.9712	0.9843

ance say σ^2. Similar types of prior distributions are used in Ibrahim et al. (2001), Sahu et al. (1997) and Santos and Achcar (2010). So, in our study also, for Model G-III and Model IG-III, we use same prior for θ and β's. Since we do not have any prior information about baseline parameters, λ_1, λ_2, and λ_3, prior distributions are assumed to be informative. For baseline parameters λ_1, λ_2, and λ_3, the prior is $\Gamma(a, b)$, for the frailty parameter θ, the prior is $\Gamma(\phi, \phi)$, and for regression coefficients β_i, $(i = 1, \ldots, 2)$, the prior is $N(0, \sigma^2)$ for both shared frailty models. Here $\Gamma(a, b)$ is gamma distribution with shape parameter a and scale parameter b. All the hyperparameters ϕ, a, b, and σ^2 are known. We set hyperparameters as $\phi = 0.00001$, $a = 0.0001$; $b = 0.0001$, and $\sigma^2 = 10^5$ for both shared frailty models Model G-III and Model IG-III.

The Bayesian estimators were obtained through the Metropolis–Hastings algorithm within Gibbs sampling scheme already described in earlier sections. To estimate the parameters, we run two parallel Markov chains with the different starting points for large number of iterations to obtain reasonable information about the posterior

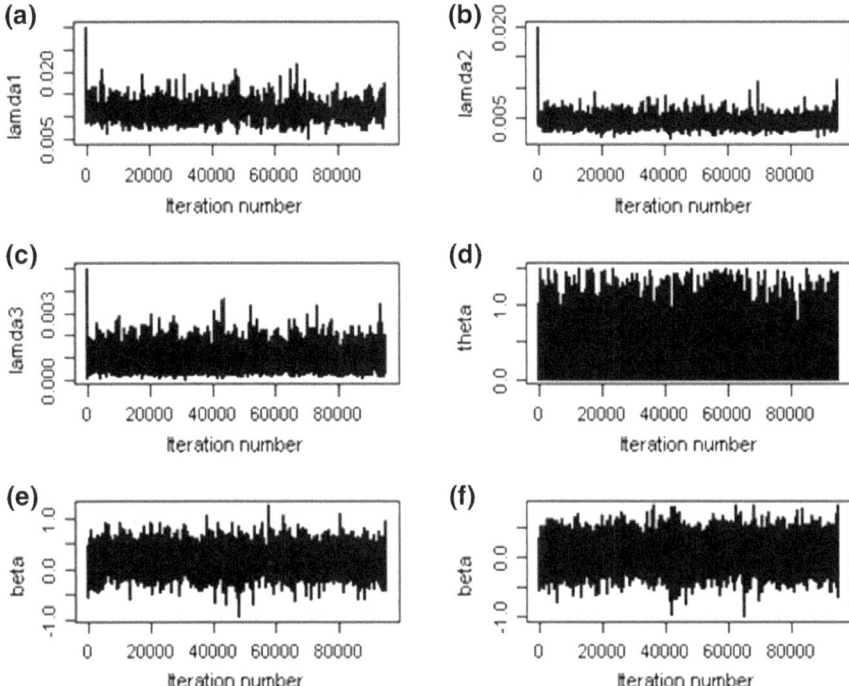

Fig. 11.10 Posterior for Model G-III: time series plots of the posterior samples for diabetic retinopathy data

distribution of parameters. We iterate both the chains for 95,000 times and discard 2,000 observations as burn-in period for both Model G-III and Model IG-III. As in the simulation, here also, results for chain I and chain II are similar, so we present result for only one chain (i.e., chain I) with $\Gamma(a, b)$ as prior for baseline parameters.

Graphs for time series (or trace) plot, coupling from past plots, and sample autocorrelation plot with thinning (i.e., after considering lag shown in figures) for the parameters for chain I are shown in Figs. 11.10, 11.11, and 11.12 for Model G-III. Due to lack of space, we present these graphs for Model G-III only. For chain II, these graphs have similar pattern, so we are not presenting graphs for chain II. Trace plots for all the parameters show zigzag pattern which indicates that parameters move more freely. Thus, it seems that the Markov chain has reached the stationary state. Simulated values of parameters have autocorrelation of lag k value given below each plot in Fig. 11.12 for Model G-III, so every kth iteration is selected as sample to thin the chain and discarding the rest. The autocorrelation of parameters becomes almost negligible after the defined lag, given in figures.

We can also use running mean plots to check how well our chains are mixing. Running mean plots display a time series of the running mean for each parameter in each chain, as shown in Fig. 11.13 for Model G-III. It can be observed from these

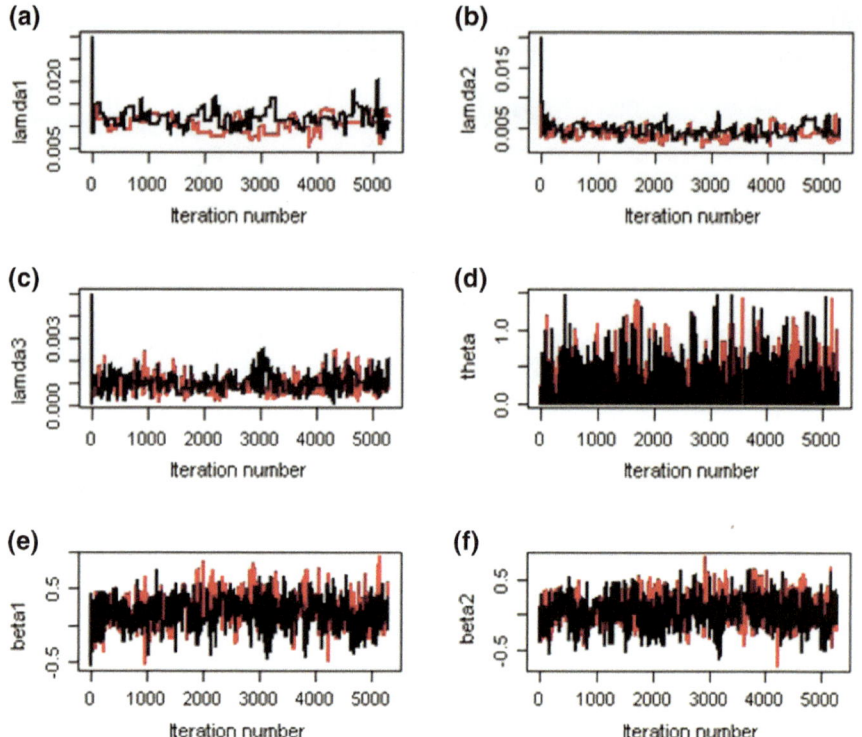

Fig. 11.11 Posterior for Model G-III: coupling from past plots of the posterior samples for diabetic retinopathy data

figures that running mean plot for each parameter is converging to the posterior mean of the parameter, and thus represents a good mixing of chain. Thus, our diagnostic plots suggest that the MCMC chains are mixing very well.

Tables 11.19 and 11.20 present the posterior mean, standard deviation, and 95% credible intervals for all baseline parameters, frailty variance along with Gelman–Rubin convergence statistic values, and Geweke test statistic values with corresponding p-values for Model V and Model VI, respectively. Monitoring convergence of the chains has been done via the Brooks and Gelman (1998) convergence diagnostic. Hence, once convergence has been achieved, 93,000 observations are taken from each chain after the burn-in period for both shared frailty models. On inspection of the Brooks and Gelman's diagnostic, we find the Brooks and Gelman ratio (BGR) convergent to one, and this shows that the convergence for regression coefficients β, variance of frailty θ, and other parameters have been obtained. Also, the Geweke test statistic values, given in Tables 11.19 and 11.20, are quite small and corresponding p-values are large enough to say the chains attain stationary distribution.

The posterior mean of all estimated parameters for Model G-III, given in Table 11.19, are 0.01112, 0.00439, 0.00097, 0.06587, 0.18897, and 0.06610. The posterior

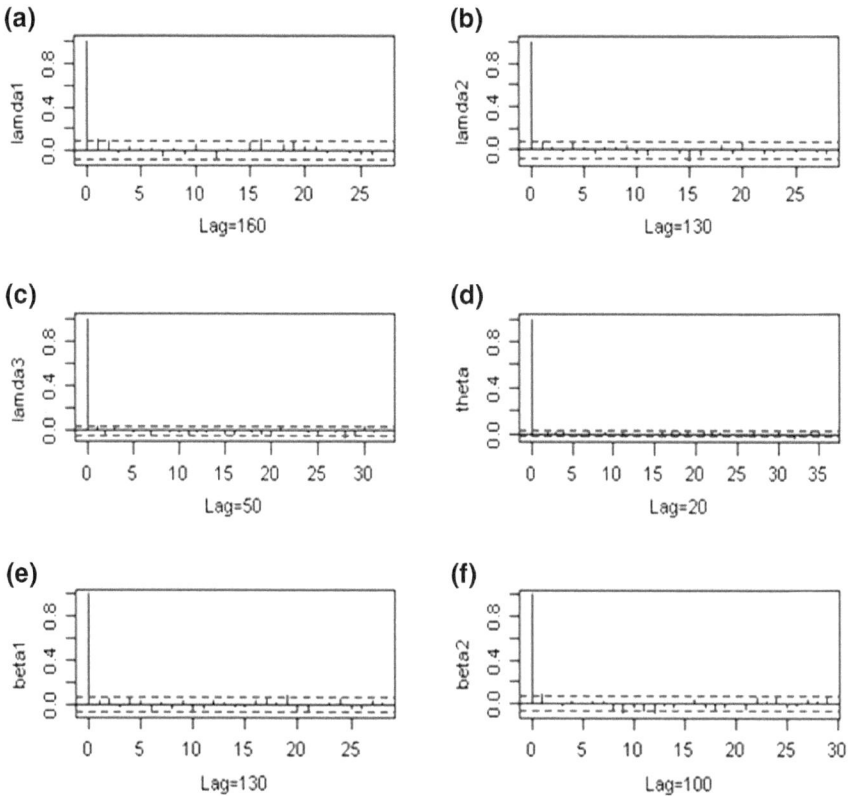

Fig. 11.12 Plots of autocorrelations with thinning number lag (given below the figure) of the posterior samples for diabetic retinopathy data for Model G-III

mean of all estimated parameters for Model IG-III, given in Table 11.20, are 0.01097, 0.00436, 0.00097, 0.06422, 0.20614, and 0.08403. As we can see, posterior mean of Model G-III and Model IG-III are somewhat close for all baseline parameters λ_1, λ_2, and λ_3, and also for frailty variance θ, whereas posterior estimates of β_1 and β_2 are not so much close for both shared frailty models.

Now, we see the treatment effect by considering λ_1 and λ_2. On the average, λ_1 is greater than λ_2 for both models. This is attributed to the treatment effect. Also, the sample mean of the survival time for the treated eye is 38.87 months while the same for the untreated eye is 32.29 months. This may indicate a possible treatment effect. Thus, it is concluded that the untreated eye is likely to fail before the treated eye. The parameter λ_3 relates to the intensity of failure of both eyes at the same time. We see that its posterior mean is 0.00097 for both models, showing that there is positive probability of simultaneous failure. We also see that the two survival times cannot be treated independently as λ_3 and θ are estimated to be positive. Also, λ_3 and θ are significantly different from zero based on information criteria AIC, BIC, and DICs

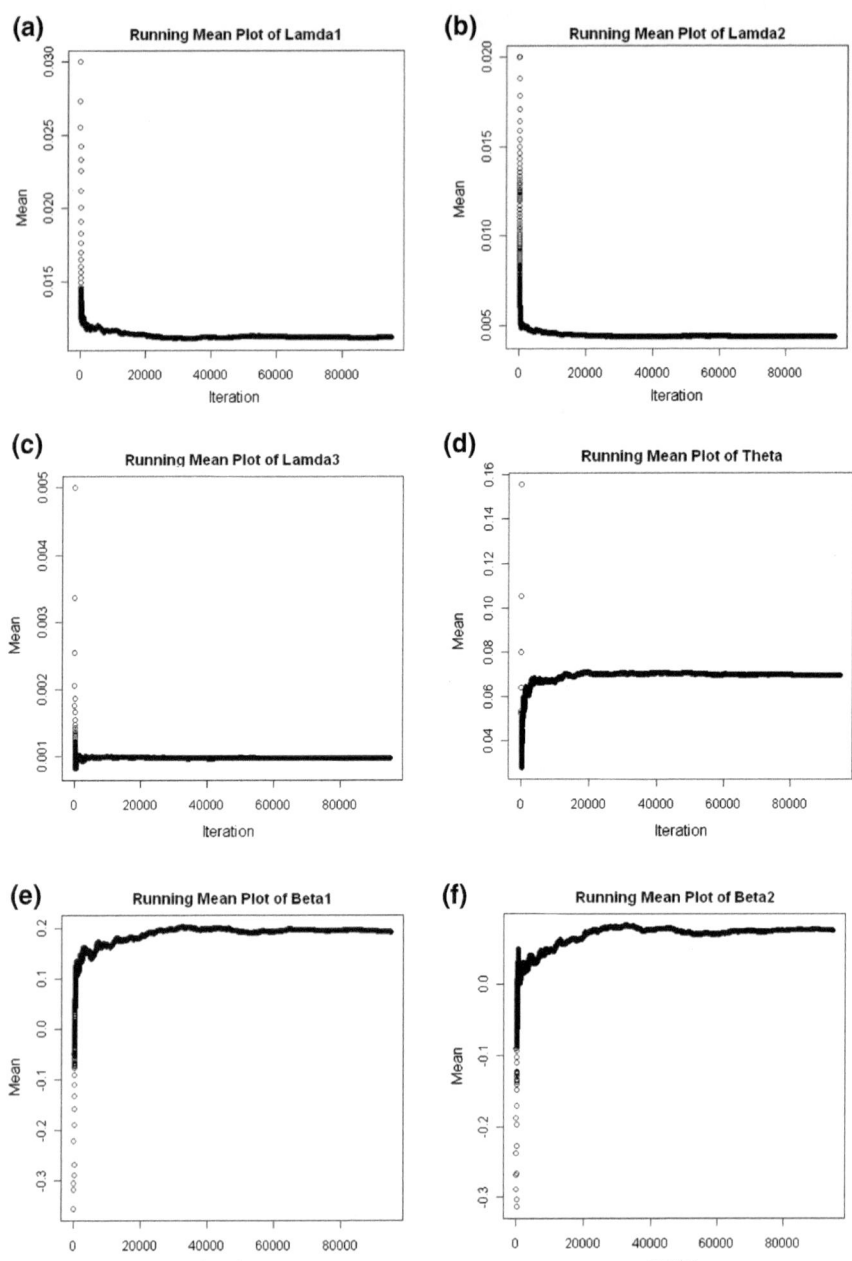

Fig. 11.13 Graphs of running mean plots for diabetic retinopathy data for Model G-III

Table 11.19 Posterior summary for diabetic retinopathy data set for Model G-III

Par	BGR	Geweke test		Estimate	S.E.	Credible lower limit	Interval upper limit
		Test-stat	p-value				
λ_1	1.03958	−0.01108	0.49557	0.01112	0.00201	0.00761	0.01528
λ_2	1.02401	−0.01103	0.49559	0.00439	0.00095	0.00281	0.00653
λ_3	1.00119	0.00154	0.50061	0.00097	0.00041	0.00036	0.00193
θ	0.99998	0.00103	0.50041	0.06587	0.15726	5.831e-06	0.59613
β_1	1.02312	0.01808	0.50721	0.18897	0.19843	−0.22829	0.58189
β_2	1.00847	0.00557	0.50222	0.06610	0.20338	−0.32123	0.47764

Table 11.20 Posterior summary for diabetic retinopathy data set for Model IG-III

Par	BGR	Geweke test		Estimate	S.E.	Credible lower limit	Interval upper limit
		Test-stat	p-value				
λ_1	1.064056	0.01815	0.50724	0.01097	0.00196	0.00731	0.01518
λ_2	1.001659	0.01515	0.50604	0.00436	0.00098	0.00276	0.00693
λ_3	1.018196	0.00362	0.50144	0.00097	0.00041	0.00034	0.00195
θ	1.000203	0.00861	0.50343	0.06422	0.14996	6.546e-06	0.57938
β_1	1.042331	−0.01339	0.49465	0.20614	0.19401	−0.15915	0.57846
β_2	1.000111	−0.01707	0.49318	0.08403	0.19847	−0.29637	0.47688

values given in Table 11.21 for Model G-III as well as for Model IG-III. Hence, it is concluded that there is positive association between the two survival times. Sahu and Dey (2000) also analyzed the same data and observed that Kendall's τ was 0.385 and the Pearsons product moment correlation between the log of the event times was 0.395, indicating positive dependence between the survival times of the two eyes.

The covariates laser type has mean 0.1889799 with standard deviation 0.1984392 and the 95% credible region is (−0.228292, 0.5818944) for Model V and mean 0.20614 with standard deviation 0.19401 and the 95% credible region is (−0.15915, 0.57846) for Model VI. It seems to be insignificant since the 95% credible region includes zero for both models. Since the posterior mean of β_1 is positive, we can conclude that the patients treated with argon laser type have higher but insignificant risk of blindness as compared to the patients treated with xenon laser type. To investigate the effect of age as estimated by the frailty model, we consider the posterior distribution of β_2. The posterior mean of β_2 is 0.06610 with standard deviation 0.20338 and the 95% credible region is (−0.32123, 0.47764) for Model G-III and 0.08403 with standard deviation 0.19847 and the 95% credible region is (−0.29637, 0.47688) for Model IG-III. Recall that the age covariate has value 1 for adult and 0 for the juvenile patients. Since the posterior mean is positive, this shows that the effect of the laser type and age covariate is only slight on the positive side. Thus, we can conclude that the hazard for the adult patients is higher but not significant than the hazard for the juveniles on average. Therneau and Grambsch (2000) also analyzed this data using semiparametric gamma and Gaussian frailty models. Similar results have obtained there also.

The posterior estimate of dispersion of random effects, i.e., $\theta = 0.06587243$ for proposed model Model G-III and $\theta = 0.06422$ for other proposed model Model IG-III, shows that there exists significant heterogeneity in population. Thus, there is a dependence within the eyes of a patient. Since estimate of θ is not very large and close to zero, we test the significance of frailty.

Testing of Significance of Frailty and Independence

To test significance of frailty, we compared two models. One with shared gamma frailty model as Model G-III; shared inverse Gaussian frailty model as Model IG-III, and without frailty model as Model MO. As it is observed from Table 11.21, there is no significant difference between the values of the information criteria AIC, BIC, DIC, and $-2\mathrm{log}L$ (-2log-likelihood) of Model IG-III and Model MO (without frailty) and these values are approximately same for IG-III and MO. Thus, these information criteria are not able to discriminate between the models with frailty and without frailty for proposed Model IG-III.

For Model G-III, there is significant difference between the values of the information criteria AIC, BIC, DIC, and $-2\mathrm{log}L$ of model with frailty Model G-III and model without frailty (Model MO) and even these values (given in Table 11.21) are minimum for Model G-III as compared to Model MO. Since these information criteria are able to discriminate between the models with frailty and without frailty and Model G-III is better model compared to other two models, it is observed from the results that frailty variable, i.e., patient effect is very highly significantly related to the blindness time of eyes.

Another test to test the significance of independence, i.e., T_1 and T_2 are independent if and only if $\lambda_3 = 0$ and $\theta = 0$. In most of the frailty models, we considered in this book, we note that the test for no frailty is equivalent to test for independence of T_1 and T_2. The model with independence is noted as Model MOI. As it is observed from Table 11.21, there is significant difference between the values of the information criteria AIC, BIC, DIC, and $-2\mathrm{log}L$ of three models (G-III, IG-III, and MO) and model with independence Model MOI (independence) and even these values are minimum for models with dependency structure. Hence, the models with dependence structure are better than the models with independence (MOI). This shows there is clear evidence that T_1 and T_2 are dependent.

Table 11.21 AIC, BIC, and DIC values for test for frailty and independence for diabetic retinopathy data set

Models	AIC	BIC	DIC	$-2\mathrm{log}L$
G-III	1715.535	1742.041	1717.149	1703.5352
IG-III	1723.679	1750.612	1726.147	1711.6788
MO	1723.205	1744.969	1723.901	1713.2054
MOI	1742.173	1759.022	1741.606	1734.1728

References

Ahuja, J.C., Nash, S.W.: The generalized Gompertz Verhulst family distributions. Sankhya A **29**, 141–156 (1979)

Barlow, R.E., Proschan, F.: Statistical Theory of Reliability and Life Testing: Probability Models. Holt, Rinehart & Winston, New York (1975)

Bennett, S.: Log-logistic regression model for survival data. Appl. Stat. **32**(2), 165–171 (1983)

Brooks, S.P., Gelman, A.: Alternative methods for monitoring convergence of iterative simulations. J. Comput. Graph. Stat. **7**, 434–455 (1998)

Cox, D.R.: The Analysis of Binary Data. Methenn & Co., London (1970)

Cox, D.R.: Regression models and life tables (with discussions). J. R. Stat. Soc. B **34**, 187–220 (1972)

Cox, D.R., Oakes, D.: Analysis of Survival Data. Chapman & Hall, London (1984)

Freireich, E.J., Gehan, E., Frei, E., Schroeder, L.R., Wolman, I.J., Anbari, R., Burgert, E.O., Mills, S.D., Pinkel, D., Selawry, O.S., Moon, J.H., Gendel, B.R., Spurr, C.L., Storrs, R., Haurani, F., Hoogstraten, B., Lee, S.: The effect of 6-Mercaptopurine on the duration of steroid-induced remissions in acute leukemia: a model for evaluation of other potential useful therapy. Blood **21**, 699–716 (1963)

Gompertz, B.: On the nature of the function expressive of the law of human mortality, and the new mode of determining the value of life contingencies. Philos. Trans. Roy. Soc. London, **115**, 513–585 (1825)

Gupta, R.C., Akman, O., Lvin, S.: A study of log-logistic model in survival analysis. Biom. J. **41**(4), 431–443 (1999)

Hanagal, D.D., Kale, B.K.: Large sample tests of λ_3 in the bivariate exponential distribution. Stat. Probab. Lett. **12**(4), 311–313 (1991)

Hanagal, D.D., Sharma, R.: A bivariate Gompertz regression model with shared gamma frailty for censored data. Model Assist. Stat. Appl. **7**, 161–168 (2012a)

Hanagal, D.D., Sharma, R.: Analysis of tumorigenesis data using shared gamma frailty models via Bayesian approach. Int. J. Stat. Manag. Syst. **7**, 105–135 (2012c)

Hanagal, D.D., Sharma, R.: Analysis of tumorigenesis data using shared inverse Gaussian frailty models via Bayesian approach. J. Indian Soc. Probab. Stat. **14**, 76–102 (2013b)

Hanagal, D.D., Sharma, R.: Bayesian estimation of parameters for bivariate Gompertz model with shared gamma shared gamma frailty under random censoring. Stat. Probab. Lett. **82**, 1310–1317 (2012b)

Hanagal, D.D., Sharma, R.: Bayesian inference in Marshall-Olkin bivariate exponential shared gamma frailty regression model under random censoring. Commun. Stat.: Theory Methods **44**(1), 24–47 (2015a)

Hanagal, D.D., Sharma, R.: Comparison of frailty models for acute leukaemia data under Gompertz baseline distribution. Commun. Stat.: Theory Methods **44**(7), 1338–1350 (2015b)

Hanagal, D.D., Sharma, R.: Modeling heterogeneity for bivariate survival data by shared gamma frailty regression model. Model Assist. Stat. Appl. **8**, 85–102 (2013a)

Hanagal, D.D.: Inference procedures in some bivariate exponential models under hybrid random censoring. Stat. Pap. **38**(2), 169–189 (1997)

Hanagal, D.D.: Selection of a better component in bivariate exponential models. Stat. Methods Appl. **5**(2), 229–238 (1996)

Hanagal, D.D.: Some inference results in bivariate exponential distributions based on censored samples. Commun. Stat. Theory Methods **21**(5), 1273–1295 (1992)

Hanagal, D.D.: Testing reliability in a bivariate exponential stress-strength model. J. Indian Stat. Assoc. **33**, 41–45 (1995)

Hanagal, D.D.: Modeling Survival Data Using Frailty Models. Chapman and Hall, New York (2011)

Hanagal, D.D., Kale, B.K.: Large sample tests for testing symmetry and independence in some bivariate exponential models. Commun. Stat. Theory Methods **21**(9), 2625–2643 (1992)

Harris, R.: Reliability applications of a bivariate exponential distribution. J. Oper. Res. Soc. Am. **16**, 18–27 (1968)

Hougaard, P.: Analysis of Multivariate Survival Data. Springer, New York (2000)

Ibrahim, J.G., Chen, M.H., Sinha, D.: Bayesian Survival Analysis. Springer, New York (2001)

Langlands, A.O., Pocock, S.J., Kerr, G.R., Gore, S.M.: Long-term survival of patients with breast cancer: a study of the curability of the disease. Br. Med. J. **2**, 1247–1251 (1979)

Mantel, N., Bohidar, N.R., Ciminera, J.L.: Mantel-Haenzel anlysis of litter-matched time-to-response data, with modifications for recovery of interlitter information. Cancer Res. **37**, 3863–3868 (1977)

Marshall, A.W., Olkin, I.: A multivariate exponential distribution. J. Am. Stat. Assoc. **62**, 30–44 (1967)

O'Quigley, J., Struthers, L.: Survival models based upon the logistic and loglogistic distributions. Comput. Programs Biomed. Res. **15**, 3–12 (1982)

Osman, M.I.: A new model for analyzing the survival of heterogeneous data. Ph.D. thesis, Case Western Reserve University, USA (1987)

Sahu, S.K., Dey, D.K.: A comparison of frailty and other models for bivariate survival data. Lifetime data anal. **6**, 207–228 (2000)

Sahu, S.K., Dey, D.K., Aslanidou, H., Sinha, D.: A Weibull regression model with gamma frailties for multivariate survival data. Life Time Data Anal. **3**, 123–137 (1997)

Santos, C.A., Achcar, J.A.: A Bayesian analysis for multivariate survival data in the presence of covariates. Jr. Stat. Theor. Appl. **9**, 233–253 (2010)

Spiegelhalter, D.J., Best, N.G., Carlin, B.P., Van der Linde, A.: Bayesian measure of model complexity and fit (with discussion). J. R. Stat. Soc. B **64**, 583–639 (2002)

Therneau, T.M., Grambsch, P.M.: Modeling Survival Data: Extending the Cox Model. Springer, New York (2000)

Part III
Correlated Frailty Models
for Survival Data

Chapter 12
Correlated Frailty Models

12.1 Introduction

Frailty models are becoming increasingly popular in multivariate survival analysis. Shared frailty models, in particular, are often used despite their limitations. To overcome their disadvantages, numerous correlated frailty models were established during the last decade. In the present study, we examine correlated frailty models, and especially the behavior of the parameter estimates when using different estimation strategies.

Shared frailty models explain correlations within groups (family, litter, or clinic) or for recurrent events facing the same individual. However, this approach does have limitations. First, it forces unobserved factors to be the same within the cluster, which is not generally acceptable. For example, sometimes it may be inappropriate to assume that both partners in a twin pair share all of their unobserved risks. Second, the dependence between survival times within the cluster is based on their marginal distributions. To see this, when covariates are present in a proportional hazard model with a gamma-distributed frailty, the dependence parameter and the population heterogeneity are confounded (see Clayton and Cuzick 1985), implying that the multivariate distribution of the lifetimes can be identified from the marginal distributions of these lifetimes (see Hougaard 1986a). Elbers and Rider (1982) show that this problem applies to any univariate frailty distribution with a finite mean. Third, in most cases, shared frailty will only induce a positive association within the group. However, there are some situations in which survival times for subjects within the same cluster are negatively associated. For example, this applies to growth rates for animals in the same litter that have a limited food supply.

To avoid these limitations, correlated frailty models are being developed for the analysis of multivariate failure time data, in which associated random variables are used to characterize the frailty effect for each cluster. In twin pairs, for example, one random variable is assigned to twin 1 and another to twin 2, so that they are no longer constrained to have a common frailty. These two variables are associated and jointly distributed, therefore, knowing one of them does not automatically imply the other.

© Springer Nature Singapore Pte Ltd. 2019
D. D. Hanagal, *Modeling Survival Data Using Frailty Models*,
Industrial and Applied Mathematics, https://doi.org/10.1007/978-981-15-1181-3_12

Also, these two variables certainly can be negatively associated, which would then induce a negative association between survival times.

Correlated frailty models provide not only variance parameters of the frailties as in shared frailty models, but they also contain additional parameter for modeling the correlation between frailties in each group.

Frequently one is interested in construction of a bivariate extension of some univariate family distributions (e.g., gamma). For example, for the purpose of genetic analysis of frailty, one might be interested in estimation of correlation of frailty. It turns out that it is possible to carry out such extension for the class of infinitely divisible distributions (Iachine 1995a, b). In this case, an additional parameter representing the correlation coefficient of the bivariate frailty distribution is introduced.

12.2   Correlated Gamma Frailty Model

The gamma distribution (we use notation $\Gamma(k, l)$ for the two-parameter distribution with shape parameter k and scale parameter l) is one of the most popular frailty distributions. Frailty cannot be negative. The gamma distribution is, along with the lognormal distribution, one of the most commonly used distributions to model variables that are necessarily positive. Furthermore, it turns out that the assumption that frailty at birth is gamma distributed yielding some useful mathematical results which include the following:

- Frailty among the survivors at any time t is gamma distributed with the same value of the shape parameter k as at birth. The value of the second parameter, however, k is now given by $l(t) = l + H_0(t)$, where $H_0(t)$ denotes the cumulative baseline hazard function.
- Frailty among those who die at any age t is also gamma distributed, with the same parameter $l(t)$ as among those surviving to age t but with shape parameter $k + 1$.
- The Laplace transform of a gamma-distributed random variable $Z \sim \Gamma(k, l)$ is of a very simple form: $L_Z(s) = Ee^{-Zs} = (1 + \frac{s}{l})^{-k}$.

To make sure that the model can be identified, it makes sense to use the parameter restriction $EZ = 1$, which results in $k = l$ for the gamma distribution. Denoting the variance of the frailty variable by $\sigma^2 = \frac{1}{l}$, the univariate survival function is represented by

$$S(t) = \mathbf{L}(H_0(t)) = (1 + \sigma^2 H_0(t))^{-\frac{1}{\sigma^2}},$$

where $H_0(t)$ denotes the cumulative baseline hazard function.

The correlated gamma frailty model is developed by Yashin and Iachine (1994), Pickles and Crouchley (1994), and Petersen (1998) for the analysis of multivariate failure time data, in which two associated random variables are used to characterize the frailty effect for each cluster. For example, one random variable is assigned to twin 1 and another to twin 2 so that they are no longer constrained to having a common frailty as in the shared frailty model.

Correlated gamma frailty model was introduced by Yashin et al. (1993a, 1995) and applied to related lifetimes in many different settings, for example, by Pickles et al. (1994). The model has a very convenient representation of the survival function in closed-form expressions, which allows nice interpretation of the model parameters. Kheiri et al. (2005) have suggested correlated gamma frailty model for the data on graft rejection in bilateral grafts in Keratoconus. Here we restrict again to the bivariate model.

Let k_0, k_1, k_2 be some nonnegative real-valued numbers. Set $v_1 = k_0 + k_1$ and $v_2 = k_0 + k_2$. Let Y_0, Y_1, Y_2 be independent, gamma-distributed random variables with parameters $Y_0 \sim \Gamma(k_0, v_0)$, $Y_1 \sim \Gamma(k_1, v_1)$, and $Y_2 \sim \Gamma(k_2, v_2)$. Consequently,

$$Z_1 = \frac{v_0}{v_1} Y_0 + Y_1 \sim \Gamma(k_0 + k_1, v_1),$$

$$Z_2 = \frac{v_0}{v_2} Y_0 + Y_2 \sim \Gamma(k_0 + k_2, v_2),$$

and $E(Z_1) = E(Z_2) = 1$, $V(Z_1) = \frac{1}{v_1} = \sigma_1^2$, $V(Z_2) = \frac{1}{v_2} = \sigma_2^2$. Then the following relation holds:

$$Cov(Z_1, Z_2) = Cov\left(\frac{v_0}{v_1} Y_0 + Y_1, \frac{v_0}{v_2} Y_0 + Y_2\right)$$

$$= \frac{v_0^2}{v_1 v_2} V(Y_0) = \frac{v_0^2}{v_1 v_2} \frac{k_0}{v_0^2}$$

$$= \frac{k_0}{(k_0 + k_1)(k_0 + k_2)}.$$

This leads to the following correlation:

$$\rho = \frac{Cov(Z_1, Z_2)}{\sqrt{V(Z_1)V(Z_2)}} = \frac{k_0}{\sqrt{(k_0 + k_1)(k_0 + k_2)}}.$$

(See Wienke 2011).

Consequently, because of the relation $k_0 + k_i = v_i = \frac{1}{\sigma_i^2} (i = 1, 2)$, and it holds that $k_0 = \frac{\rho}{\sigma_1 \sigma_2}$ and $k_i = \frac{1}{\sigma_i^2} - k_0 = \frac{1 - \frac{\sigma_i}{\sigma_j}\rho}{\sigma_i^2} (i, j = 1, 2; i \neq j)$. Now we can derive the unconditional survival function, applying the Laplace transform of gamma-distributed random variables. Hence,

$$S(t_1, t_2) = E[S(t_1, t_2 | Z_1, Z_2)] = E[S_1(t_1 | Z_1)][S_2(t_2 | Z_2)]$$

$$= \left(1 + \eta_j \sigma_1^2 H_{01}(t_1) + \eta_j \sigma_2^2 H_{02}(t_2)\right)^{\frac{-\rho}{\sigma_1 \sigma_2}} \times \left(1 + \eta_j \sigma_1^2 H_{01}(t_1)\right)^{\frac{-1 + \frac{\sigma_1}{\sigma_2}\rho}{\sigma_1^2}}$$

$$\left(1 + \eta_j \sigma_2^2 H_{02}(t_2)\right)^{\frac{-1 + \frac{\sigma_2}{\sigma_1}\rho}{\sigma_2^2}}, \tag{12.1}$$

which results in the following representation of the gamma correlated frailty model:

$$S(t_1, t_2) = \frac{S_1(t_1)^{1 - \frac{\sigma_1}{\sigma_2}\rho} S_2(t_2)^{1 - \frac{\sigma_2}{\sigma_1}\rho}}{\left(S_1(t_1)^{-\sigma_1^2} + S_2(t_2)^{-\sigma_2^2} - 1\right)^{\frac{\rho}{\sigma_1 \sigma_2}}},$$

using independence of the gamma-distributed variables Y_0, Y_1, Y_2 and the unconditional survival function of t_1 and t_2. This representation is called here the copula representation, because it reveals that the correlated gamma frailty model can be considered as a copula, but this copula is not an Archimedian copula as in the shared gamma frailty model. Copula representations allow separation of the marginal part of the model (univariate distributions) from the correlation structure of the model. Besides the fact that frailty models and copulas look very similar, it is important to note that there are also differences between both approaches that are often overlooked.

This model was first applied to the analysis of Danish twin survival data (Yashin et al. 1993a, b; Yashin and Iachine 1995a, b, c, 1997). Later, similar analyses have been performed for Swedish, Finnish, and Danish data (Yashin et al. 1999; Iachine et al. 1998). The properties of the correlated gamma frailty model were also studied by Pickles and Crouchley (1994). The properties of the correlated frailty model are discussed by Yashin et al. (1993b) and Yashin and Iachine (1993a, b). Methods of parametric estimation related to the correlated frailty model are discussed by Yashin and Iachine (1994).

The possible range of the correlation between frailties depends on the values of σ_1 and σ_2,

$$0 \leq \rho \leq min \left\{ \frac{\sigma_1}{\sigma_2}, \frac{\sigma_2}{\sigma_1} \right\}.$$

Hence, if $\sigma_1 \neq \sigma_2$, the correlation between the frailties is always less than one.

According to different assumptions on the baseline distributions, we get different correlated gamma frailty models.

12.3   Correlated Lognormal Model

Assume that the two frailties of individuals in a pair are given by

$$\begin{pmatrix} Z_{i1} \\ Z_{i2} \end{pmatrix} \sim Log \ N \left(\begin{pmatrix} m \\ m \end{pmatrix}, \begin{pmatrix} s^2 & rs^2 \\ rs^2 & s^2 \end{pmatrix} \right),$$

where $Log\ N$ denotes the (bivariate) lognormal distribution. Here m, s^2 and r denote the mean, variance, and correlation of the respective normal distribution. Mean, variance, and correlation of the frailties are related to these parameters as follows:

$$\mu = \mathbf{E} Z_{ij} = e^{m+\frac{s^2}{2}},$$

$$\sigma^2 = \mathbf{V}(z_{ij}) = e^{2m+s^2}(e^{s^2} - 1),$$

$$\rho = corr(Z_{i1}, Z_{i2}) = \frac{e^{rs^2} - 1}{e^{s^2} - 1}.$$

(See Wienke 2011).

Two different types of lognormal frailty models arise from two restrictions on the parameters of frailty distribution. First, one can use the restriction $m = 0$. This means that the logarithm of frailty has a mean of zero. In this case, a "standard" individual has the logarithm of a hazard rate which is equal to ln $h_0(t)$. Any individual in a population has the logarithm of the hazard rate distorted by some random variables $W_{ij} = \ln Z_{ij}$. This value is added to the "true" logarithm of hazard rate ln $h_0(t)$ to provide the logarithm of the hazard rate of the individual. In this interpretation, it is natural to assume that the distortions W_{ij} have a normal distribution with a mean of zero. Such a model is called Model 2.

Second, following the usual definition of frailty by Clayton (1978) and Vaupel et al. (1979), one can use $\mu = 1$ and in this case

$$m = \mathbf{E} \ln Z_{ij} = -\frac{1}{2}s^2,$$

$$s^2 = \mathbf{V}(\ln Z_{ij}) = \ln(1 + \sigma^2).$$

In this model, a "standard" individual has the hazard rate $h_0(t)$. Individual j in the ith pair has the hazard rate of a "standard" individual multiplied by the frailty Z_{ij}. The above restriction on μ means that the average frailty in a population equals 1 (at the beginning of the follow-up). We refer to this model as Model 3.

Estimation Strategies

Parameter estimation in the gamma model is straightforward. The frailty term can be integrated out and an explicit representation of the unconditional bivariate survival function exists (12.1), which can be used to derive the likelihood function.

Several estimation methods for bivariate lognormal frailty models in consequence have been suggested to be used within a non-Bayesian framework. Various modifications of the maximum likelihood procedure are applicable to the bivariate frailty models. Ripatti and Palmgren (2000) derived an estimating algorithm based on the penalized partial likelihood (PPL). Xue and Brookmeyer (1996) suggested a modified EM algorithm for the bivariate lognormal frailty models. Sastry (1997) developed the modified EM algorithm for the multiplicative two-level gamma frailty model.

The same method can be applied to bivariate lognormal frailty models. Ripatti and Palmgren (2000) present yet another method to deal with EM-like algorithms in a bivariate lognormal frailty model.

Wienke et al. (2005) use numerical integration procedures. Integrals over the univariate and multivariate normal distributions can be approximated in different ways. One possibility is to use Gauss–Hermite quadratures by Naylor and Smith (1982) and Smith et al. (1987). Similar ideas are employed in various applications of random effect models in event history analysis by Lillard (1993), Lillard et al. (1995), and Panis and Lillard (1995). The methods are implemented in the aML software package (aML version 1, see Lillard and Panis 2000). Both methods were used to estimate parameters of the bivariate lognormal frailty models for simulated data.

Several studies on the application of Bayesian methods to multivariate frailty models exist. An example of a Bayesian approach to the gamma frailty model is found in Bolstad and Manda (2001). Gibbs' sampling scheme for the bivariate lognormal frailty model with an exponential baseline hazard is given in Xue and Ding (1999). Korsgaard and Andersen (1998) present a Bayesian inference in the lognormal frailty model with a semiparametric hazard.

12.4   Correlated Compound Poisson Frailty

Moger and Aalen (2005) developed correlated compound Poisson frailty model for the survival time of the two individuals in a family. Let Z_1 and Z_2 be the frailty variables of two individuals in a family with joint distribution $f_{Y_1,Y_2}(y_1, y_2)$. Let their marginal distribution given ρ, $f_{Y_1}(y_1|\rho)$ and $f_{Y_2}(y_2|\rho)$ be independent identically distributed compound Poisson with parameters η and ν. The parameter ρ, which is common for both Z_1 and Z_2, is assumed to be PVF distributed with parameters α, ϵ, and θ. The joint discrete part of (Z_1, Z_2) is

$$P(Z_1 = 0, Z_2 = 0) = E_\rho[\exp(-2\rho)] = L_\rho(2). \tag{12.2}$$

The joint density of the continuous part of the distribution can be found analogously to (12.2), by using the ρ, in the distributions $f_{Z_1|\rho}(z_1|\rho)$ and $f_{Z_2|\rho}(z_2|\rho)$ to get derivatives of $L_\rho(s)$. It is given by

$$f_{Z_1,Z_2}(z_1, z_2; \eta, \nu, \alpha, \theta, \epsilon) =$$
$$\frac{1}{z_1 z_2} \exp[-\nu(z_1 + z_2)] \sum_{n=2}^{\infty} (-1)^n L_\rho^{(n)}(2) \times \sum_{k=1}^{n-1} \frac{\nu u^{n\eta} z_1^{(n-k)\eta} z_2^{k\eta}}{\Gamma((n-k)\eta)\Gamma(k\eta)(n-k)!k!}, \tag{12.3}$$

where $L_\rho^{(n)}(s)$ is defined in (12.3). Since the marginal distributions are compound Poisson given ρ, the joint distribution has an interesting feature: it is possible to have two related individuals where one has zero frailty and the other has a positive frailty. The probability is given by

$$P(Z_1 = 0, Z_2 > 0) = E_\rho[\exp(-\rho) - \exp(-2\rho)] = L_\rho(1) - L_\rho(2). \quad (12.4)$$

In some situations, this is an aspect that may make the model fit better than a shared frailty model. Also, it is interesting for the interpretation. For instance, testicular cancer is hypothesized to be caused by some sort of damage in fetal life (Henderson et al. 1988). This damage could be due to genetics, mothers, or pregnancies. If there is a mother effect, it may not be natural with the possibility of $Z_1 = 0$ and $Z_2 > 0$.

By using (12.4), one easily finds their joint Laplace transform

$$L_{Z_1, Z_2}(s, t) = L_\rho\left(2 - \left(\frac{v}{v+s}\right)^\eta - \left(\frac{v}{v+t}\right)^\eta\right),$$

which in the case of PVF distributed ρ is

$$L_{Z_1, Z_2}(s, t) = \begin{cases} \exp\left(-\frac{\epsilon}{\alpha}\left\{\left[\theta + 2 - \left(\frac{v}{v+s}\right)^\eta - \left(\frac{v}{v+t}\right)^\eta\right]^\alpha - \theta^\alpha\right\}\right) \\ \qquad\qquad \text{if } \alpha \le 1, \alpha \ne 0, \\ \left[\frac{\theta}{\theta+2-\left(\frac{v}{v+s}\right)^\eta-\left(\frac{v}{v+t}\right)^\eta}\right]^\epsilon \quad \text{if } \alpha = 0. \end{cases} \quad (12.5)$$

Note that the univariate Laplace transform in (12.5) appears by setting $t = 0$.

By noting that $Cov(Z_1, Z_2) = COV(E(Z_1|\rho), E(Z_2|\rho))$ and using the correlation coefficient between frailties of two individuals in a family obtained by Moger and Aalen (2005) is

$$Corr(Z_1, Z_2) = \frac{\eta(1 - \alpha)}{\theta + \eta(1 - \alpha + \theta)} \quad \text{if } \theta > 0.$$

The parameter θ determines the degree of correlation. Since none of the moments exists (when $\theta = 0$), the correlation coefficient cannot be used as a measure of dependence for the compound Poisson-positive stable distribution. For values of θ close to zero, the correlation between two related individuals is approaching one. It is evident that the correlation has to be larger than zero, so the model cannot handle negative dependencies.

Let T_1 and T_2 be the lifetimes of the two individuals which are independent. The survival function of (T_1, T_2) given the two dependent frailties (Z_1, Z_2) is given by

$$S_{T_1, T_2|Z_1, Z_2}(t_1, t_2|z_1, z_2) = \exp(-H_1(t_1)z_1 - H_2(t_2)z_2).$$

The unconditional survival function of (T_1, T_2) is obtained by integrating (Z_1, Z_2) out

$$S_{T_1, T_2}(t_1, t_2) = E(\exp(-H_1(t_1)Z_1 - H_2(t_2)Z_2))$$

$$
= \begin{cases} \exp\left(-\frac{\epsilon}{\alpha}\left\{\left[\theta + 2 - \left(\frac{v}{v+M_1(t_1)}\right)^{\eta} - \left(\frac{v}{v+M_2(t_2)}\right)^{\eta}\right]^{\alpha} - \theta^{\alpha}\right\}\right) \\ \qquad\qquad \text{if } \alpha \le 1, \alpha \ne 0, \\[2ex] \left[\dfrac{\theta}{\theta+2-\left(\frac{v}{v+M_1(t_1)}\right)^{\eta}-\left(\frac{v}{v+M_2(t_2)}\right)^{\eta}}\right]^{\epsilon} \quad \text{if } \alpha = 0. \end{cases}
$$

Let (T_1, T_2) are independent Weibull distributions with $W(\lambda_1, c_1)$ and $W(\lambda_2, c_2)$, respectively, where λ_i's are scale parameters and c_i's are shape parameters of Weibull distributions. The survival function of T_i is

$$
S_{T_i}(t_i) = \exp(-\lambda_i t_i^{c_i}).
$$

Now the unconditional survival function of (T_1, T_2) with correlated compound Poisson frailties is given by

$$
S_{T_1,T_2}(t_1, t_2) = \begin{cases} \exp\left(-\frac{\epsilon}{\alpha}\left\{\left[\theta + 2 - \left(\frac{v}{v+\lambda_1 t_1^{c_1}}\right)^{\eta} - \left(\frac{v}{v+\lambda_2 t_2^{c_2}}\right)^{\eta}\right]^{\alpha} - \theta^{\alpha}\right\}\right) \\ \qquad\qquad \text{if } \alpha \le 1, \alpha \ne 0, \\[2ex] \left[\dfrac{\theta}{\theta+2-\left(\frac{v}{v+\lambda_1 t_1^{c_1}}\right)^{\eta}-\left(\frac{v}{v+\lambda_2 t_2^{c_2}}\right)^{\eta}}\right]^{\epsilon} \quad \text{if } \alpha = 0. \end{cases}
$$

In order to solve the identifiability problem, we assume a mean of 1 for the frailty distributions. For the gamma distribution, this can be achieved by setting $\theta = \epsilon$. In the shared PVF model, $E(Z) = 1$ is achieved by setting $\epsilon = \theta^{1-\alpha}$. The shared frailty models are compared to a compound Poisson model where ρ is gamma distributed, yielding a compound Poisson–gamma model. To secure a unit mean for the frailty, we get $\epsilon = v\theta/\eta$.

Hanagal (2010a) assumed the distribution of frailty as compound Poisson–gamma (with $\alpha = 0$) distribution for the bivariate survival data. The bivariate survival function based on this frailty is given by

$$
S(t_1, t_2) = \left[\frac{\theta}{\theta + 2 - \left(\frac{v}{v+\lambda_1 t_1^{c_1}}\right)^{\eta} - \left(\frac{v}{v+\lambda_2 t_2^{c_2}}\right)^{\eta}}\right]^{v\theta/\eta}.
$$

Hanagal (2010a) obtained the estimation of parameters in correlated compound Poisson frailty with Weibull distributions as baseline models based on the censored samples. He did a simulation study based on 100 samples of sizes from bivariate Weibull baseline and obtained MLEs of the parameters.

12.5 Correlated Power Variance Function Frailty Model

To investigate the sensitivity of heritability estimates to the choice of the frailty distribution, the correlated frailty model was extended by applying the ideas of correlated frailty to the power variance function (PVF) family of frailty distributions. The univariate version of this distribution was introduced to frailty modeling by Hougaard (1986b).

In the correlated PVF family model, the marginal distributions of (Z_1, Z_2) satisfy $Z_i \sim \mathrm{PVF}(\alpha, \delta = (\frac{1-\alpha}{\sigma^2})^{1-\alpha}, \theta = \frac{1-\alpha}{\sigma^2})$, i.e., Z_i is PVF distributed with mean 1, variance σ^2, and Laplace transform

$$L(s; \alpha, \sigma^2) = \exp\left\{ -\frac{1-\alpha}{\alpha\sigma^2} \left(\left(1 + \frac{\sigma^2}{1-\alpha}s\right)^{\alpha} - 1 \right) \right\}.$$

The bivariate Laplace transform for the correlated PVF frailty model is given by

$$
\begin{aligned}
L(s_1, s_2; \alpha, \sigma^2, \rho) = {} & \exp\left\{ -\rho\frac{1-\alpha}{\alpha\sigma^2} \left(\left(1 + \frac{\sigma^2}{1-\alpha}(s_1 + s_2)\right)^{\alpha} - 1 \right) \right\} \times \\
& \exp\left\{ -(1-\rho)\frac{1-\alpha}{\alpha\sigma^2} \left(\left(1 + \frac{\sigma^2}{1-\alpha}s_1\right)^{\alpha} - 1 \right) \right\} \times \\
& \exp\left\{ -(1-\rho)\frac{1-\alpha}{\alpha\sigma^2} \left(\left(1 + \frac{\sigma^2}{1-\alpha}s_2\right)^{\alpha} - 1 \right) \right\},
\end{aligned}
$$

where $\mathrm{corr}(Z_1, Z_2) = \rho$.

The correlated frailty model with PVF frailty distribution is characterized by the bivariate survival function of the following form:

$$
\begin{aligned}
S(t_1, t_2) = {} & S(t_1)^{1-\rho} S(t_2)^{1-\rho} \exp\left(\frac{\rho(1-\alpha)}{\alpha\sigma^2}\left[1 - \left(\left(1 - \frac{\alpha\sigma^2}{1-\alpha}\ln S(t_1)\right)^{\frac{1}{\alpha}} \right. \right.\right. \\
& \left.\left.\left. + \left(1 - \frac{\alpha\sigma^2}{1-\alpha}\ln S(t_2)\right)^{\frac{1}{\alpha}} - 1 \right)^{\alpha} \right] \right).
\end{aligned}
\tag{12.6}
$$

This model has been used in the analysis of the Danish Twin survival data by Yashin et al. (1999). The results confirm the presence of genetic influence on frailty. Note that the bivariate gamma distribution (used in the correlated gamma frailty model) and the inverse Gaussian distribution are special cases of the three-parameter bivariate frailty distribution. This gives us the opportunity to compare the analysis of the same data using different frailty models. The results show that the gamma frailty model and the extended PVF model fit the Danish twin data equally well.

The presence of a parameter representing the correlation between the frailty variables is crucial for genetic analysis of frailty, in particular, for heritability estimation, since standard twin analysis methods of quantitative genetics are based on the analysis of correlations for MZ and DZ twins (Falconer 1965). The idea of genetic analysis of frailty using twin data is presented in more detail in Yashin and Iachine (1995a) and Iachine et al. (1998).

12.6 Other Correlated Frailty Models

Iachine (2001) gave a general formula to formulate correlated frailty models which is stated in the following theorem.

Theorem 12.1 *Let Z be an infinitely divisible frailty variable with Laplace transformation $L_Z(s)$. Let $\rho \in [0, 1]$, then there exist random variables Z_1, Z_2 each with univariate Laplace transform $L_Z(s)$ such that the Laplace transform of Z_1, Z_2 is given by*

$$L(s_1, s_2) = L_Z^{\rho}(s_1 + s_2)L_Z^{1-\rho}(s_1)L_Z^{1-\rho}(s_2).$$

If Z has a variance, the $Corr(Z_1, Z_2) = \rho$.

In terms of cumulative hazard function, the bivariate Laplace transform is given by

$$L(H_1(t_1), H_2(t_2)) = L_Z^{\rho}(H_1(t_1) + H_2(t_2))L_Z^{1-\rho}(H_1(t_1))L_Z^{1-\rho}(H_2(t_2))$$
$$= S(t_1, t_2). \tag{12.7}$$

The respective bivariate survival model is identifiable under mild regularity conditions on Z provided that $\rho > 0$. The case $\rho = 1$ is known as the shared frailty model. If $\rho = 0$, Z_1 and Z_2 are independent. Versions of shared frailty model were analyzed by Clayton and Cuzick (1985), Vaupel et al. (1992) in the case of gamma frailty, and Hougaard (1987) in the case of positive stable frailty, among others. The above theorem gives the expression for the bivariate Laplace transform in terms of univariate Laplace transform with different arguments. This will solve the problem of obtaining bivariate survival function through the bivariate Laplace transform. For every univariate survival, one can find bivariate survival function.

Equation (12.7) can be extended to multivariate case ($\rho > 0$) as given below:

$$L[H_1(t_1), \ldots, H_k(t_k)] = L_Z^{\rho}[H_1(t_1) + \cdots + H_k(t_k)]L_Z^{1-\rho}[H_1(t_1)]\ldots L_Z^{1-\rho}[H_k(t_k)]$$
$$= S(t_1, \ldots, t_k).$$

The case $\rho = 1$ leads to shared frailty. If $\rho = 0$, $Z_1, \ldots, Z_k$ are mutually independent.

12.6.1 Correlated Inverse Gaussian Frailty Model

The univariate Laplace transform of inverse Gaussian frailty distribution is

$$L_Z(H_1(t_1)) = \exp\left[\frac{1 - (1 + 2\sigma^2 H_1(t_1))^{\frac{1}{2}}}{\sigma^2}\right]$$
$$= S_1(t_1).$$

Now $H_1(t_1)$ can be expressed in terms of survival function as

$$H_1(t_1) = \frac{[1 - \sigma^2 \ln S_1(t_1)]^2 - 1}{2\sigma^2}.$$

Using the bivariate Laplace transform given in Eq. (12.7), we obtain the bivariate survival function with correlated inverse Gaussian frailty in terms of cumulative hazard functions which is given by

$$S(t_1, t_2) = \exp\left\{\frac{[1 - (1 + 2\sigma^2(H_1(t_1) + H_2(t_2)))^{\frac{1}{2}}]}{\sigma^2}\rho\right\}$$
$$\times \exp\left\{\frac{[1 - (1 + 2\sigma^2 H_1(t_1))^{\frac{1}{2}}]}{\sigma^2}(1 - \rho)\right\}$$
$$\times \exp\left\{\frac{[-(1 + 2\sigma^2 H_2(t_2))^{\frac{1}{2}}]}{\sigma^2}(1 - \rho)\right\}. \qquad (12.8)$$

Now the bivariate survival function with correlated inverse Gaussian frailty in terms of univariate survival functions is given by

$$S(t_1, t_2) = \exp\left[\frac{\{1 - \{1 - \sigma^2 \ln S_1(t_1)\}^2 + \{1 - \sigma^2 \ln S_2(t_2)\}^2 - 1\}^{\frac{1}{2}}\rho}{\sigma^2}\right]$$
$$\times S_1(t_1)^{1-\rho} S_2(t_2)^{1-\rho}.$$

12.6.2 Correlated Positive Stable Frailty Model

The univariate Laplace transform of positive stable frailty distribution is

$$L_Z(H_1(t_1)) = \exp[-H_1(t_1)^\alpha]$$
$$= S_1(t_1).$$

Now $H_1(t_1)$ can be expressed in terms of survival function as

$$H_1(t_1) = [-\ln S_1(t_1)]^{\frac{1}{\alpha}}.$$

Using the bivariate Laplace transform given in Eq. (12.7), we obtain the bivariate survival function with correlated positive stable frailty in terms of cumulative hazard functions which is given by

$$S(t_1, t_2) = \exp[-(H_1(t_1) + H_2(t_2))^\alpha \rho] \exp[-H_1(t_1)^\alpha (1 - \rho)]$$
$$\times \exp[-H_2(t_2)^\alpha (1 - \rho)].$$

Now the bivariate survival function with correlated positive stable frailty in terms of univariate survival functions is given by

$$S(t_1, t_2) = \exp[-\{(-\ln S_1(t_1))^{\frac{1}{\alpha}} + (-\ln S_1(t_1))^{\frac{1}{\alpha}}\}^\alpha \rho]$$
$$\times S_1(t_1)^{1-\rho} S_2(t_2)^{1-\rho}.$$

12.6.3   Correlated PVF Frailty Model

In the correlated PVF family model, the marginal distributions (Z_1, Z_2) satisfy $Z_i \sim PVF(\alpha, \delta, \theta)$, where $\theta = \frac{1-\alpha}{\sigma^2}$ and $\delta = \theta^{1-\alpha}$ then Z_i is PVF with mean one and variance σ^2. The Laplace transform of Z is

$$S_1(t_1) = L_Z(H_1(t_1)) = \exp\left\{-\frac{1-\alpha}{\alpha\sigma^2}\left(\left(1 + \frac{\sigma^2}{1-\alpha}H_1(t_1)\right)^\alpha - 1\right)\right\}.$$

Using the bivariate Laplace transform given in Eq. (12.7), we obtain bivariate survival function with correlated PVF frailty in terms of cumulative hazard function models as follows:

$$S(t_1, t_2) = \exp\left\{-\rho\frac{(1-\alpha)}{\alpha\sigma^2}\left(\left(1 + \frac{\sigma^2}{1-\alpha}(H_1(t_1) + H_2(t_2))\right)^\alpha - 1\right)\right\}$$
$$\times \exp\left\{-(1-\rho)\frac{(1-\alpha)}{\alpha\sigma^2}\left(\left(1 + \frac{\sigma^2}{1-\alpha}H_1(t_1)\right)^\alpha - 1\right)\right\}$$
$$\times \exp\left\{-(1-\rho)\frac{(1-\alpha)}{\alpha\sigma^2}\left(\left(1 + \frac{\sigma^2}{1-\alpha}H_2(t_2)\right)^\alpha - 1\right)\right\},$$

we obtain bivariate survival function with correlated PVF frailty in terms of univariate survival function models as follows:

$$S(t_1, t_2) = \exp\left\{-\rho\frac{(1-\alpha)}{\alpha\sigma^2}\left[\left(1 - \frac{\alpha\sigma^2}{1-\alpha}\ln S_1(t_1)\right)^{\frac{1}{\alpha}} + \left(1 - \frac{\alpha\sigma^2}{1-\alpha}\ln S_2(t_2)\right)^{\frac{1}{\alpha}} - 1\right]\right\}$$
$$\times S_1(t_1)^{1-\rho} S_2(t_2)^{1-\rho},$$

the expression is the same as the expression given in Eq. (12.6). One can obtain the correlated gamma frailty from Eq. (12.7) which will lead to the correlation gamma frailty discussed in Sect. 12.2 which is left as an exercise.

12.6.4 Correlated Compound Poisson Frailty Model

The correlated compound Poisson has been already discussed in Sect. 12.4. There exists one more version of correlated compound Poisson frailty based on Eq. (12.7). The Laplace transform of univariate compound Poisson frailty is

$$L_Z(H_1(t_1)) = S_1(t_1) = \exp\left\{-\mu\left[1 - \left(1 + \frac{H_1(t_1)}{\mu\gamma}\right)^{-\gamma}\right]\right\}.$$

Using the bivariate Laplace transform given in Eq. (12.7), we obtain bivariate survival function with correlated compound Poisson frailty in terms of cumulative hazard functions model as follows:

$$S(t_1, t_2) = \exp\left\{-\rho\mu\left[1 - \left(1 + \frac{H_1(t_1) + H_2(t_2)}{\mu\gamma}\right)^{-\gamma}\right]\right\}$$
$$\times \exp\left\{-\mu(1-\rho)\left[1 - \left(1 + \frac{H_1(t_1)}{\mu\gamma}\right)^{-\gamma}\right]\right\}$$
$$\times \exp\left\{-\mu(1-\rho)\left[1 - \left(1 + \frac{H_2(t_2)}{\mu\gamma}\right)^{-\gamma}\right]\right\}.$$

We obtain bivariate survival function with correlated compound Poisson frailty in terms of univariate survival functions model as follows:

$$S(t_1, t_2) = \exp\left\{-\rho\mu\left[1 - \left\{\left(1 + \frac{1}{\mu}\ln S_1(t_1)\right)^{-\frac{1}{\gamma}} + \left(1 + \frac{1}{\mu}\ln S_2(t_2)\right)^{-\frac{1}{\gamma}} - 1\right\}^{-\gamma}\right]\right\}$$
$$\times S_1(t_1)^{1-\rho} S_2(t_2)^{1-\rho}.$$

12.6.5 Correlated Compound Negative Binomial Frailty Model

The Laplace transform of univariate compound negative binomial frailty is

$$L_Z(H_1(t_1)) = S_1(t_1) = \left[\frac{p}{1 - q \left(1 + \frac{H_1(t_1)}{\nu}\right)^{-\gamma}} \right]^r.$$

Using the bivariate Laplace transform given in Eq. (12.7), we obtain bivariate survival function with correlated compound negative binomial frailty in terms of cumulative hazard functions model as follows:

$$S(t_1, t_2) = \left[\frac{p}{1 - q \left(1 + \frac{H_1(t_1)+H_2(t_2)}{\nu}\right)^{-\gamma}} \right]^{r\rho} \left[\frac{p}{1 - q \left(1 + \frac{H_1(t_1)}{\nu}\right)^{-\gamma}} \right]^{r(1-\rho)}$$

$$\times \left[\frac{p}{1 - q(1 + \frac{H_2(t_2)}{\nu})^{-\gamma}} \right]^{r(1-\rho)}.$$

We obtain bivariate survival function with correlated compound negative binomial frailty in terms of univariate survival functions model as follows:

$$S(t_1, t_2) = \left[\frac{p}{1 - q \left\{ \left[\frac{1}{q}\left(1 - \frac{p}{S_1(t_1)^{1/r}}\right)\right]^{-1/\gamma} + \left[\frac{1}{q}\left(1 - \frac{p}{S_2(t_2)^{1/r}}\right)\right]^{-1/\gamma} - 1 \right\}^{-\gamma}} \right]^{r\rho}$$

$$\times S_1(t_1)^{1-\rho} S_2(t_2)^{1-\rho}.$$

12.7 Applications

Commenges and Gadda (1997) presented a family of tests based on correlated random effects models which provides a synthesis and generalization of tests for homogeneity. In these models, each subject has a particular random effect, but the random effects between subjects are correlated. They derive the general form of the score statistic for testing that the random effects have a variance equal to zero. They applied this result to both parametric and semiparametric models. In both cases, they showed that under certain conditions, the score statistic has an asymptotic normal distribution. They considered several applications of this theory, including overdispersion, heterogeneity between groups, spatial correlations, and genetic linkage.

Zahl (1997) analyzed two data sets, one is based on malignant melanoma patients with cancer and another is based on cancer using correlated gamma frailty model. He used bivariate frailty variables $Z_1 = X_1 + X_2$ and $Z_2 = \alpha(X_1 + X_3)$, where X_1, X_2, and X_3 are three independent gamma variables and α is scaling parameter.

Viswanathan and Manatunga (2001) compared two frailty distributions, gamma and positive stable, based on the diagnostic plots. These plots are capable of differentiating between the two frailty models when strong association is present between two frailty models. They analyzed diabetic retinopathy data and a reasonable fit to the gamma frailty model is found.

Giard et al. (2002) suggested that multivariate frailty model can be used in the genetic analysis of the aging process as a whole, simplified to consisting of the states such as healthy, disabled, and deceased. They evaluated simultaneously the relative magnitude of genetic and environmental influences on frailty variables corresponding to the period of good health and to the life span. The frailty variables can be interpreted as susceptibility to illness or death. The model can be applied to data on groups of related individuals (twins, siblings, a litter). One of the major advantages of this model is that it allows one to include groups of individuals where some or all members of the group are already deceased at the time of observation. They discussed the estimation procedures and analyzed twin data on prostate cancer.

Wienke et al. (2003) suggested a cure-mixture model to analyze bivariate time-to-event data using correlated gamma frailty model. They obtained the model for left-truncated and right-censored data, and accounts for heterogeneity, as well as for an insusceptible (cure) fraction in the study population. They obtained estimation procedures and applied it to breast cancer incidence data for 5857 Swedish female monozygotic and dizygotic twin pairs from the cohort of the Swedish Twin Registry. They estimated the size of the susceptible fraction and the correlation between the frailties of the twin partners.

Finkelstein and Esaulova (2006) considered correlated frailty model under the assumption of conditional independence of components. They also discussed two examples based on their results.

Wienke et al. (2006) used three correlated frailty models to analyze bivariate survival data by assuming gamma, lognormal, and compound Poisson distributed frailty. All approaches allow to deal with right-censored lifetime data and account for heterogeneity as well as for a non-susceptible (cure) fraction in the study population. In the gamma and compound Poisson model, traditional ML estimation methods are used, whereas in the lognormal model, MCMC methods are applied. Breast cancer incidence data of Swedish twin pairs illustrate the practical relevance of the models, which are used to estimate the size of the susceptible fraction and the correlation between the frailties of the twin partners.

Garibotti et al. (2006) applied Cox proportional hazards models to data from three-generation pedigrees in the Utah Population Database using two different frailty specification schemes that account for common environments (shared frailty) and genetic effects (correlated frailty). In a model that includes measures of familial history of longevity and both frailty effects, they find that the variance component due to genetic factors is comparable to the one attributable to shared environments.

Congdon (2008) considered a model for survival data with a permanent survival fraction and non-monotonic failure rates and evaluate the gain in model fit, and effects on inference, from adding frailty. An application considers age at first maternity using data from the 2002 German General Social Survey, with permanent survival amounting to childlessness. Regressions are used to explain both the failure time of the event (here age at first maternity) and the permanent survival mechanism (susceptibility to undergo maternity or not). Additive correlated effects are included in the linked models defining these regressions and relate to two types of frailty: influences on the event rate itself and influences on the probability of susceptibility. A hierarchical Bayesian approach is adopted with likelihood conditional on bivariate random frailty effects, and a second stage prior defining the density of those effects. A Bayesian approach facilitates modeling with multivariate random effects, whereas frequentist approaches based on marginal likelihoods with random effects integrated out using numerical methods may become infeasible or unreliable when there are many random parameters (Tutz and Kauermann 2003; Kim et al. 2002). Monte Carlo Markov Chain (MCMC) methods are used for estimation via the WINBUGS package (Lunn et al. 2000), and generate samples from the posterior distribution without the form of the posterior density being known analytically (Gilks et al. 1996). This is useful in summarizing possibly non-normal densities relating to model functionals (e.g., modal ages at maternity) and in obtaining posterior probabilities relating to hypotheses on such functionals, e.g., that the modal age for women with low education years is lower than the modal age for women with extended education.

References

Bolstad, W.M., Manda, S.O.: Investigating child mortality in Malawi using family and community random effects: a Bayesian analysis. J. Am. Stat. Assoc. **96**, 12 (2001)

Clayton, D.G.: A model for association in bivariate life tables and its application in epidemiological studies of familial tendency in chronic disease incidence. Biometrika **65**, 141–151 (1978)

Clayton, D.G., Cuzick, J.: Multivariate generalizations of the proportional hazard model (with discussion). J. R. Stat. Soc. A **148**, 82–117 (1985)

Commenges, H., Gadda, H.J.: Generalized score test of homogeneity based on correlated random effects models. J. R. Stat. Soc. B **59**(1), 157–171 (1997)

Congdon, P.: A bivariate frailty model for events with a permanent survivor fraction and non-monotonic hazards; with an application to age at first maternity. Comput. Stat. Data Anal. **52**, 4346–4356 (2008)

Elbers, C., Rider, G.: True and spurious duration dependence: the identifiability of the proportional hazard model. Rev. Econ. Stud. **49**, 403–409 (1982). Enky, D.G., Noufaily, A., Farrington, P.: A time-varying shared frailty model with application to infectious diseases. Ann. Appl. Stat. **8**(1), 3430–3447

Falconer, D.S.: The inheritance of liability to certain diseases estimated from the incidence among relatives. Ann. Hum. Genet. **29**, 51–76 (1965)

Finkelstein, M., Esaulova, V.: On asymptotic failure rates in bivariate frailty competing risk models. Maxplanck Institute, Rostock, Germany (Preprint) (2006)

Garibotti, G., Smith, K.R., Kerber, R.A., Boucher, K.M.: Longevity and correlated frailty in multi-generational families. J. Gerontol. **61A**(12), 1253–1261 (2006)

Giard, N., Lichtenstein, P., Yashin, A.I.: A multistate model for the genetic analysis of the aging process. Stat. Med. **21**, 2511–2526 (2002)

Gilks, W., Richardson, S., Spiegelhalter, D.: Markov Chain Monte Carlo in Practice. Chapman & Hall, New York (1996)

Hanagal, D.D.: Correlated compound Poisson frailty model for the bivariate survival data. Int. J. Stat. Manag. Syst. **5**, 127–140 (2010a)

Henderson, B.E., Ross, R., Bernstein, L.: Estrogens as a cause of human cancer: The Richard and Hinda Rosenthal Foundation Award lecture. Cancer Res. **48**, 246–253 (1988)

Hougaard, P.: A class of multivariate failure time distributions. Biometrika **73**, 671–678 (1986a)

Hougaard, P.: Survival models for hetrogeneous populations derived from stable distributions. Biometrika **73**, 387–396 (1986b)

Hougaard, P.: Modeling multivariate survival. Scand. J. Stat. **14**, 291–304 (1987)

Iachine, I.A.: Correlated frailty concept in the analysis of bivariate survival data. Bachelor project, Department of Mathematics and Computer Science, Odense University, Denmark (1995a)

Iachine, I.A.: Parameter estimation in the bivariate correlated frailty model with observed covariates via the EM-algorithm. Working Paper Series: Population Studies of Aging 16, CHS, Odense University, Denmark (1995b)

Iachine, I.A.: The use of twin and family survival data in the population studies of aging: statistical methods based on multivariate survival data. Ph.D. thesis, Department of Statistics and Demography, University of Southern Denmark, Denmark (2001)

Iachine, I.A., Holm, N.V., Harris, J.R., Begun, A.Z., Iachina, M.K., Laitinen, M., Kaprio, J., Yashin, A.I.: How heritable is individual susceptibility to death? The results of an analysis of survival data on Danish, Swedish and Finnish twins. Twin Res. **1**(4), 196–205 (1998)

Kheiri, S., Meshkani, M.R., Faghihzadeh, S.: A correlated frailty model for analyzing risk factors in bilateral corneal fraft rejection for Keratoconus: a Bayesian approach. Stat. Med. **24**, 2681–2693 (2005)

Kim, H., Sun, D., Tsutakawa, R.: Lognormal vs. gamma: extra variations. Biom. J. **44**, 305–323 (2002)

Korsgaard, I.R., Andersen, A.H.: The additive genetic gamma frailty model. Scand. J. Stat. **25**(2), 255–269 (1998)

Lillard, L.A., Panis, C.W.A.: AML User's Guide and Reference Manual. EconWare, Los Angeles (2000)

Lillard, L.A.: Simultaneous equations for hazards: marriage duration and fertility timing. J. Econ. **56**, 189–217 (1993)

Lillard, L.A., Brien, M.J., Waite, L.J.: Premarital cohabitation and subsequent marital dissolution: a matter of self-selection? Demography **32**, 437–457 (1995)

Lunn, D., Thomas, A., Best, N., Spiegelhalter, D.: WinBUGS - A Bayesian modelling framework: concepts, structure, and extensibility. Stat. Comput. **10**, 325–337 (2000)

Moger, T.A., Aalen, O.O.: A distribution for multivariate frailty based on the compound Poisson distribution with random scale. Lifetime Data Anal. **11**, 41–59 (2005)

Naylor, J.C., Smith, A.F.M.: Applications of a method for the efficient computation of posterior distribution. J. Appl. Stat. **31**, 214–225 (1982)

Panis, C.W.A., Lillard, L.A.: Child mortality in Malaysia: explaining ethnic differences and the recent decline. Popul. Stud. **49**, 463–479 (1995)

Petersen, J.H.: An additive frailty model for correlated life times. Biometrics **54**, 646–661 (1998)

Pickles, A., Crouchley, R.: A simple frailty model for family studies with covariates. Stat. Med. **3**, 263–278 (1994)

Pickles, A., Crouchley, R., Simonoff, E., Eaves, L., Meyer, J., Rutter, M., Hewit, J., Silberg, J.: Survival models for developmental genetic data: age at onset of puberty and antisocial behaviour in twins. Genet. Epidemiol. **11**, 155–170 (1994)

Ripatti, S., Palmgren, J.: Estimation of multivariate frailty models using penalized likelihood. Biometrics **56**, 1016–1022 (2000)

Sastry, N.: A nest frailty model for survival data with an application to the study of child survival in Northeast Brazil. J. Am. Stat. Assoc. **92**, 426–435 (1997)

Smith, A.F.M., Skene, A.M., Shaw, J.E.H., Naylor, J.C.: Progress with numerical and graphical methods for practical Bayesian statistics. Statistician **36**, 75–82 (1987)

Tutz, G., Kauermann, G.: Generalized linear random effects models with varying coefficients. Comput. Stat. Data Anal. **43**, 13–28 (2003)

Vaupel, J.W., Yashin, A.I., Hauge, M., Harvald, B., Holm, N.Y., Xue, L.: Survival analysis in genetics: Danish twins data applied to gerontological question. In: Klein, J.P., Goel, P.K. (eds.) Survival Analysis: State of Art. Kluwer, Dordrecht (1992)

Vaupel, J.W., Manton, K.G., Stallard, E.: The impact of heterogeneity on individual frailty in the dynamic of mortality. Demography **16**(3), 439–454 (1979)

Viswanathan, B., Manatunga, A.K.: Diagnostic plots for assessing the frailty distribution in multi-variate survival data. Lifetime Data Anal. **7**, 143–155 (2001)

Wienke, A., Lichtenstein, P., Yashin, A.I.: A bivariate frailty model with a cure fraction for modeling familial correlations in diseases. Biometrics. **59**, 1178–1183 (2003)

Wienke, A.: Frailty Models in Survival Analysis. CRC Press, New York (2011)

Wienke, A., Arbeev, K.G.A., Locantelli, I., Yashin, A.I.: A comparison of different bivariate corre-lated frailty models and estimation strategies. Math. Sci. **198**(1), 1–13 (2005)

Wienke, A., Locantelli, I., Yashin, A.I.: The modeling of a cure fraction in bivariate time-to-event data. Austrian J. Stat. **35**(1), 67–76 (2006)

Xue, S., Brookmeyer, R.: Bivariate frailty model for the analysis of multivariate survival time. Lifetime Data Anal. **2**, 277–290 (1996)

Xue, X., Ding, Y.: Assessing heterogeneity and correlation of paired failure times with the bivariate frailty model. Stat. Med. **18**, 907–918 (1999)

Yashin, A.I., Iachine, I.A., Harris, J.R.: Half of variation in susceptibility is gentic: findings from Swedish twin survival data. Behav. Genet. **29**(1), 11–19 (1999)

Yashin, A.I., Iachine, I.A.: Environment determines 50% of variability in individual frailty: results from Dansih twin study. Research report, Population Studies of Aging, 10, Odense University, Denmark (1994)

Yashin, A.I., Iachine, I.A.: Genetic analysis of durations: correlated frailty model applied to survival of Dansih twins. Genet. Epidemiol. **12**, 529–538 (1995a)

Yashin, A.I., Iachine, I.A.: How long can humans live? Lower bound for biological limit of human longevity calculated from Danish twin data using correlated frailty model. Mech. Aging Dev. **80**, 147–169 (1995b)

Yashin, A.I., Iachine, I.A.: How to reduce standard errors analyzing bivariate survival data. An approach based on correlated frailty model. Research report, Population Studies of Aging, 9, Odense University, Denmark (1993b)

Yashin, A.I., Iachine, I.A.: Survival of related individuals: an extension of some fundamental results of heterogeneity analysis. Research report, Population Studies of Aging, 8, Odense University, Denmark (1993a)

Yashin, A.I., Vaupel, J.W., Iachine, I.A.: Correlated individual frailty: an advantageous approach to survival analysis of bivariate data. Working Paper Series: Population Studies of Aging 7, CHS, Odense University, Denmark (1993a)

Yashin, A.I., Vaupel, J.W., Iachine, I.A.: Duality of aging: the equivalence of mortality models based on radically different concepts. Mech. Aging Dev. **74**, 1–14 (1993b)

Yashin, A.I., Iachine, I.A.: How frailty models can be used in the analysis of mortality and longevity limits. Demography **34**, 31–48 (1997)

Yashin, A.I., Vaupel, J.W., Iachine, I.A.: Correlated individual frailty: an advantages approach to survival analysis of bivariate data. Math. Popul. Stud. **5**, 145–159 (1995)

Zahl, P.H.: Frailty modelling for the excess hazard. Stat. Med. **16**, 1573–1585 (1997)

Chapter 13
Correlated Gamma and Inverse Gaussian Frailty Models

13.1 Introduction

Shared frailty explains correlations between subjects within clusters. However, it does have some limitations. First, it forces the unobserved factors to be the same within the cluster, which may not always reflect reality. For example, at times, it may be inappropriate to assume that all partners in a cluster share all their unobserved risk factors. Second, the dependence between survival times within the cluster is based on marginal distributions of survival times. However, when covariates are present in a proportional hazards model with gamma-distributed frailty, the dependence parameter and the population heterogeneity are confounded (Clayton and Cuzick 1985). This implies that the joint distribution can be identified from the marginal distributions (Hougaard 1986). Third, in most cases, a one-dimensional frailty can only induce positive association within the cluster. However, there are some situations in which the survival times for subjects within the same cluster are negatively associated. For example, in the Stanford Heart Transplantation Study, generally the longer an individual must wait for an available heart, the shorter he or she is likely to survive after the transplantation. Therefore, the waiting time and the survival time afterward may be negatively associated.

To avoid these limitations, correlated frailty models are being developed for the analysis of multivariate failure time data, in which associated random variables are used to characterize the frailty effect for each cluster. Correlated frailty models provide not only variance parameters of the frailties as in shared frailty models, but they also contain additional parameter for modeling the correlation between frailties in each group. Frequently one is interested in construction of a bivariate extension of some univariate family distributions (e.g., gamma). For example, for the purpose of genetic analysis of frailty, one might be interested in estimation of correlation of frailty. It turns out that it is possible to carry out such extension for the class of infinitely divisible distributions (Iachine 1995a, b). In this case, an additional parameter representing the correlation coefficient of the bivariate frailty distribution is introduced. Hens et al. (2009) studied the behavior of the bivariate-correlated

© Springer Nature Singapore Pte Ltd. 2019
D. D. Hanagal, *Modeling Survival Data Using Frailty Models*,
Industrial and Applied Mathematics, https://doi.org/10.1007/978-981-15-1181-3_13

gamma frailty model for type I interval-censored data, better known as current status data. They showed that applying a shared rather than a correlated frailty model to cross-sectionally collected serological data on hepatitis A and B leads to biased estimates for the baseline hazard and variance parameters. Hanagal (2010) proposed correlated compound Poisson frailty model for bivariate survival data. Hanagal and Pandey (2019) and Hanagal et al. (2017) analyzed kidney infection data using correlated gamma and correlated inverse Gaussian frailty models for the multiplicative models.

13.2 Correlated Frailty Models with Baseline Distributions

In Chap. 12, we obtained correlated gamma frailty and correlated inverse Gaussian distribution as follows:

$$S(t_1, t_2) = \left(1 + \eta_j \sigma_1^2 H_{01}(t_1) + \eta_j \sigma_2^2 H_{02}(t_2)\right)^{\frac{-\rho}{\sigma_1 \sigma_2}} \times \left(1 + \eta_j \sigma_1^2 H_{01}(t_1)\right)^{\frac{-1 + \frac{\sigma_1}{\sigma_2}\rho}{\sigma_1^2}}$$
$$\left(1 + \eta_j \sigma_2^2 H_{02}(t_2)\right)^{\frac{-1 + \frac{\sigma_2}{\sigma_1}\rho}{\sigma_2^2}}$$

$$S(t_1, t_2) = \exp\left\{\frac{[1 - (1 + 2\sigma^2(H_1(t_1) + H_2(t_2)))^{\frac{1}{2}}]}{\sigma^2}\rho\right\}$$
$$\times \exp\left\{\frac{[1 - (1 + 2\sigma^2 H_1(t_1))^{\frac{1}{2}}]}{\sigma^2}(1 - \rho)\right\}$$
$$\times \exp\left\{\frac{[1 - (1 + 2\sigma^2 H_2(t_2))^{\frac{1}{2}}]}{\sigma^2}(1 - \rho)\right\}.$$

Substituting cumulative hazard function for generalized Weibull and the generalized log-logistic type II baseline distributions with the distribution function in the above equations, we get the unconditional bivariate survival functions at time $t_{1j} > 0$ and $t_{2j} > 0$ corresponding to correlated gamma frailty and correlated inverse Gaussian frailty as

$$S(t_{1j}, t_{2j}) =$$
$$\left(1 - \eta_j \sigma_1^2 ln\left(1 - (1 - e^{-\lambda_1 t_{1j}^{\gamma_1}})^{\alpha_1}\right) - \eta_j \sigma_2^2 ln\left(1 - (1 - e^{-\lambda_2 t_{2j}^{\gamma_2}})^{\alpha_2}\right)\right)^{\frac{-\rho}{\sigma_1 \sigma_2}}$$
$$\times \left(1 - \eta_j \sigma_1^2 ln\left(1 - (1 - e^{-\lambda_1 t_{1j}^{\gamma_1}})^{\alpha_1}\right)\right)^{\frac{-1 + \frac{\sigma_1}{\sigma_2}\rho}{\sigma_1^2}}$$
$$\times \left(1 - \eta_j \sigma_2^2 ln\left(1 - (1 - e^{-\lambda_2 t_{2j}^{\gamma_2}})^{\alpha_2}\right)\right)^{\frac{-1 + \frac{\sigma_2}{\sigma_1}\rho}{\sigma_2^2}} \tag{13.1}$$

$$S(t_{1j}, t_{2j}) = \left(1 + \eta_j \sigma_1^2 \alpha_1 ln(1 + (\lambda_1 t_{1j})^{\gamma_1}) + \eta_j \sigma_2^2 \alpha_2 ln(1 + (\lambda_2 t_{2j})^{\gamma_2})\right)^{\frac{-\rho}{\sigma_1 \sigma_2}}$$

$$\times \left(1 + \eta_j \sigma_1^2 \alpha_1 ln(1 + (\lambda_1 t_{1j})^{\gamma_1})\right)^{\frac{-1 + \frac{\sigma_1}{\sigma_2}\rho}{\sigma_1^2}} \times \left(1 + \eta_j \sigma_2^2 \alpha_2 ln(1 + (\lambda_2 t_{2j})^{\gamma_2})\right)^{\frac{-1 + \frac{\sigma_2}{\sigma_1}\rho}{\sigma_2^2}}$$

$$(13.2)$$

$$S(t, t_{2j}) =$$

$$\exp\left[\rho \frac{1 - (1 - 2\sigma^2 \eta_j (ln[1 - (1 - e^{-\lambda_1 t_{1j}^{\gamma_1}})^{\alpha_1}] + ln[1 - (1 - e^{-\lambda_2 t_{2j}^{\gamma_2}})^{\alpha_2}]))^{\frac{1}{2}}}{\sigma^2}\right]$$

$$\times \exp\left[(1-\rho) \frac{1 - (1 - 2\sigma^2 \eta_j (ln[1 - (1 - e^{-\lambda_1 t_{1j}^{\gamma_1}})^{\alpha_1}]))^{\frac{1}{2}}}{\sigma^2}\right]$$

$$\times \exp\left[(1-\rho) \frac{1 - (1 - 2\sigma^2 \eta_j (ln[1 - (1 - e^{-\lambda_2 t_{2j}^{\gamma_2}})^{\alpha_2}]))^{\frac{1}{2}}}{\sigma^2}\right]$$

$$(13.3)$$

$$S(t_{1j}, t_{2j}) =$$

$$\exp\left[\rho \frac{1 - (1 + 2\sigma^2 \eta_j (\{\alpha_1 ln(1 + (\lambda_1 t_{1j})^{\gamma_1}) + \alpha_2 ln(1 + (\lambda_2 t_{2j})^{\gamma_2})\}))^{\frac{1}{2}}}{\sigma^2}\right]$$

$$\times \exp\left[(1-\rho) \frac{1 - (1 + 2\sigma^2 \eta_j (\alpha_1 ln(1 + (\lambda_1 t_{1j})^{\gamma_1})))^{\frac{1}{2}}}{\sigma^2}\right]$$

$$\times \exp\left[(1-\rho) \frac{1 - (1 + 2\sigma^2 \eta_j (\alpha_2 ln(1 + (\lambda_2 t_{2j})^{\gamma_2})))^{\frac{1}{2}}}{\sigma^2}\right].$$

$$(13.4)$$

Here onward, we call Eqs. (13.1)–(13.4) as Model XI, Model XII, Model XIII, and Model XIV, respectively. Model XI and Model XII are correlated gamma frailty with the generalized Weibull and generalized log-logistic type II distribution as baseline distributions. Model XIII and Model XIV are correlated inverse Gaussian frailty with the generalized Weibull and generalized log-logistic type II distribution as baseline distributions. Model VI and Model VII are without frailty with respective baseline distribution which are defined in Chap. 9.

13.3 Likelihood Specification and Bayesian Estimation of Parameters

Suppose there are n individuals under study, whose first and second observed failure times are represented by (t_{1j}, t_{2j}). Let c_{1j} and c_{2j} be the observed censoring times for the jth individual ($j = 1, 2, 3, \ldots, n$) for the first and the second recurrence times, respectively. We also assume that independence between the censoring time and the lifetimes of individuals.

The contribution of the bivariate lifetime random variable of the jth individual in likelihood function is given by

$$
L_j(t_{1j}, t_{2j}) = \begin{cases}
f_1(t_{1j}, t_{2j}), & t_{1j} < c_{1j}, t_{2j} < c_{2j}, \\
f_2(t_{1j}, c_{2j}), & t_{1j} < c_{1j}, t_{2j} > c_{2j}, \\
f_3(c_{1j}, t_{2j}), & t_{1j} > c_{1j}, t_{2j} < c_{2j}, \\
f_4(c_{1j}, c_{2j}), & t_{1j} > c_{1j}, t_{2j} > c_{2j},
\end{cases}
$$

and the likelihood function is

$$
L(\underline{\psi}, \underline{\beta}, \theta) = \prod_{j=1}^{n_1} f_1(t_{1j}, t_{2j}) \prod_{j=1}^{n_2} f_2(t_{1j}, c_{2j}) \prod_{j=1}^{n_3} f_3(c_{1j}, t_{2j}) \prod_{j=1}^{n_4} f_4(c_{1j}, c_{2j}),
$$

$$(13.5)$$

where θ, ψ, and β are, respectively, the frailty parameter $(\sigma_1, \sigma_2, \rho)$, the vector of baseline parameters, and the vector of regression coefficients.

The counts n_1, n_2, n_3, and n_4 are the numbers of individuals for which the first and the second failure times (t_{1j}, t_{2j}) lie in the ranges $t_{1j} < c_{1j}, t_{2j} < c_{2j}$; $t_{1j} < c_{1j}, t_{2j} > c_{2j}$; $t_{1j} > c_{1j}, t_{2j} < c_{2j}$; and $t_{1j} > c_{1j}, t_{2j} > c_{2j}$, respectively.

Substituting cumulative hazard functions $H_{01}(t_{1j})$, $H_{02}(t_{2j})$ hazard functions $h_{01}(t_{1j})$, $h_{02}(t_{2j})$, and survival function $S(t_{1j}, t_{2j})$ for four correlated frailty models into the likelihood equation, we get the likelihood function given by Eq. (13.5) for Model XI, Model XII, Model XII, and Model XIV.

Unfortunately, computing the maximum likelihood estimators (MLEs) involves solving a 14-dimensional optimization problem for Model V and Model VI and 11-dimensional optimization problem for Model II and Model IV. As the method of maximum likelihood fails to estimate the parameters due to convergence problem in the iterative procedure, we use the Bayesian approach. The traditional maximum likelihood approach to estimation is commonly used in survival analysis, but it can encounter difficulties with frailty models. Moreover, standard maximum likelihood based inference methods may not be suitable for small sample sizes or situations in which there is heavy censoring (see Kheiri et al. 2007). Thus, in our problem, a Bayesian approach, which does not suffer from these difficulties, is a natural one, even though it is relatively computationally intensive. The detailed discussion on the simulation study based on Bayesian approach is given in Hanagal et al. (2017) and Hanagal and Pandey (2019).

13.4 Analysis of Kidney Infection Data

To illustrate the Bayesian estimation procedure, we use kidney infection data of McGilchrist and Aisbett (1991). These data are already analyzed in Chap. 9 with shared gamma frailty models. These data are partially presented in Chap. 1. Now we analyze these data using correlated frailty models. We run two parallel chains for both models using two sets of prior distributions (uniform and gamma priors) with the different starting points using the Metropolis–Hastings algorithm and the Gibbs sampler based on normal transition kernels. We iterate both the chains for 1,00,000 times. We got nearly the same estimates of parameters for two different sets of prior, so estimates are not dependent on the different prior distributions. The convergence rate of the Gibbs sampler for both the prior sets is almost the same. Also, both the chains show somewhat similar results, so we present here the analysis for only one chain with $G(a_1, a_2)$ as prior for the baseline parameters, for all four models.

The trace plots for all the parameters show zigzag pattern which indicates that parameters move and mix more freely. Thus, it seems that the Markov chain has reached the stationary state. Burn-in period is decided by using coupling from the past plot. However, a sequence of draws after burn-in period may have the autocorrelation. Because of the autocorrelation, consecutive draws may not be random, but values at widely separated time points are approximately independent. So, a pseudorandom sample from the posterior distribution can be found by taking values from a single run of the Markov chain at widely spaced time points (autocorrelation lag) after burn-in period. The autocorrelation of the parameters becomes almost negligible after the certain lag. ACF plot after thinning shows that observations are independent. We can also use running mean plots to check how well our chains are mixing. A running mean plot is a plot of the iterations against the mean of the draws up to each iteration. In fact, running mean plots display a time series of the running mean for each parameter in each chain. These plots should be converging to a value. Running mean plot for each parameter is converging to the posterior mean of the parameter, and thus represents a good mixing of chain. Thus, our diagnostic plots suggest that the MCMC chains are mixing very well. Due to lack of space, we are not able to present the trace plots, the coupling from the past plots, the autocorrelation plots after thinning, and the running mean plots for the parameters. The detailed discussion on the simulation study based on Bayesian approach is given in Hanagal et al. (2017).

To check goodness of fit of kidney data set, we consider Kolmogorov–Smirnov (K–S) test for two baseline distributions.

Table 13.1 gives the p-values of goodness-of-fit test for Model XI to Model XIV. Thus, from p-values of K–S test, we can say that there is no statistical evidence to reject the hypothesis that data are from these models in the marginal case and we assume that they also fit for bivariate case.

The Gelman–Rubin convergence statistic values are nearly equal to one and the Geweke test statistic values are quite small and the corresponding p-values are large enough to say that the chains attain stationary distribution. The posterior mean and the standard error with 95% credible intervals, the Gelman–Rubin statistics values,

Table 13.1 p-values of K–S statistics for goodness-of-fit test for kidney infection data set

Distribution	Recurrence time	
	First	Second
Model XI	0.44755	0.70024
Model XII	0.33158	0.68668
Model XIII	0.77412	0.69595
Model XIV	0.61466	0.71815

Table 13.2 Posterior summary for kidney infarction data set Model XI

Parameter	Estimate	Standard error	Lower credible limit	Upper credible limit	Geweke values	p-values	Gelman and Rubin values
Burn-in period = 3150;	Autocorrelation lag = 300						
α_1	2.0115	0.30116	1.4137	2.63607	−0.000156	0.49993	0.9999
λ_1	0.0998	0.02584	0.0555	0.14729	0.008087	0.50322	1.0046
γ_1	0.8259	0.08308	0.6709	0.97540	−0.008807	0.49648	1.0001
α_2	2.5602	0.28182	2.0214	3.02306	−0.011038	0.49559	1.0108
λ_2	0.0669	0.01935	0.0327	0.10706	−0.014303	0.49429	1.0013
γ_2	0.9183	0.07771	0.7415	1.06258	0.012442	0.50496	1.0014
ρ	0.0481	0.02405	0.0054	0.09611	−0.006141	0.49755	1.0096
σ_1	0.2774	0.11552	0.0401	0.47946	−0.021687	0.49134	1.0175
σ_2	0.6613	0.11406	0.4380	0.86395	−0.009812	0.49608	1.0049
β_1	0.0121	0.00891	−0.0046	0.03053	−0.002711	0.49891	1.0031
β_2	−2.0482	0.39737	−2.8252	−1.30207	0.003592	0.50143	1.0011
β_3	−0.1092	0.18939	−0.5304	0.22123	0.000254	0.50010	1.0009
β_4	−0.0211	0.02982	−0.0746	0.03599	0.007755	0.50309	1.0005
β_5	−1.6225	0.66843	−2.8982	−0.45800	−0.001066	0.49957	1.0012

and the Geweke test values with p-values for Model XI to Model XIV are presented in Tables 13.2, 13.3, 13.4, and 13.5. The AIC, BIC, and DIC values for models with frailty, i.e., Models XI to XIV and without frailty, i.e., Models VI and VII are given in Table 13.6. The models without frailty are discussed in Chap. 9. The Bayesian test-based Bayes factors to test frailty for all four models are given in Table 13.7.

The comparison between four proposed models is done using AIC, BIC, and DIC values given in Table 13.6. The smallest AIC value is Model XIII (generalized Weibull baseline distribution with inverse Gaussian frailty). Same result holds for BIC and DIC values. From Tables 13.6 and 13.7, we can observe that Model XIII is the best.

The Bayesian test based on the Bayes factors for Model XI against Model VII is 11.34, Model XII against Model VI is 9.76, Model XIII against Model VII is 10.4, and Model XIV against Model VI is 8.32 which are high and strongly support

Table 13.3 Posterior summary for kidney infarction data set Model XII

Parameter	Estimate	Standard error	Lower credible limit	Upper credible limit	Geweke values	p-values	Gelman and Rubin values
Burn-in period = 3500; Autocorrelation lag = 300							
α_1	2.3595	0.30998	1.7492	2.8886	−0.00190	0.4992	0.9999
λ_1	0.0041	0.00064	0.0030	0.00525	−0.00557	0.4977	1.0013
γ_1	1.3661	0.10954	1.1985	1.5869	−0.00556	0.4977	1.0262
α_2	3.4975	0.12780	3.2726	3.7367	0.00469	0.5018	1.0089
λ_2	0.0013	0.00045	0.0005	0.00216	−0.00229	0.4990	1.0002
γ_2	1.4344	0.09695	1.2310	1.6039	−0.00641	0.4974	1.0082
ρ	0.0405	0.02103	0.0027	0.0802	0.01443	0.5057	1.0003
σ_1	0.1176	0.06230	0.0064	0.2383	0.00695	0.5027	1.0008
σ_2	0.4888	0.08252	0.3326	0.6392	0.00258	0.5010	1.0003
β_1	0.0136	0.00698	0.0006	0.0271	0.00377	0.5015	1.0041
β_2	−1.6716	0.30527	−2.2963	−1.1075	0.00333	0.5013	1.0004
β_3	−0.0812	0.18504	−0.4920	0.2504	0.00431	0.5017	1.0018
β_4	−0.0176	0.03058	−0.0735	0.0346	0.00219	0.5008	1.0011
β_5	−1.4999	0.60591	−2.8066	−0.4345	0.00341	0.5013	1.0025

Table 13.4 Posterior summary for kidney infection data set Model XIII

Parameter	Estimate	Standard error	Lower credible limit	Upper credible limit	Geweke values	p-values	Gelman and Rubin values
Burn-in period = 3150; Autocorrelation lag = 300							
α_1	1.8151	0.32204	1.2217	2.44162	0.005102	0.50203	1.0014
λ_1	17.6474	0.53979	16.7111	18.59658	−0.001360	0.49945	1.0089
γ_1	0.9514	0.05163	0.6709	0.85537	−0.013566	0.49458	1.0041
α_2	2.8186	0.10723	2.6334	3.01025	−0.003313	0.49867	1.0043
λ_2	20.4053	0.56331	19.4496	21.36722	−0.014091	0.49437	0.9999
γ_2	0.9585	0.05438	0.8677	1.05631	−0.008583	0.49657	1.0024
ρ	0.6594	0.05703	0.5540	0.76740	−0.018870	0.49247	1.0009
σ	0.6009	0.04958	0.5072	0.69349	−0.004090	0.49836	1.0008
β_1	0.0123	0.00802	−0.0022	0.02820	−0.003226	0.49871	0.9999
β_2	−2.0570	0.41285	−2.8688	−1.31025	0.005089	0.50203	1.0008
β_3	−0.1542	0.22927	−0.5472	0.30237	0.006850	0.50273	1.2086
β_4	−0.0231	0.03882	−0.0940	0.04252	−0.002433	0.49902	1.0013
β_5	−1.7523	0.67155	−3.1208	−0.41960	0.005508	0.50219	0.9999

Table 13.5 Posterior summary for kidney infection data set Model XIV

Parameter	Estimate	Standard error	Lower credible limit	Upper credible limit	Geweke values	p-values	Gelman and Rubin values
Burn-in period = 3500; Autocorrelation lag = 300							
α_1	31.8017	1.59643	28.72178	34.6363	0.00874	0.5034	1.0010
λ_1	551.5971	82.61825	413.0491	688.895	−0.00126	0.4994	1.0089
γ_1	1.2349	0.13353	0.98610	1.5265	−0.00481	0.4980	0.9999
α_2	28.7922	7.04799	16.04439	41.0204	−0.00242	0.4990	1.0064
λ_2	540.5013	76.5729	410.8869	683.2429	−0.00082	0.4996	1.0110
γ_2	1.4066	0.15208	1.10940	1.7230	−0.00641	0.4974	1.0010
ρ	0.8053	0.09019	0.62666	0.9720	0.00595	0.5023	1.0005
σ	0.7014	0.30422	0.16458	1.2912	−0.00405	0.4983	1.0026
β_1	0.0166	0.00960	−0.00129	0.0345	−0.00481	0.4980	1.0041
β_2	−1.9902	0.37287	−2.71766	−1.2694	0.00942	0.5037	1.0002
β_3	−0.1867	0.21856	−0.56428	0.2257	−0.01161	0.4953	1.0015
β_4	−0.0234	0.03457	−0.08878	0.0388	−0.02241	0.4910	1.0058
β_5	−1.7901	0.72743	−3.14538	−0.3748	0.00394	0.5015	0.9999

Table 13.6 Comparison of AIC, BIC, and DIC

Models	AIC	BIC	DIC
Moeel XI	683.7014	706.6276	669.5544
Model XII	692.1532	715.0794	674.5276
Model XIII	682.7512	704.0398	666.1273
Model XIV	686.4115	707.7002	673.2021
Model VII	690.2814	708.2949	678.103
Model VI	696.9474	714.9608	683.9278

Table 13.7 Bayesian test based on Bayes factor to test the frailty for kidney infection data set

Numerator model against denominator model	$2log(B_{jk})$	Range	Evidence against model in denominator
Model XI against Model VII	11.34	>10	Very strong
Model XII against Model VI	9.76	6–10	Strong
Model XI against Model XII	6.22	6–10	Strong
Model XIII against Model VII	10.40	>10	Very strong
Model XIV against Model VI	8.32	6–10	Strong
Model XIII against Model XIV	2.39	2–6	Moderate

Model XI to Model XIV for kidney infection data set compared to their corresponding models without frailty ($\sigma_1 = \sigma_2 = 0$) and frailty is significant in Model XI and Model XIV. The estimates of the correlation coefficient, ρ, are 0.0481, 0.0405, 0.6594, and 0.8053 for the Model XI, Model XII, Model XIII, and Model XIV, respectively. The estimates of the correlation coefficient are low for Model XI and Model XII but the corresponding estimates in Model XIII and Model IX are high. This shows there is a correlation between the pairs of twins and the correlation is significant for the Model XIII and Model XIV.

Some patients are expected to be very prone to infection compared to others with same covariate value. This is not surprising, as seen in the data set there is a male patient with infection time 8 and 16, and there is also male patient with infection time 152 and 562. Table 13.7 shows that frailty models are better than without frailty models.

We can observe that the regression coefficients for all the models are different. The credible interval of the regression coefficients of β_2 and β_5 in the models from Model XI to Model XIV does not contain zero, which is significant. Negative value of β_2 indicates that the female patients have a slightly lower risk for infection. Negative value of β_5, the regression coefficient corresponding to the covariate X_5 (the disease type PKD), indicates that the absence of the disease type PKD in the patients has lower risk of infection in Model XI to Model XIV. If we compare all the values of AIC, BIC, DIC, and Bayes factors for shared frailty and correlated frailty models discussed in Chap. 9 and this chapter, the Model XIII (correlated inverse Gaussian frailty with generalized Weibull baseline) is best, more suitable, and performs better among all 14 models for modeling kidney infection data.

References

Clayton, D.G., Cuzick, J.: Multivariate generalizations of the proportional hazard model (with discussion). J. Roy. Stat. Soc. A, **148**, 82–117 (1985)

Hanagal, D.D.: Correlated compound Poisoon frailty model for the bivariate survival data. Int. J. Stat. Manag. Syst. **5**, 127–140 (2010)

Hanagal, D.D., Pandey, A.: Correlated inverse Gaussian frailty model for bivariate survival data. Commun. Stat. Theory Methods **48**, (to appear) (2019)

Hanagal, D.D., Pandey, A., Ganguly, A.: Correlated gamma frailty models for bivariate survival data. Commun. Stat.: Simul. Comput. **46**(5), 3627–3644 (2017)

Hens, N., Wienke, A., Aerts, M., Molenberghs, G.: The correlated and shared frailty model for bivariate current status data: an illustration for cross-sectional serological data. Stat. Med. **28**(22), 2785–2800 (2009)

Hougaard, P.: Survival models for hetrogeneous populations derived from stable distributions. Biometrika **73**, 387–396 (1986)

Iachine, I.A.: Correlated frailty concept in the analysis of bivariate survival data. Bachelor project, Department of Mathematics and Computer Science, Odense University, Denmark (1995a)

Iachine, I.A.: Parameter estimation in the bivariate correlated frailty model with observed covariates via the EM-algorithm. Working Paper Series: Population Studies of Aging 16, CHS, Odense University, Denmark (1995b)

Kheiri, S., Kimber, A., Meshkani, M.R.: Bayesian analysis of an inverse Gaussian correlated frailty model. Comput. Stat. Data Anal. **51**, 5317–5326 (2007)

McGilchrist, C.A., Aisbett, C.W.: Regression with frailty in survival analysis. Biometrics **47**, 461–466 (1991)

Chapter 14
Correlated Frailty Models Based on Reversed Hazard

14.1 Introduction

The correlated frailty model is the important concept in the area of multivariate frailty models. In the 13th chapter, we have discussed the properties of the correlated gamma frailty and correlated inverse Gaussian frailty models based on hazard rate. Now, in this chapter, we will discuss correlated gamma frailty models based on reversed hazard rate with three different baseline distributions and also applied to Australian twin data. Hanagal and Pandey (2017) and Hanagal (2019) analyzed Australian twin data using correlated gamma and correlated inverse Gaussian frailty models based on reversed hazard rate for the multiplicative model. In the correlated frailty model, the frailties of individuals in a cluster are correlated but not necessarily shared. It enables the inclusion of additional correlation parameters, which then allows the addressing of questions about associations between event times. Furthermore, associations are no longer forced to be the same for all pairs of individuals in a cluster. This makes the model especially appropriate for situations where the association between event times is of special interest, for example, genetic studies of event times in families. The conditional distribution function in the bivariate case (here without observed covariates) looks like

$$F(t_1, t_2|Z_1, Z_2) = F_1(t_1|Z_1) F_2(t_2|Z_2) = e^{-Z_1 M_{01}(t_1)} e^{-Z_2 M_{02}(t2)}, \qquad (14.1)$$

where Z_1 and Z_2 are two correlated frailties and $M_{0i}(t_i)$, $(i = 1, 2)$ is cumulative reversed hazard rate. The distribution of the random vector (Z_1, Z_2) needs to be specified and determines the association structure of the event times in the model.

In the (bivariate) correlated frailty model, the frailty of each individual in a pair is defined by a measure of relative risk, that is, exactly as it was defined in the univariate case. For two individuals in a pair, frailties are not necessarily the same, as they are in the shared frailty model. We are assuming that the frailties are acting multiplicatively on the baseline hazard function (proportional hazards model) and that the observations in a pair are conditionally independent, given the frailties.

© Springer Nature Singapore Pte Ltd. 2019
D. D. Hanagal, *Modeling Survival Data Using Frailty Models*,
Industrial and Applied Mathematics, https://doi.org/10.1007/978-981-15-1181-3_14

Hence, the reversed hazard of the individual $i(i = 1, 2)$ in pair $j(i = j, \ldots, n)$ has the following form:

$$m(t|X_{ij}, Z_{ij}) = Z_{ij}m_{0i}(t)e^{\beta' X_{ij}},$$

where t denotes age or time, X_{ij} is a vector of observed covariates, β is a vector of regression parameters describing the effect of the covariates X_{ij}, $m_{0i}(.)$ are baseline reversed hazard functions, and Z_{ij} are frailties. Bivariate-correlated frailty models are characterized by the joint distribution of a two-dimensional vector of frailties (Z_{1j}, Z_{2j}). If the two frailties are independent, the resulting lifetimes are independent, and no clustering is present in the model. If the two frailties are equal, the shared frailty model is obtained as a special case of the correlated frailty model with correlation one between the frailties (Wienke 2011).

In order to derive a marginal likelihood function, the assumption of conditional independence of life spans, given the frailty, is used. Let δ_{ij} be a censoring indicator for individual $i(i = 1, 2)$ in pair $j(j = 1, \ldots, n)$. Indicator δ_{ij} is 1 if the individual has experienced the event of interest, and 0 otherwise. According to (14.1), the conditional distribution function of the ith individual in the jth pair is

$$F(t|X_{ij}, Z_{ij}) = e^{-Z_{ij}M_{0i}(t)}e^{\beta' X_{ij}},$$

with $M_{0i}(t)$ denoting the cumulative baseline hazard function. Here and in the following, F is used as a generic symbol for a distribution function. The contribution of individual $i(i = 1, 2)$ in pair $j(j = 1, \ldots, n)$ to the conditional likelihood is given by

$$\left[Z_{ij}m_{0i}(t)e^{\beta' X_{ij}} \right]^{\delta_{ij}} e^{-Z_{ij}M_{0i}(t_{ij})}e^{\beta' X_{ij}},$$

where t_{ij} stands for observation time of individual i from pair j. Assuming the conditional independence of life spans, given the frailty, and integrating out the frailty, we obtain the marginal likelihood function,

$$\prod_{j=1}^{n} \int_{R\times} \int_{R} \left[u_{1j}m_{01}(t_{1j})e^{\beta' X_{1j}} \right]^{\delta_{1j}} e^{-z_{1j}M_{01}(t_{1j})}e^{\beta' X_{1j}}$$

$$\left[u_{2j}m_{02}(t_{2j})e^{\beta' X_{2j}} \right]^{\delta_{2j}} e^{-z_{2j}M_{02}(t_{2j})}e^{\beta' X_{2j}} f(z_{1j}, z_{2j})dz_{1j}dz_{2j},$$

where $f(.,.)$ is the probability density function of the corresponding frailty distribution. All these formulas can be easily extended to the multivariate case, but need a specification of the correlation structure between individuals in a cluster in terms of the multivariate density function, which complicates analysis. For more details, see Hanagal (2011) and Wienke (2011).

14.2 Correlated Frailty Models Based on Reversed Hazard with Baseline Distributions

This model was introduced by Yashin et al. (1993, 1995) and applied to related life-times in many different settings, for example, by Pickles et al. (1994). The model has a very convenient representation of the survival function in closed-form expressions, which allows nice interpretation of the model parameters. Here we restrict again to the bivariate model first.

Now we can derive the unconditional distribution function for $\sigma_1 = \sigma_2 = \sigma$, applying the Laplace transform of gamma-distributed random variables. Hence,

$$
\begin{aligned}
F(t_1, t_2) &= E\left[F(t_1, t_2 | Z_1, Z_2)\right] = E\left[F_1(t_1 | Z_1)\right]\left[F_2(t_2 | Z_2)\right] \\
&= \left(1 + \sigma^2 M_{01}(t_1) + \sigma^2 M_{02}(t_2)\right)^{\frac{-\rho}{\sigma^2}} \left(1 + \sigma^2 M_{01}(t_1)\right)^{\frac{-1+\rho}{\sigma^2}} \\
&\quad \times \left(1 + \sigma^2 M_{02}(t_2)\right)^{\frac{-1+\rho}{\sigma^2}},
\end{aligned}
\tag{14.2}
$$

which results in the following representation of the gamma correlated frailty model:

$$
F(t_1, t_2) = \frac{F_1(t_1)^{1-\rho} F_2(t_2)^{1-\rho}}{\left(F_1(t_1)^{-\sigma^2} + F_2(t_2)^{-\sigma^2} - 1\right)^{\frac{\rho}{\sigma^2}}}
$$

using independence of the gamma-distributed variables Y_0, Y_1, Y_2 and the unconditional distribution function of t_1 and t_2. This representation is called here the copula representation, because it reveals that the correlated gamma frailty model can be considered as a copula, but this copula is not an Archimedian copula as in the shared gamma frailty model. Copula representations allow separation of the marginal part of the model (univariate distributions) from the correlation structure of the model. Besides the fact that frailty models and copulas look very similar, it is important to note that there are also differences between both approaches that are often overlooked.

Let Z be an infinitely divisible frailty variable with Laplace transformation $L_Z(s)$ and $\rho \in [0, 1]$, then there exist random variables Z_1, Z_2 each with univariate Laplace transform $L_Z(s)$ such that the Laplace transform of Z_1, Z_2 is given by

$$
L(s_1, s_2) = L_Z^{\rho}(s_1 + s_2) L_Z^{1-\rho}(s_1) L_Z^{1-\rho}(s_2).
$$

If Z has a variance, the $Corr(Z_1, Z_2) = \rho$.

The respective bivariate survival model is identifiable under mild regularity conditions on Z provided that $\rho > 0$. The case $\rho = 1$ is known as the shared frailty model.

Let Z_i be the inverse Gaussian distributed with mean 1, variance σ^2, and Laplace transform

$$
L(s_i, \sigma^2) = \exp\left[\frac{1 - (1 + 2\sigma^2 s_i)^{\frac{1}{2}}}{\sigma^2}\right].
$$

The bivariate Laplace transform for the correlated inverse Gaussian frailty model is given by

$$L(s_1, s_2, \sigma^2, \rho) = \exp\left[\rho\frac{1 - (1 + 2\sigma^2(s_1 + s_2))^{\frac{1}{2}}}{\sigma^2}\right]$$

$$\exp\left[(1 - \rho)\frac{1 - (1 + 2\sigma^2 s_1)^{\frac{1}{2}}}{\sigma^2}\right]$$

$$\exp\left[(1 - \rho)\frac{1 - (1 + 2\sigma^2 s_2)^{\frac{1}{2}}}{\sigma^2}\right]$$

where $Corr(Z_1, Z_2) = \rho$.

The correlated inverse Gaussian frailty model in the presence of covariates is characterized by the bivariate distribution function of the following form:

$$F(t_{1j}, t_{2j}) = \exp\left[\rho\frac{1 - (1 + 2\sigma^2\eta_j(M_{01}(t_{1j}) + M_{02}(t_{2j})))^{\frac{1}{2}}}{\sigma^2}\right]$$

$$\exp\left[(1 - \rho)\frac{1 - (1 + 2\sigma^2\eta_j M_{01}(t_{1j}))^{\frac{1}{2}}}{\sigma^2}\right]$$

$$\exp\left[(1 - \rho)\frac{1 - (1 + 2\sigma^2\eta_j M_{02}(t_{2j}))^{\frac{1}{2}}}{\sigma^2}\right], \tag{14.3}$$

where $M_{01}(t_{1j})$ and $M_{02}(t_{2j})$ are the cumulative baseline hazard functions of the lifetime random variables T_{1j} and T_{2j}, respectively.

The bivariate distribution in the presence of covariates, when the frailty variable is degenerate is given by

$$F(t_{1j}, t_{2j}) = \exp\left[-\left(\eta_j\left\{(M_{01}(t_{1j}) + M_{02}(t_{2j}))\right\}\right)\right].$$

According to different assumptions on the baseline distributions, we get different correlated frailty models.

Substituting cumulative reversed hazard function for the modified inverse Weibull baseline distribution, generalized log-logistic distribution type I and generalized log-logistic distribution type II in Eqs. (14.2) and (14.3), we get following six correlated frailty models based on reversed hazard:

$$F(t_1, t_2) = \left(1 + \sigma^2\eta_{0j}\left(\eta_{1j}\alpha_1 ln\left(\frac{1 + (\lambda_1 t_{1j})^{\gamma_1}}{(\lambda_1 t_{1j})^{\gamma_1}}\right) + \eta_{2j}\alpha_2 ln\left(\frac{1 + (\lambda_2 t_{2j})^{\gamma_2}}{(\lambda_2 t_{2j})^{\gamma}}\right)\right)\right)^{\frac{-\rho}{\sigma^2}}$$

$$\times \left(1 + \sigma^2\eta_{0j}\eta_{1j}\alpha_1 ln\left(\frac{1 + (\lambda_1 t_{1j})^{\gamma_1}}{(\lambda_1 t_{1j})^{\gamma_1}}\right)\right)^{\frac{-1+\rho}{\sigma^2}}$$

$$\left(1 + \sigma^2 \eta_{0j} \eta_{2j} \alpha_2 ln \left(\frac{1 + (\lambda_2 t_{2j})^{\gamma_1}}{(\lambda_2 t_{2j})^{\gamma_2}}\right)\right)^{\frac{-1+\rho}{\sigma^2}}, \tag{14.4}$$

$$F(t_1, t_2) = \left(1 - \sigma^2 \eta_{0j} (\eta_{1j} ln(1 - (1 + (\lambda_1 t_{1j})^{\gamma_1})^{-\alpha_1}) + \eta_{2j} ln(1 - (1 + (\lambda_2 t_{2j})^{\gamma_2 j})^{-\alpha_2})))^{\frac{-\rho}{\sigma^2}}$$
$$\times \left(1 - \sigma^2 \eta_{0j} \eta_{1j} ln(1 - (1 + (\lambda_1 t_{1j})^{\gamma_1})^{-\alpha_1})\right)^{\frac{-1+\rho}{\sigma^2}}$$
$$\left(1 - \sigma^2 \eta_{0j} \eta_{2j} ln(1 - (1 + (\lambda_2 t_{2j})^{\gamma_2})^{-\alpha_2})\right)^{\frac{-1+\rho}{\sigma^2}}, \tag{14.5}$$

$$F(t_{1j}, t_{2j}) = \left(1 + \sigma^2 \eta_{0j} (\eta_{1j} \alpha_1 t_{1j}^{-\lambda_1} e^{-\gamma_1 t_{1j}} + \eta_{2j} \alpha_2 t_{2j}^{-\lambda_2} e^{-\gamma_2 t_{2j}})\right)^{\frac{-\rho}{\sigma^2}}$$
$$\times \left(1 + \sigma^2 \eta_{0j} \eta_{1j} \alpha_1 t_{1j}^{-\lambda_1} e^{-\gamma_1 t_{1j}}\right)^{\frac{-1+\rho}{\sigma^2}} \left(1 + \sigma^2 \eta_{0j} \eta_{2j} \alpha_2 t_{2j}^{-\lambda_2} e^{-\gamma_2 t_{2j}}\right)^{\frac{-1+\rho}{\sigma^2}}, \tag{14.6}$$

$$F(t_{1j}, t_{2j}) = \exp\left[\rho \frac{1 - (1 + 2\sigma^2 \eta_{0j} (\eta_{1j} \alpha_1 \ln(1 + 1/(\lambda_1 t_{1j})^{\gamma_1}) + \eta_{2j} \alpha_2 \ln(1 + 1/(\lambda_2 t_{2j})^{\gamma_2})))^{\frac{1}{2}}}{\sigma^2}\right]$$
$$\exp\left[(1 - \rho) \frac{1 - (1 + 2\sigma^2 \eta_{0j} \eta_{1j} \alpha_1 \ln(1 + 1/(\lambda_1 t_{1j})^{\gamma_1}))^{\frac{1}{2}}}{\sigma^2}\right]$$
$$\exp\left[(1 - \rho) \frac{1 - (1 + 2\sigma^2 \eta_{0j} \eta_{2j} \alpha_2 \ln(1 + 1/(\lambda_2 t_{2j})^{\gamma_2}))^{\frac{1}{2}}}{\sigma^2}\right], \tag{14.7}$$

$$F(t_{1j}, t_{2j}) = \exp\left[\rho \frac{1 - (1 + 2\sigma^2 \eta_{0j} (\eta_{1j} \ln(1 - (1 + 1(\lambda_1 t_{1j})^{\gamma_1})^{-\alpha_1}) + \eta_{2j} \ln(1 - (1 + 1(\lambda_2 t_{2j})^{\gamma_2})^{-\alpha_2})))^{\frac{1}{2}}}{\sigma^2}\right]$$
$$\exp\left[(1 - \rho) \frac{1 - (1 + 2\sigma^2 \eta_{0j} \eta_{1j} \ln(1 - (1 + 1(\lambda_1 t_{1j})^{\gamma_1})^{-\alpha_1}))^{\frac{1}{2}}}{\sigma^2}\right]$$
$$\exp\left[(1 - \rho) \frac{1 - (1 + 2\sigma^2 \eta_{0j} \eta_{2j} \ln(1 - (1 + 1(\lambda_2 t_{2j})^{\gamma_2})^{-\alpha_2}))^{\frac{1}{2}}}{\sigma^2}\right], and \tag{14.8}$$

$$F(t_{1j}, t_{2j}) = \exp\left[\rho \frac{1 - (1 + 2\sigma^2 \eta_{0j} (\eta_{1j} \alpha_1 t_{1j}^{-\lambda_1} e^{-\gamma_1 t_{1j}} + \eta_{2j} \alpha_2 t_{2j}^{-\lambda_2} e^{-\gamma_2 t_{2j}}))^{\frac{1}{2}}}{\sigma^2}\right]$$
$$\exp\left[(1 - \rho) \frac{1 - (1 + 2\sigma^2 \eta_{0j} \eta_{1j} \alpha_1 t_{1j}^{-\lambda_1} e^{-\gamma_1 t_{1j}})^{\frac{1}{2}}}{\sigma^2}\right]$$
$$\exp\left[(1 - \rho) \frac{1 - (1 + 2\sigma^2 \eta_{0j} \eta_{2j} \alpha_2 t_{2j}^{-\lambda_2} e^{-\gamma_2 t_{2j}})^{\frac{1}{2}}}{\sigma^2}\right]. \tag{14.9}$$

Here onward, we call Eqs. (14.4)–(14.9) as Model RH-XI, Model RH-XII, Model RH-XIII, Model RH-XIV, Model RH-XV, and Model RH-XVI, respectively. Model RH-XI, Model RH-XII, and Model RH-XIII are generalized log-logistic baseline distribution type I, generalized log-logistic baseline distribution type II, and the modified inverse Weibull baseline distribution with gamma frailty and Model RH-XIV, Model RH-XV, and Model RH-XVI are generalized log-logistic baseline distribution type I, generalized log-logistic baseline distribution type II, and the modified inverse Weibull baseline distribution with inverse Gaussian frailty. Model RH-VI, Model RH-VII, and Model RH-IX are without frailty models with baseline distributions, the generalized log-logistic type I, generalized log-logistic type II, and modified inverse Weibull distribution, respectively, are defined in Chap. 10.

14.3   Likelihood Specification and Bayesian Estimation of Parameters

Suppose there are n individuals under study, whose first and second observed failure times are represented by (t_{1j}, t_{2j}). Let c_{1j} and c_{2j} be the observed censoring times for the jth individual ($j = 1, 2, 3, \ldots, n$) for the first and the second recurrence times, respectively. We use the left censoring scheme. Also, we assume independence between the censoring scheme and the lifetimes of individuals.

The contribution of the bivariate lifetime random variable of the jth individual in likelihood function is given by

$$L_j(t_{1j}, t_{2j}) = \begin{cases} f_1(t_{1j}, t_{2j}), & ; t_{1j} > c_{1j}, t_{2j} > c_{2j}, \\ f_2(t_{1j}, c_{2j}), & ; t_{1j} > c_{1j}, t_{2j} < c_{2j}, \\ f_3(c_{1j}, t_{2j}), & ; t_{1j} < c_{1j}, t_{2j} > c_{2j}, \\ f_4(c_{1j}, c_{2j}), & ; t_{1j} < c_{1j}, t_{2j} < c_{2j}, \end{cases}$$

and likelihood function is

$$L(\underline{\psi}, \underline{\beta}, \theta) = \prod_{j=1}^{n_1} f_1(t_{1j}, t_{2j}) \prod_{j=1}^{n_2} f_2(t_{1j}, c_{2j}) \prod_{j=1}^{n_3} f_3(c_{1j}, t_{2j}) \prod_{j=1}^{n_4} f_4(c_{1j}, c_{2j}),$$

(14.10)

where θ, $\underline{\psi}$, and $\underline{\beta}$ are, respectively, the frailty parameter (σ, ρ), the vector of baseline parameters, and the vector of regression coefficients. For without frailty model, likelihood function is

$$L(\underline{\psi}, \underline{\beta}) = \prod_{j=1}^{n_1} f_1(t_{1j}, t_{2j}) \prod_{j=1}^{n_2} f_2(t_{1j}, c_{2j}) \prod_{j=1}^{n_3} f_3(c_{1j}, t_{2j}) \prod_{j=1}^{n_4} f_4(c_{1j}, c_{2j}). \quad (14.11)$$

The counts n_1, n_2, n_3, and n_4 be the number of individuals for which first and second failure times (t_{1j}, t_{2j}) lie in the ranges $t_{1j} > c_{1j}, t_{2j} > c_{2j}; t_{1j} > c_{1j}, t_{2j} < c_{2j}; t_{1j} < c_{1j}, t_{2j} > c_{2j}$; and $t_{1j} < c_{1j}, t_{2j} < c_{2j}$, respectively, and

$$f_1(t_{1j}, t_{2j}) = \frac{\partial^2 F(t_{1j}, t_{2j})}{\partial t_{1j} \partial t_{2j}},$$

$$f_2(t_{1j}, c_{2j}) = \frac{\partial F(t_{1j}, c_{2j})}{\partial t_{1j}},$$

$$f_3(c_{1j}, t_{2j}) = \frac{\partial F(c_{1j}, t_{2j})}{\partial t_{2j}}, \text{ and}$$

$$f_4(c_{1j}, c_{2j}) = F(c_{1j}, c_{2j}).$$

Substituting cumulative reversed hazard rate $M_{01}(t_{1j})$, $M_{02}(t_{2j})$ reversed hazard rate $m_{01}(t_{1j})$, $m_{02}(t_{2j})$, and distribution function $F(c_{1j}, c_{2j})$ for above models into the last relations, we get the likelihood function given by Eq. (14.10) for Model RH-XI, Model RH-XII, Model RH-XIII, Model XIV, Model XV, and Model XVI and Eq. (14.11) for Model RH-VI, Model RH-VII, and Model RH-IX.

Computing the maximum likelihood estimators (MLEs) involves solving a 11-dimensional optimization problem for Model RH-XI, Model RH-XII, Model RH-XIII, Model RH-XIV, Model RH-XV, and Model RH-XVI and nine-dimensional optimization problem for Model RH-VI, Model RH-VII, and Model RH-IX. As the method of maximum likelihood fails to estimate the parameters due to convergence problem in the iterative procedure, we use the Bayesian approach. The traditional maximum likelihood approach to estimation is commonly used in survival analysis, but it can encounter difficulties with frailty models. Moreover, standard maximum likelihood based inference methods may not be suitable for small sample sizes or situations in which there is heavy censoring (see Kheiri et al. 2007). Thus, in our problem, a Bayesian approach, which does not suffer from these difficulties, is a natural one, even though it is relatively computationally intensive. To estimate parameters of the model, the Bayesian approach is now popularly used, because computation of the Bayesian analysis becomes feasible due to advances in computing technology. The detailed discussion on the simulation study based on Bayesian approach is given in Hanagal and Pandey (2017).

14.4 Analysis of Australian Twin Data

Now we apply all the models to the Australian twin data given in Duffy et al. (1990). This data is partially presented in Chap. 1. In Chap. 10, the Australian twin data is analyzed using shared gamma frailty model. Now this data is analyzed using

Table 14.1 p-values of K–S statistics for goodness-of-fit test for Australian twin data set

Distribution	Recurrence time	
	First	Second
Model RH-XI	0.83243	0.7584
Model RH-XII	0.99957	0.99647
Model RH-XIII	0.54102	0.57488
Model RH-XIV	0.85443	0.7794
Model RH-XV	0.99977	0.99787
Model RH-XVI	0.57402	0.59688

correlated frailty models based on reversed hazard rate. To check goodness of fit of Australian twin data set, we obtain Kolmogorov–Smirnov (K–S) statistics and their p-values for T_1 and T_2. Table 14.1 gives the p-values of K–S test for Model RH-XI to Model RH-XVI. The p-values of K–S test are quite high. Hence, we can say that there is no statistical evidence to reject the hypothesis that data are from these six models.

We run two parallel chains for both models using two sets of prior distributions (uniform and gamma priors) with the different starting points using the Metropolis–Hastings algorithm and the Gibbs sampler based on normal transition kernels. We iterate both the chains for 1,00,000 times. We got nearly the same estimates of parameters for two different sets of prior, so estimates are not dependent on the different prior distributions. The convergence rate of the Gibbs sampler for both the prior sets is almost the same. Also, both the chains show somewhat similar results, so we present here the analysis for only one chain with $G(a_1, a_2)$ as prior for the baseline parameters, for all six models. Trace plots for all the parameters show zigzag pattern which indicates that parameters move and mix more freely. Thus, it seems that the Markov chain has reached the stationary state. Burn-in period is decided by using coupling from the past plot. However, a sequence of draws after burn-in period may have autocorrelation. Because of autocorrelation, consecutive draws may not be random, but values at widely separated time points are approximately independent. So, a pseudorandom sample from the posterior distribution can be found by taking values from a single run of the Markov chain at widely spaced time points (autocorrelation lag) after burn-in period. The autocorrelation of parameters becomes almost negligible after a certain lag. The detailed discussion on the simulation study based on Bayesian approach is given in Hanagal and Pandey (2017).

The Gelman–Rubin convergence statistic values are nearly equal to one and the Geweke test statistic values are quite small and corresponding p-values are large enough to say the chains attain stationary distribution. The posterior mean and standard error with 95% credible intervals for baseline parameters, frailty parameter, and regression coefficients are presented in Tables 14.2, 14.3, 14.4, 14.5, 14.6, and 14.7. The posterior summery of the Model RH-XI, Model RH-XII, Model RH-XIII, Model

Table 14.2 Posterior summary for Australian twin data set Model RH-XI

Parameter	Estimate	Standard error	Lower credible limit	Upper credible limit	Geweke values	p-values	Gelman and Rubin values
Burn-in period = 7500; Autocorrelation lag = 1100							
α_1	16.5475	0.2850	16.0600	16.9640	0.0015	0.5006	1.0004
λ_1	0.0601	0.0014	0.0575	0.0625	-0.0259	0.4896	1.0095
γ_1	21.1861	0.2169	20.6769	21.4879	-0.0056	0.4977	1.0000
α_2	16.0086	0.5575	15.0466	16.9802	0.0022	0.5008	1.0003
λ_2	0.0601	0.0015	0.0574	0.0629	-0.0254	0.4898	1.0149
γ_2	21.1054	0.2381	20.6751	21.4480	-0.0043	0.4982	1.0026
ρ	0.8925	0.0160	0.8631	0.9171	0.0026	0.5010	0.9999
σ	4.7745	0.1175	4.5326	4.9504	-0.0061	0.4975	1.0039
β_0	0.8265	0.0310	0.7668	0.8786	-0.0235	0.4906	1.0083
β_1	-0.0517	0.0297	-0.1072	-0.0042	0.0042	0.5017	1.0134
β_2	-0.0173	0.0334	-0.0746	0.0463	0.0113	0.5045	1.0321

RH-XIV, Model RH-XV, and Model RH-XVI are given in Tables 14.2, 14.3, 14.4, 14.5, 14.6, and 14.7. Tables 14.2, 14.3, 14.4, 14.5, 14.6, and 14.7 present estimates, credible intervals, Geweke test, and Gelman–Rubin statistics for all the parameters of the Model RH-XI, Model RH-XII, Model RH-XIII, Model RH-XIV, Model RH-XV, and Model RH-XVI, respectively, based on Australian twin data. For Model RH-XI, Model RH-XII, Model RH-XIII, Model RH-XIV, Model RH-XV, and Model RH-XVI, the estimates of frailty parameter σ^2 are, respectively, 4.7745, 1.6686, 0.6096, 5.7845, 4.7686, and 5.6081. This shows that there is a heterogeneity between the pairs of twins. Bayes factor is also a Bayesian test for testing $\sigma^2 = 0$ against $\sigma^2 > 0$ and which supports the alternative hypothesis, i.e., models with frailty fit better. The estimates of the correlation coefficient, ρ are 0.8925, 0.8814, 0.9284, 0.8941, 0.8824, and 0.9294 for the Model RH-XI, Model RH-XII, Model RH-XIII, Model RH-XIV, Model RH-V, and Model RH-VI, respectively. This shows there is a correlation between the pairs of twins and the correlation is significant. The credible interval of regression coefficient β_0 does not contain zero for all models. The credible interval of regression coefficient β_1 does not contain zero for all models except Model RH-XII and Model RH-XV. The credible interval of regression coefficient β_2 contains zero for all models. Hence, age is the significant covariate for all the models. The convergence rate of Gibbs sampling algorithm does not depend on these choices of prior distributions in our proposed model for Australian twin data. The Geweke test values are near to zero and corresponding p-values are quite high and the Gelman–Rubin statistics for all the parameters of all models based on data are very close to one.

Table 14.3 Posterior summary for Australian twin data set Model RH-XII

Parameter	Estimate	Standard error	Lower credible limit	Upper credible limit	Geweke values	p-values	Gelman and Rubin values
Burn-in period = 6500; Autocorrelation lag = 300							
α_1	0.0857	0.0028	0.0791	0.0897	−0.00066	0.4997	1.0002
λ_1	0.0506	0.0014	0.0485	0.0524	−0.00274	0.4989	1.0004
γ_1	57.4383	1.1477	54.8765	59.2271	0.00761	0.5030	1.0026
α_2	0.0851	0.0029	0.0796	0.0909	0.00678	0.5027	1.0069
λ_2	0.0506	0.0015	0.0487	0.0528	−0.00166	0.4993	1.0012
γ_2	57.1274	1.6205	53.7728	60.0354	−0.00435	0.4983	1.0057
ρ	0.8814	0.0252	0.8266	0.9263	0.00041	0.5001	0.9999
σ	1.6686	0.0705	1.5395	1.8069	0.00315	0.5012	0.9999
β_0	0.0685	0.0067	0.0551	0.0813	0.00317	0.5012	1.0002
β_1	−0.0512	0.0242	−0.1029	−0.0078	0.01608	0.5064	1.0018
β_2	−0.0244	0.0257	−0.0715	0.0244	−0.00370	0.4985	1.0136

Table 14.4 Posterior summary for Australian twin data set Model RH-XIII

Parameter	Estimate	Standard error	Lower credible limit	Upper credible limit	Geweke values	p-values	Gelman and Rubin values
Burn-in period = 7500; Autocorrelation lag = 1300							
α_1	41.1861	2.9877	35.2212	45.7319	0.01771	0.5070	1.0068
λ_1	0.4432	0.0313	0.3816	0.4877	−0.00162	0.4993	1.0341
γ_1	0.1027	0.0052	0.0905	0.1115	−0.00224	0.4991	1.0034
α_2	39.1301	3.0285	33.917	44.3825	0.00857	0.5034	1.0192
λ_2	0.4374	0.0229	0.3866	0.4759	0.00243	0.5009	1.0041
γ_2	0.1011	0.0045	0.0923	0.1103	−0.01221	0.4951	1.0066
ρ	0.9284	0.0474	0.8124	0.9875	−0.00069	0.4997	1.0099
σ	0.6096	0.0758	0.4473	0.7775	−0.01036	0.4958	1.0054
β_0	0.0109	0.0043	0.0033	0.0204	−0.01873	0.4925	1.0000
β_1	−0.0639	0.0844	−0.2587	0.1240	−0.00320	0.4987	1.0086
β_2	−0.0202	0.0305	−0.0864	0.0368	−0.00684	0.4972	1.0045

   To compare all models, we first use AIC, BIC, and DIC values which are given in Table 14.8 and Bayes factor in Table 14.9. The AIC, BIC, and DIC values for Model RH-XV are least among all the models. On the basis of AIC, BIC, and DIC values, Model RH-XV is the best among all the models. Similarly, the Bayes factor shows that models with frailty(Model RH-XI, Model RH-XII, Model RH-XIII, Model RH-XIV,

Table 14.5 Posterior summary for Australian twin data set Model RH-XIV

Parameter	Estimate	Standard error	Lower credible limit	Upper credible limit	Geweke values	p-values	Gelman and Rubin values
Burn-in period = 7500; Autocorrelation lag = 1100							
α_1	18.5175	0.2150	18.0612	18.8641	0.0015	0.5006	1.0004
λ_1	0.0701	0.0012	0.0676	0.0722	−0.0259	0.4896	1.0095
γ_1	23.1861	0.2119	22.6789	23.4689	−0.0056	0.4977	1.0000
α_2	18.0016	0.5215	17.1468	18.1801	0.0022	0.5008	1.0003
λ_2	0.0801	0.0012	0.0771	0.0823	−0.0254	0.4898	1.0149
γ_2	24.1014	0.2182	23.6952	24.4461	−0.0043	0.4982	1.0026
ρ	0.8941	0.0151	0.8721	0.9078	0.0026	0.5010	0.9999
σ	5.7845	0.1155	5.5526	5.9101	−0.0061	0.4975	1.0039
β_0	0.8465	0.0290	0.8161	0.8722	−0.0235	0.4906	1.0083
β_1	−0.0507	0.0277	−0.0971	−0.0052	0.0042	0.5017	1.0134
β_2	−0.0143	0.0314	−0.0426	0.0413	0.0113	0.5045	1.0321

Table 14.6 Posterior summary for Australian twin data set Model RH-XV

Parameter	Estimate	Standard error	Lower credible limit	Upper credible limit	Geweke values	p-values	Gelman and Rubin values
Burn-in period = 6500; Autocorrelation lag = 300							
α_1	0.2817	0.0032	0.2781	0.2877	−0.00066	0.4997	1.0002
λ_1	0.0701	0.0025	0.0585	0.0724	−0.00274	0.4989	1.0004
γ_1	55.4383	1.1412	52.9768	57.2222	0.00761	0.5030	1.0026
α_2	0.1051	0.0031	0.0891	0.1108	0.00678	0.5027	1.0069
λ_2	0.0706	0.0012	0.0687	0.0728	−0.00166	0.4993	1.0012
γ_2	58.6274	1.6105	55.7728	61.0344	−0.00435	0.4983	1.0057
ρ	0.8824	0.0242	0.8461	0.9165	0.00041	0.5001	0.9999
σ	4.7686	0.0505	4.5495	4.8869	0.00315	0.5012	0.9999
β_0	0.0785	0.0057	0.0751	0.0903	0.00317	0.5012	1.0002
β_1	−0.0412	0.0202	−0.0819	−0.0051	0.01608	0.5064	1.0018
β_2	−0.0214	0.0247	−0.0615	0.0221	−0.00370	0.4985	1.0136

Model RH-XV, and Model RH-XVI) are better than the models without frailty(Model RH-VI, Model RH-VII, and Model RH-IX). From Tables 14.8 and 14.9, Model RH-XV, the correlated inverse Gaussian frailty based on reversed hazard rate with generalized log-logistic type II baseline is the best and the frailty is significant.

Table 14.7   Posterior summary for Australian twin data set Model RH-XVI

Parameter	Estimate	Standard error	Lower credible limit	Upper credible limit	Geweke values	p-values	Gelman and Rubin values
Burn-in period $= 7500$; Autocorrelation lag $= 1300$							
α_1	44.1762	2.7887	39.12322	48.7418	0.01771	0.5070	1.0068
λ_1	0.4632	0.0311	0.4111	0.5071	-0.00162	0.4993	1.0341
γ_1	0.1227	0.0042	0.1106	0.1312	-0.00224	0.4991	1.0034
α_2	41.1201	2.9285	35.816	46.3785	0.00857	0.5034	1.0192
λ_2	0.4574	0.0217	0.4161	0.4989	0.00243	0.5009	1.0041
γ_2	0.2011	0.0035	0.1913	0.2112	-0.01221	0.4951	1.0066
ρ	0.9294	0.0414	0.8424	0.9978	-0.00069	0.4997	1.0099
σ	5.6081	0.0651	5.4172	5.7571	-0.01036	0.4958	1.0054
β_0	0.0209	0.0023	0.0133	0.0304	-0.01873	0.4925	1.0000
β_1	-0.0742	0.0641	-0.2287	0.1041	-0.00320	0.4987	1.0086
β_2	-0.0312	0.0204	-0.0564	0.0161	-0.00684	0.4972	1.0045

Table 14.8   AIC, BIC, and DIC comparison

Model	AIC	BIC	DIC
Model RH-XI	5078.679	5102.252	5067.799
Model RH-XII	5046.704	5070.908	5037.085
Model RH-XIII	5355.413	5378.613	5343.785
Model RH-XV	5071.699	5082.212	5057.809
Model RH-XVI	5016.714	5018.908	5003.093
Model RH-XIV	5155.713	5188.813	5113.985

Table 14.9   Bayes factor values and decision for models fitted to Australian twin data set

Numerator model against denominator model	$2log(B_{jk})$	Range	Evidence against model in denominator
Model RH-XI against Model RH-XIII	278.09	>10	Very strong
Model RH-XII against Model RH-XIII	306.78	>10	Very strong
Model RH-XII against Model RH-XI	028.69	>10	Very strong
Model RH-XI against Model RH-VI	282.48	> 10	Very strong
Model RH-XII against Model RH-VII	1601.32	>10	Very strong
Model RH-XIII against Model RH-IX	029.80	>10	Very strong
Model RH-XV against Model RH-XIV	032.79	>10	Very strong
Model RH-XV against Model RH-XVI	336.81	>10	Very strong
Model RH-XIV against Model RH-XVI	302.08	>10	Very strong
Model RH-XIV against Model RH-VI	298.41	>10	Very strong
Model RH-XV against Model RH-VII	1704.12	>10	Very strong
Model RH-XVI against Model RH-IX	032.80	>10	Very strong

14.5 Conclusion

Our main aim of the study is to examine the role of the bivariate-correlated frailty model based on the reversed hazard rate in survival studies. For this, we used the correlated gamma frailty model with the modified inverse Weibull distribution, generalized log-logistic type I, and generalized log-logistic type II as a baseline distribution and these models are compared with their baseline model based on reversed hazard rate. We also found that the correlated gamma frailty models are better models as compared to their baseline model on the basis of AIC, BIC, and DIC values for Australian twin data set. Bayes factor support the correlated frailty models.

Initially, we thought to use the method of maximum likelihood to estimate the parameters but likelihood equations do not converge and the method of maximum likelihood fails to estimate the parameters so we used the Bayesian approach. In this study, the model is specified in a Bayesian framework and estimated with the MCMC algorithms. We have discussed the Bayesian estimation procedure including Gibbs sampling for computing the estimation of the unknown parameters by simulating samples of size 25. We have clearly written the steps involved in the iteration procedure. The entire estimation procedure using the Bayesian approach took large amount of computational time. The estimates of the parameters are not dependent on the different prior distributions.

Two different chains were run for the proposed models from different starting points using the Metropolis–Hastings algorithm within Gibbs sampler. We have provided 1,00,000 iterations to perform the simulation study. Estimates were calculated after discarding a burn-in interval for each chain. Trace plots for all the parameters show zigzag pattern which indicates that parameters move freely. The quality of convergence was checked by Gelman–Rubin statistics. The values of the Gelman–Rubin statistics in this case are quite close to one and also the Geweke test values are small with large p-values. Thus, the sample can be considered to have arisen from stationary distribution and descriptive statistics can be seen as valid estimates of unknown parameters. The simulation results indicate that the performance of the Bayesian estimation method is quite satisfactory. Bayes factor is used to test the frailty parameter $\sigma^2 = 0$ and it is observed that the frailty parameter is highly significant in all frailty models. From Table 14.8, it is clear that the models with frailty fit better than without frailty models and Model RH-XV is best among all the six models. Age is significant for all the models.

The choice of the best model for Australian twin data is based on AIC, BIC, DIC, and Bayes factor values. We found that Model RH-XV is a better model on the basis of AIC, BIC, DIC, and Bayes factor values. The age is the significant covariate for all models. Correlated frailty models (Model RH-XI, Model RH-XII, Model RH-XIII, Model RH-XIV, Model RH-XV, and Model RH-XVI) are better than their baseline models. If we compare all the values of AIC, BIC, DIC, and Bayes factors for shared frailty and correlated frailty models based on reversed hazard rate discussed in Chap. 10 and this chapter, the Model RH-XV (correlated inverse Gaussian frailty based on reversed hazard rate with generalized log-logistic type II baseline) is best, more suitable, and performs better among all 16 models for modeling Australian twin data set, with left-censored data.

References

Duffy, D.L., Martin, N.G., Mathews, J.D.: Appendectomy in Australian twins. Aust. J. Hum. Genet. **47**(3), 590–592 (1990)

Hanagal, D.D.: Modeling Survival Data Using Frailty Models. Chapman and Hall, New York (2011)

Hanagal, D.D.: Correlated inverse Gaussian frailty models based on reversed hazard rate. Preprint, unpublished work (2019)

Hanagal, D.D., Pandey, A.: Correlated gamma frailty models for bivariate survival data based on reversed hazard rate. Int. J. Data Sci. **2**(4), 301–324 (2017)

Kheiri, S., Kimber, A., Meshkani, M.R.: Bayesian analysis of an inverse Gaussian correlated frailty model. Comput. Stat. Data Anal. **51**, 5317–5326 (2007)

Pickles, A., Crouchley, R., Simonoff, E., Eaves, L., Meyer, J., Rutter, M., Hewit, J., Silberg, J.: Survival models for developmental genetic data: age at onset of puberty and antisocial behaviour in twins. Genet. Epidemiol. **11**, 155–170 (1994)

Wienke, A.: Frailty Models in Survival Analysis. CRC Press, New York (2011)

Yashin, A.I., Vaupel, J.W., Iachine, I.A.: Correlated individual frailty: an advantageous approach to survival analysis of bivariate data. Working Paper Series: Population Studies of Aging 7, CHS, Odense University, Denmark (1993)

Index

© Springer Nature Singapore Pte Ltd. 2019
D. D. Hanagal, *Modeling Survival Data Using Frailty Models*,
Industrial and Applied Mathematics, https://doi.org/10.1007/978-981-15-1181-3

Diabetic retinopathy data, 9, 213
Diagnostic plots, 224
Dizygotic, 77, 265

E

EM algorithm, 126, 128, 129, 131, 132, 255
Erlang distribution, 28
Exponential marginals, 216
Exponentiated Gumbel, 195, 198, 199
Extended Weibull, 171, 172

G

Gamma distribution, 87
Gamma frailty, 123, 135, 140, 141, 143, 147, 149, 165
Gaussian distribution, 137
Gaussian frailty, 135, 140, 141, 143, 145, 149
Geiger counters, 216
Gelman and Rubin Diagnostics, 45
Gelman–Rubin convergence statistic, 231
Gelman–Rubin statistics, 181, 203, 273, 287, 291
Generalized additive models, 107
Generalized exponential, 86, 114, 124
Generalized gamma, 86, 115
Generalized gamma frailty, 86
Generalized inverse Rayleigh, 196, 198, 199
Generalized linear mixed model, 106
Generalized linear model, 75, 106, 107
Generalized log-logistic distribution, 167, 168, 199, 282
Generalized log-logistic type I, 168, 194, 197, 198
Generalized log-logistic type II, 168, 172, 195, 197, 198, 270
Generalized Rayleigh, 169, 172, 196
Generalized Weibull, 168, 172, 270, 271, 274
Geometric distribution, 99
Geweke test, 46, 176, 181, 203, 205, 231, 273, 286, 287, 291
Gibbs sampler, 43, 176, 180, 201, 273, 286, 291
Gibbs sampling, 222
Gompertz distribution, 214, 228
Goodness-of-fit, 228

H

Hepatitis, 270
Hierarchical Bayesian approach, 266

Hierarchical likelihood, 106, 108

I

Identifiability, 80, 81, 87, 93, 106
Integrated quasi-likelihood, 107
Interval censored, 16
Inverse Gaussian, 86, 89, 90, 93, 103, 213
Inverse Gaussian frailty, 291

K

Kaplan–Meier estimate, 57, 58
Kidney dialysis, 6–9, 39, 141
Kidney infection, 7, 59, 145, 153, 159–161
Kidney infection data, 7, 165, 178, 183, 273, 276
KM–EM algorithm, 130
Kolmogorov–Smirnov test, 222, 228

L

Lack of memory property, 216
Least Absolute Shrinkage and Selection Operator (LASSO), 124
Lévy–Khinchin formula, 116
Lévy processes, 116, 117
Litters of rats, 8, 147
Litters of rats data, 8, 213
Log-logistic distribution, 216, 228
Log-normal, 86
Lognormal distribution, 215
Logrank test, 49, 66, 153, 156
Log-skew-normal frailty, 85
Loss of memory property, 20

M

Marginal quasi-likelihood, 107
Markov Chain Monte Carlo (MCMC), 40, 181, 273, 291
Marshall–Olkin bivariate exponential, 216
Maximum likelihood estimate, 215
MCMC chains, 224
MCMC methods, 265
Mean time to fail, 20, 21
Metropolis algorithm, 42
Metropolis–Hastings algorithm, 42, 176, 180, 201, 222, 273, 286, 291
Mixture distributions, 108
Modified inverse Weibull, 192, 196–199, 282, 284
Monozygotic, 77, 265
Mortality ratio, 214
Mortgage termination risks, 85